DIET-RELATED DISEASES

DIET-RELATED DISEASES

THE MODERN EPIDEMIC

Stephen Seely, BSc,
Department of Bacteriology and Virology,
University of Manchester Medical School

David L. J. Freed, MD,
Department of Immunology,
University of Manchester Medical School

Gerald A. Silverstone, PhD,
Department of Chemistry,
University of Manchester

and

Vicky Rippere, PhD,
Department of Clinical Psychology,
Institute of Psychiatry, University of London

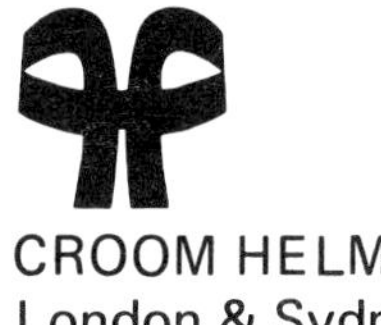

CROOM HELM
London & Sydney

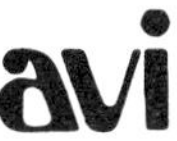

THE AVI PUBLISHING COMPANY, INC.
Westport, Connecticut 1985

Croom Helm Ltd, Provident House, Burrell Row,
Beckenham, Kent BR3 1AT

Croom Helm Australia Pty Ltd, First Floor, 139 King Street,
Sydney, NSW 2001, Australia

British Library Cataloguing in Publication Data

Seely, Stephen
Diet-related diseases: the modern epidemic.
1. Diet
I. Title
613.2 RA784

ISBN 0-7099-3364-9
ISBN 0-7099-3365-7 Pbk

Published in the United States and dependencies, Canada,
Mexico, Central and South America 1985 by

The AVI Publishing Company, Inc.
250 Post Road East, P.O. Box 831
Westport, Connecticut 06881, USA

ISBN 0-87055-503-0

Typeset by Mayhew Typesetting, Bristol, UK
Printed and bound in Great Britain
by Billing & Sons Limited, Worcester.

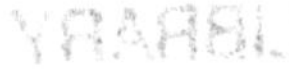

CONTENTS

FIGURES

TABLES

PREFACE

When talking of food-related diseases, we are primarily concerned with such diseases in advanced countries, not with those due to starvation or malnutrition. From the biological point of view prosperity means abundance and variety of food, greater understanding of the nutritional needs of the body, stricter measures in avoiding spoilage and contamination of nutrients. At the same time nutritional needs are reduced by low energy expenditure. This is due partly to the use of machines which reduce the need for physical exertion, and partly to the use of clothing and the heating of dwellings which reduce the energy needed for maintaining constant body temperature. Additional benefits of prosperity assist the individual in ill health and in old age. In a nutshell, members of an affluent society live in a more benign environment than their ancestors and contemporaries in poorer countries, and in an incomparably more benign environment than that provided by nature for wild animals.

It is obviously easier to survive in a benign than in a hostile environment. Thus the primary consequence of prosperity is the prolongation of life.

It is all the more puzzling to find that, in spite of the obvious advantages, affluence is not entirely beneficial. While, on one hand, it eradicates many ailments which have plagued humanity in the past or do so in less advanced countries at present, in its wake come new plagues, specific to advanced communities. Diseases of the circulatory system, for example, are virtually unknown in the poorer parts of the world, but kill more people in some prosperous countries than all other diseases combined. Cancers present a more varied picture. Some are prevalent in poor, others in rich countries.

Richer or poorer, we all have to die of some cause. As the inhabitants of rich countries live longer than those of poor countries, is it possible that the new diseases appearing in affluent society are simply diseases of old age? If we eliminated them, would other old age diseases appear to take their place a few years later in life? Prosperity-related diseases do, in fact, take their greatest toll in old age, but they are not necessarily and exclusively old age diseases. Mortality from coronary disease in prosperous countries, for example, begins long before old age, in the thirties and forties. Mortality from such diseases is high in advanced countries even in comparison with people in the same age group in poor countries. Hence it seems necessary to assume that prosperity for some reason, promotes certain diseases or reduces resistance to them. Let us consider a few possible reasons for this.

The animal body has been designed for survival in a hostile environment, and may not be in a hurry to adapt itself to less abrasive conditions which, in biological terms, may only be transitory. It must have happened many times in biological history that an evolutionary novelty gave a species some decisive advantage against its competitors for limited resources. For that species survival ceased to be a struggle for a while, and nature, always smiling on success, ceased to be hostile. After a while the new species fills the biological niche for which it has adapted itself. Competition gradually reappears and survival, once more, becomes the reward of fitness.

Some aspects of affluence are such as to make certain biological stratagems superfluous and counterproductive. The life of a long-lived animal, under natural conditions, consists of periods of abundance interspersed with lean seasons. Various biological stratagems, such as hibernation or the accumulation of fat, are employed to see the animal through periods of starvation. An elaborate rationing system exists to ensure that when food is scarce, essential organs have first claim to available resources, and dispensable tissues, if necessary, have to starve and possibly perish. The rationing authority is the pancreas and the system works by virtue of the fact that some tissues or organs, like the brain, can draw glucose from the circulation in the absence of insulin, others only in its presence, and low priority tissues may require more insulin than others higher on the priority list. Another regulator is the thyroid which influences oxygen uptake by various tissues and thus controls the general level of physical activity. Under conditions of uninterrupted abundance these organs work under unnatural conditions and their possible malfunctions may be involved in the pathogenesis of certain disorders. Similarly, the natural thrift of the body may not always serve our best advantage and may result in overweight under conditions of affluence.

Prosperity coupled with compassion results in the perpetuation of genetic defects. In a hostile environment individuals suffering from organ or enzymal failure, like diabetes, kidney failure or cystic fibrosis, would die; in a compassionate society they survive and impart their defects to their progeny. In spite of the treatment of the primary defect, diseases like diabetes or familial hypercholesterolaemia, predispose to early death from artery disease.

Probably the most important factor is the great *variety* of food consumed in prosperous countries. An animal which can collect its food from all parts of the earth from the arctic to the tropics has never before existed in biological history. There is no bartering of food in the animal world; an animal dependent on foodstuffs unobtainable in its territory would have immediately died out. Essential nutrients which the animal cannot synthesise itself (hence has to find ready-made in its environment) must, of necessity be easily available. The belief that we have to search the world for them must be clearly mistaken. On the other hand most, if not all, plants produce substances which are mildly toxic to animals. Animals, in their turn, learn to cope with these substances. It is this ability that may be exhausted or impaired by the wide variety of foods on our table.

It is these subjects which we intend to explore in this book. The connection between food and disease is still largely a matter of search. There are few certainties; in many fields we are still groping in the dark. In some subjects we do not agree with the currently fashionable views and present arguments against them. In other cases several ideas have been put forward already. If we have not done any work on that field ourselves, we try to present the conflicting views impartially, or state our views if we believe that one side has presented a better argument than the other.

Stephen Seely,
David L.J. Freed,
Gerald A. Silverstone,
Vicky Rippere.

1 DISEASES KNOWN TO BE CAUSED BY THE DIET

D.L.J. Freed and S. Seely

Probably every disease known to mankind has some connection with the diet, at least in the sense that nutritional deficiencies weaken the natural defence mechanism of the body. A serious metabolic disturbance, like diabetes, even if corrected by the administration of insulin, predisposes to unrelated diseases, like coronary disease, presumably because neither the quantity, nor the timing of the dosage is as good as the regulatory effect of the healthy pancreas. However, this book is not concerned with distant connections with diet. Nor does it discuss an obviously diet-related disease: malnutrition. Its subject is the connection between various diseases and a hygienically prepared, adequate Western diet. Such a diet, in spite of all precautions, still plays a part in the pathogenesis of some diseases, presumably because some foods are in fact mildly toxic and their cumulative effect can be pathogenic. Such mildly toxic substances in the diet can be immensely difficult to detect.

Once a dietary pathogen has been identified, the disease it causes tends to fade into insignificance. Diseases which, at one time, were the scourges of mankind, tend to yield to ridiculously simple measures once the cause is known. Bovine tuberculosis for example, was still an important disease at the beginning of the century. It was transmitted to humans mainly in cow's milk, and the comparatively simple remedial measure of heating milk to about 70°C – pasteurisation – was sufficient to cause a dramatic reduction in its prevalence.

Most diseases which are *known* to be diet-related, are therefore only of historical interest. Nevertheless, we are giving a few examples, mainly to show the work of medical detection that went into the discovery of the pathogenic agent. The object is not only to give credit to the many unsung scientists whose work saved countless people from premature death but also because the examples serve as good omens for the future. Successes in this field are soon forgotten, the failures are still with us. Recounting the successes gives some indication of the difficulties that had to be overcome and justifies the hope that what was possible in the past, can be repeated in the future.

Dietary toxins, in the usual sense, mean substances which are toxic to a normal person. However, metabolic defects which make harmless foods pathogenic to a minority population group constitute a confusing factor and appear as added difficulties. Some examples will be cited to illustrate the point.

Contaminants and Food Additives

The Sacred Flame

In the year 994 a terrible epidemic struck in the South of France. The first sign of the unknown disease was pain in the extremities, first the toes and fingers, then the feet and hands turned blue and gradually black. Ultimately gangrene set in and the victim died, slowly and painfully, of the general sepsis that followed. The epidemic is mentioned in several chronicles, one of which estimates that it caused 40,000 deaths. What there was of medical practice at the time was largely in the hands of the priests, whom the epidemic took as much by surprise as anyone else. They were quite helpless to resist its progress and named it 'ignis sacer', declaring it to be a visitation for the sins of mankind. This was probably the best explanation at the time, but it could hardly have given much succour to the ill and dying.

Similar outbreaks, sporadic and capricious in occurrence, plagued Europe for a thousand years. Besides France the main sufferers were Germany, Austria, Poland, Finland, the Balkans and Russia. There was at least one major outbreak in every century, small outbreaks considerably more often. Another bad epidemic occurred in the South of France in 1777, causing 8,000 deaths. Probably the only European country which never suffered any fatalities was England, though some people were taken ill in a minor outbreak at Wattisham, near Bury St. Edmunds, in 1762. In Norway there was only one outbreak in recorded history, while in Finland there were two as late as the nineteenth century, in 1840 and 1862, with a death toll of about 300. There were four outbreaks in the nineteenth century in France and a serious epidemic in 1857 in Hungary. The last major outbreak occurred in 1926 in Russia. More than 10,000 people were ill, 1,600 seriously, 93 died. The last small outbreak occurred in 1951 in the small French town of Pont St. Esprit where 150 people were taken ill, and four died.

It took something like 500 years after the epidemic of 994 to discover that the disease was caused by the rye fungus ergot (*Claviceps purpurea*), the overwintering fructification (the sclerotium) of which mixes with rye grain, and if ground up with it, makes the rye flour toxic with its alkaloids (Figure 1.1). Thus in the sixteenth century in

Figure 1.1: Ergot-infested Grass

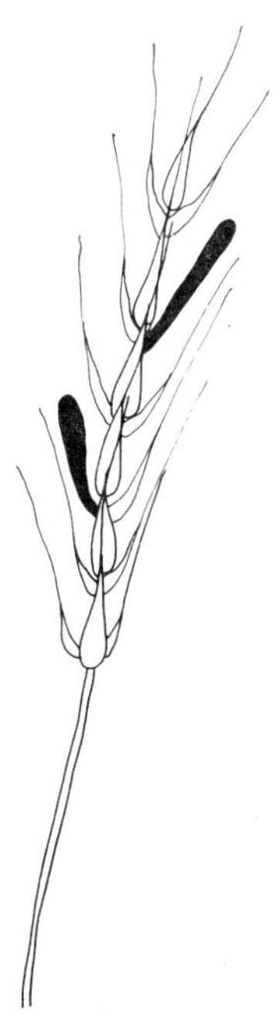

Germany sieves were used to separate the sclerotia of ergot from the grain. In other cases a flotation process was used for the separation, as the sclerotia, which are lighter than the rye grains and lighter than water, float to the surface when the mixture is immersed in water. In spite of these techniques, epidemics continued unabated, mainly because of the sporadic nature of the outbreaks. Like lightning, they seldom struck in the same place twice, and if a locality did not experience an outbreak for a century or more, farmers were invariably taken by surprise when an outbreak did occur.

The explanation of the sporadic nature of the epidemics is in the life cycle of ergot. This differs from other parasitic fungi. Instead of dispersing a multitude of individual spores, ergot produces an overwintering stage, the sclerotium. This contains a store of nutrients as well as a number of toxic alkaloids, protected by a chitinous cover. In the spring 30–40 small mushroom-like plants grow out of the sclerotium, which altogether produce about a million spores. These, unlike the spores of other parasitic fungi, like rust or mildew, which can establish themselves on the leaves of the host plant, must find their way to the stigma of a grass flower; they cannot establish themselves in any other position. There they germinate and find their way to the ovary. The fungus sequestrates the nutrients the plant produces for its seedling and the sclerotium develops in its place.

Ergot can parasitise a number of grasses, but its main hosts are rye and its wild counterparts, the rye grasses. The reason is that rye and rye grasses depend on cross fertilisation, while many other grasses are either exclusively or mainly self-pollinators. In wheat, notably, self-pollination takes place within unopened florets, so the stigma is inaccessible to fungal spores. Wheat and rye represent the two extremes, other cereals, like oats and barley are between the two, but rely mainly on self-pollination.

The ergot infestation of rye in most years is slight. One of us did some fieldwork on the subject and found that ergoted plants were not easy to find in a rye field in normal years, one had to search for them. However, rye plants growing in isolation, like self-sown plants at the roadside or among other crops, were usually heavily ergoted. The reason is that the fungal spores have to compete with the pollen of the host plant. A single floret of rye produces about 50,000 pollen grains, an ear of rye nearly as many as the spores of a sclerotium. When rye plants are growing in close proximity to each other, the competition is highly unequal in favour of the pollen. As soon as the floret is fertilised, it closes, making its stigma inaccessible to spores. The florets of isolated plants have to stay open longer, so the chance of infestation is correspondingly increased. This normal sequence of events is probably upset if heavy and prolonged rain falls at the critical time when rye pollen is released. Many pollen grains are probably beaten to the ground and washed away. The florets remaining unfertilised for longer than usual, are vulnerable to fungal spores. Such freak conditions are needed to give rise to the rare outbreaks of heavy ergot infestation.

Ergoted grass growing among other cereals, their seeds mixing with the grain, can give rise to minor outbreaks. Thus there were a few minor outbreaks in the last century in Sweden, though little if any rye is grown there. The small outbreak at Wattisham may have been caused in this manner, though ergot infestation of oats or barley might have been the possible cause. Cattle can also be affected by ergoted grass.

The most important toxic constituents of ergot are two alkaloids, ergotamine and lysergic acid diethylamide (LSD). In small quantities ergotamine is a contractor of smooth muscle. Its action on the pregnant uterus causes powerful contractions, accelerating childbirth. On the muscular layer of blood vessels it acts as a vasoconstrictor. In large doses the vasoconstrictor effect can be powerful enough to shut down peripheral circulation, causing blood-starved tissues to die of ischaemia. The other alkaloid, LSD, is a hallucinogen, a small dose of which can cause vivid visual sensations. A large, but sublethal dose, can cause epileptiform convulsions, an even larger dose is fatal.

The main reason for the disappearance of ergot epidemics is not so much that the fungus has been brought under control, but that rye, as a food plant, has largely been displaced by other foods. The cultivation of rye in Europe considerably decreased with the introduction of potatoes, and the advent of artificial fertilisers made wheat growing possible on poor soils previously suitable only for the more undemanding rye.

Butter Yellow

Coming nearer to our times, there was a serious outbreak of liver cancer in the early 1930s in the Far East. The Japanese scientist R. Kinosita,[1] investigating the outbreak, came to suspect a yellow aniline dye used to colour butter and margarine, introduced some years before in that area. Though the use of the dye was beginning to spread in Europe, it was still restricted mainly to the East when Kinosita started his investigations. He demonstrated the powerful carcinogenic effect of the dye, subsequently named butter yellow, in experiments on rats. The use of the dye was discontinued and the epidemic gradually petered out. Apart from the Far East, the timely discovery also saved Europe from a similar experience.

Pink Disease (acrodynia)[2–6]

Although the culprit agent of pink disease was not strictly a food, the story of its discovery and eradication is nicely illustrative of this kind of detective work.

Pink disease[6] was a chronic and unpleasant, occasionally fatal, illness of babies and young children that first became apparent in the late nineteenth century in Australia and soon spread to the rest of the English-speaking world and (albeit in older children) to continental Europe. By the 1940s it was quite common; most family doctors had three or four cases in their practices (especially in industrial towns) and pink disease accounted for 3–4 per cent of all paediatric hospital admissions in some cities. Within a decade, following the pinpointing of the cause, it had virtually disappeared.[5] Today's doctors have never seen a case and are not taught about it; a new epidemic of pink disease would probably catch us as unprepared as were our fathers.

Breast-fed and bottle-fed babies were equally susceptible. The child became restless and listless, unable to play, occasionally irritated by light. The arms and legs hung passively, and children who had been old enough to walk before the disease, stopped walking, although there was no true paralysis. The fingers and toes, then the palms and the soles, became swollen, cold and clammy, and assumed the dusky red colour that gave the disease its name. The cheeks and nose were often bright red. The hair fell out. The teeth loosened in inflamed gums, and there was even patchy erosion of the jawbone in some. The child lost interest in food, although it salivated excessively and was often thirsty. Most wearing of all was the dreadful insomnia, which kept child and parents awake, night after night after night. The mortality was about 10 per cent, and we can assume that some of that was due to battering, by overtired parents driven beyond breaking point.

There was no shortage of theories to explain this disease, varying from primary emotional disorder and neurosis through to endocrine or electrolyte disturbance, photosensitivity, allergy, virus infection, ergotism (see above) and arsenic or thallium poisoning. There was also no shortage of reported cures. Tonsillectomy, liver powder, vitamin supplements, hormone injections, and electrolyte adjustments all enjoyed transient popularity as first glowing claims, then negative counter-claims, appeared in the medical and lay press. Controlled clinical trials were still in their infancy, and many hopes were raised time after time, only to be cruelly dashed as the uselessness of the touted cure became obvious. Disease states similar to pink disease were induced in laboratory rats by depriving them of pyridoxine, but this vitamin proved another disappointment when tried in patients.

Then in 1945 a severely affected child was admitted to hospital in Cincinnati, Ohio, under the care of Dr Josef Warkany.[3] The disease was rare in Cincinnati, and Warkany's interest was aroused (as well as his compassion). He had a hunch that heavy metal poisoning might be implicated, so asked his laboratory to measure the levels of the common industrial heavy metals in the child's urine. The results were all negative. But one element – mercury – had not been measured as there was no adequate test for it at the time. By luck, Warkany discovered that in Cincinnati there was a young chemist, Mr Donald Hubbard, who had recently developed a reliable and sensitive method for measuring urinary mercury, so for the sake of completeness he asked Hubbard to do the measurement on his patient. The result was strongly positive. Over the next three years Warkany appealed for urine specimens from the patients of his fellow American paediatricians (pink disease was too rare in Cincinnati to allow him to do the study on his own patients), and slowly a pattern emerged. In every case of pink disease there was a history of mercury use, a positive urine mercury test or both. In a group of control patients from Warkany's own practice, urinary mercury was virtually never seen.

Mercury and its salts were, and are, commonly used in industrial processes, and prior to the introduction of effective public-health legislation in the nineteenth century cases of mercury poisoning were quite common among factory workers. The element was especially used in the manufacture of felt hats, and the touchiness and irritability of 'mad hatters' became legendary. Years later, in 1966, Warkany wryly commented[6] that if a case of pink disease had been seen by a competent eighteenth century physician, the diagnosis would have been immediately obvious. But by 1940 industrial mercury was tightly regulated by law, and frank mercury poisoning was vanishingly rare; doctors had never seen it. The only continuing source of mercury was in medicine. Mercury salts are effective against intestinal worms and syphilis, and are also effective diuretics and purgatives. In the days when nothing safer was available, these drugs were widely prescribed. In the early nineteenth century mercurous chloride also made an appearance in 'teething powders', which were given to irritable crying babies in the hopeful belief that the resulting brisk purgation would 'cleanse the system'. The more irritable the child became, the more 'teething powder' he was likely to be given. Steedman's teething powder was the most popular in Britain, containing 26.3 per cent mercurous chloride.[4] Similar powders were popular throughout the English-speaking world, though they never took hold in continental Europe.

Warkany and Hubbard published their findings in 1948, and by 1950 the hypothesis that pink disease was caused by the mercury in teething powders had become quite popular. The American Food and Drug Administration attempted (unsuccessfully) to ban the products. But there were dissenting voices. Why was pink disease rare in comparison with the enormous intake of teething powders? (Steedman's sold an incredible 7 million doses a year.) Why was it more common in some parts of the country than in others, although the sales of teething powders were the same? Why did some patients have no history of mercury exposure, in spite of intense and pointed questioning by the doctors? Why did many pharmacists swear that they had sold thousands of teething powders over the years, and had never seen a case of pink disease? (In fact, only one in 500 children exposed to the teething powders developed the disease.) In 1950 authoritative British medical opinion was still cautious about the mercury hypothesis – an understandable caution, yet responsible, as it turned out, for the prolongation of the epidemic, with uncountable cost in human and financial terms, for several years further.

But slowly the evidence was stacking up against mercury. Dimercaprol (British-anti-Lewisite; BAL) is a chelating agent developed for military use against possible gas attacks, and in the 1950s was the standard treatment for industrial mercury poisoning. Several physicians gave their pink disease patients dimercaprol, with gratifying cures. (The drug was never tested in a proper controlled clinical trial as the disease disappeared before such a trial could be organised.) Warkany and Hubbard's reports of an association between mercury exposure and the disease was confirmed by several other workers, though these later reports also noted that urinary mercury levels were often high in healthy children too. In the rare cases of industrial mercury poisoning that occurred, astute clinicians noted that in the recovery phase after the acute illness, a condition indistinguishable from pink disease could be seen for a few weeks. Clearly, if mercury was responsible for the disease, it could not be simple poisoning, or all exposed children would suffer in a dose-related manner; the children who became ill must be excessively sensitive to the poison (idiosyncrasy).

And there the matter rested, at impasse between the mercury hypothesis and the manufacturers of mercurials. In the absence of decisive evidence, Parliament declined repeated calls to ban the products (although several states in the USA and Australia did so), and the disease remained, a chronic and fearful curse. The impasse was finally broken in 1953 by Dr J.G. Dathan of Stoke-on-Trent.[4] Upset and incensed by the miserable deaths of two of his young patients, and refusing to certify the deaths as due to natural causes, he referred the cases to the coroner. The scientific cases for and against the mercury hypothesis were arrayed against each other in an English court of law – surely an unusual setting for the resolution of a scientific debate. The jury found that the deaths were caused by mercury poisoning from Steedman's teething powder – in one case by frank overdose and in the other because of unusual sensitivity of the child – and fearing litigation or Parliamentary action the manufacturers immediately removed the mercury from their preparations, and recalled all old stocks. The other manufacturers gradually followed suit. Three years later, in Sheffield, the intake of mercurials and the incidence of pink disease had both dropped sharply[5] and by 1966 Warkany, the originator of the mercury hypothesis, was able to write a final 'post-mortem' article on pink disease in the *American Journal of Diseases of Children* – a rare but well-deserved accolade for a dedicated (and lucky) medical scientist.[6]

The story illustrates the difficulty of achieving change when doctors are confronted by powerful commercial interests, and finds an echo in the 1980s in the continuing sagas of tobacco and lead. This is especially so when the companies can muster one or two experts who will say that 'the evidence is not yet decisive'. In truth it is still not proven beyond doubt that mercury caused pink disease,[2] and it is still possible that an epidemic virus, now fortunately passed, caused it. Of course that explanation is very implausible, and now that the disease is departed no-one is sufficiently interested to do more experiments. It is also true that had the world waited for 100 per cent proof of cause-and-effect, our children would probably still be ravaged by this dreadful, but preventable, scourge.

It would be dishonest to close the pink disease story without one last remark, though as scientists we are embarrassed to have to make it. Warkany and Hubbard's original 1948 study on urinary mercury levels was seriously flawed in one crucial respect (though luckily the opponents of mercury hypothesis did not notice until too late). The control subjects whose urine was free of mercury were drawn from Warkany's own practice in Cincinnati, where the disease was rare and *where teething powders were rarely used*. Had the control urines been taken from the geographical areas where patients came from, mercury would have been found in several apparently normal healthy children, thus making the association far less striking. If Warkany and Hubbard had done a scientifically impeccable trial, the cause might never have been noticed.

When the Dietary Item Itself Contains a Toxicant

Alcohol and Other Addictants

The usual reason for a toxic or noxious agent remaining undetected in food is its inconspicuousness. If the consumer knew that a tin of fish was infected by *Salmonella*, he would obviously not eat it. In other cases the toxic substance, for instance, a food additive, may be detectable, but it is thought to be harmless. In such cases the discovery that a seemingly harmless substance is pathogenic, may demand an immense amount of medical detective work.

In a different class of diet-related diseases the toxicity of the pathogen is well-known. The reason for its presence in the diet is that it is addictive. The consumer, well aware of the consequences (even if he hopes that the worst will not happen to him) is unable to abstain from its use. Fact is truly stranger than fiction. The acme of the poisoner's art in fiction is the tasteless, colourless, odourless poison; one so pleasant that the victim immediately asks for a second helping is, at least from the poisoner's point of view, too good to be true. Perhaps even more strangely, the first use of an addictive drug is often unpleasant, yet the potential victim, as often as not, gives it a second chance.

The use of addictive drugs goes back thousands of years. Remains of poppy pods have been found in the huts of the Swiss Lake Dwellers, and poppies are mentioned in Sumerian and Assyrian scripts. The Old Testament attributes the discovery of wine making to Noah, in fact the fermentation of fruit, diluted honey or grains soaked in water probably goes back to the late Stone Age. The brewing of beer was a flourishing industry in Babylon. Other drugs, like mescaline (in peyote cactus), nicotine and cocaine (in the leaves of the coca plant) were discovered by American Indians. Humanity, in fact has been poisoning itself with addictants since time immemorial.

By far the most important addictive drug, claiming more victims than all other drugs combined, is alcohol (ethanol).[7,8] It is not a highly addictive drug, in the sense that its occasional use makes disaster a virtual certainty, but it does lead to addiction in about 4-5 per cent of its users. Thus the number of alcoholics in the United States has been put at 5-7 million, about 3 per cent of the total population including abstainers.

Alcohol is a comparatively mild drug also in the sense that it does not create a craving which only rapidly increasing doses can satisfy. Tolerance to alcohol increases only slowly. Thus a chronic alcoholic needs only 2-3 times as much alcohol as a novice to induce the same degree of intoxication, while in the case of some hard drugs the factor of tolerance can be as high as 15. A heroin addict may take 10 times the dose which would be lethal to someone trying it for the first time.

In one respect, however, alcohol is the full equal of hard drugs: in the traumatic effect of its withdrawal symptoms. The cessation of taking addictive drugs is invariably followed by a withdrawal syndrome of greater or lesser severity, which may include trembling, convulsions, sleeplessness, psychotic effects, but few as severe as the *delirium tremens* of the alcohol addict. This can be fatal in otherwise healthy adults. The first stage of the alcohol withdrawal syndrome is tremulousness, weakness and profuse perspiration, which may be followed by epileptiform seizures after about 12 hours of abstinence. Delirium tremens usually begins a day (sometimes 2-3 days) after complete alcohol withdrawal. It is a state of agitated hallucinations, fever, sleeplessness, profuse sweating, sometimes complete disorientation. Death can occur from hyperthermia, vascular collapse or self-inflicted injury. In non-fatal cases delirium tremens can last for 5–7 days. In some cases recovery is not complete, the patient remains in a permanent psychotic state. The benzodiazepine drugs are now used with some success in calming such patients and alleviating the withdrawal symptoms.

Another possibly fatal consequence of chronic alcoholism is liver damage, the terminal phase of which is cirrhosis (fatty degeneration) of the liver. This can be the consequence of damage by other toxicants besides alcohol and is not the inevitable result of alcohol addiction, but alcohol is a strong predisposing factor. Some 8–10 per cent of all alcoholics ultimately develop cirrhosis of the liver.

The mechanism whereby alcohol causes intoxication is probably similar to most psychoactive drugs. The target of most (possibly all) of these are the synaptic junctions of the nervous system.[9–11] The passage of nerve impulses at synaptic junctions is mediated by a chemical transmitter, which is acetylcholine, noradrenaline or dopamine in the autonomic and sympathetic nervous systems. Not all mediators are known in the central nervous system. Beside noradrenaline and dopamine, they include adrenaline, serotonin, histamine and other polypeptides. In some (but not in all) cases the nature of the interference exercised by the drug on the nervous system is fairly well understood. Generally, they either block the release of the mediator at synaptic junctions, or compete with it, or mimic it, or cause its slow release so as to deplete its stores when it is needed. In some cases the interference affects the electrical events connected with the transmission, notably the calcium ions which trigger the release of the chemical mediator at synapses. For example, the arrow poison curare blocks acetylcholine receptors; another alkaloid, yohimbine, does the same for noradrenaline. Nicotine mimics acetylcholine, whereas mescaline bears some resemblance to adrenaline and may act as its mimic. The alkaloids of *Rauwolfia*, an Indian shrub, cause the slow release of noradrenaline. Cocaine competes for receptor sites with calcium ions.

Whereas most neurotoxins, analgesics, psychoactive drugs, etc. act essentially in a similar manner, and some of the differences between them are due to the variety of chemical mediators in the nervous system and to the different modes of attacks on them, not all factors involved in the specificity of individual drugs are understood. Anaesthetics, for instance, seem to act selectively on the superior cervical ganglion. The optic system seems the special target of many drugs. Alcohol, for instance, can induce double vision (amblyopia), its close relative, methyl alcohol (methanol) has a particularly damaging effect on vision. Hallucinogens, like mescaline or LSD, cause vivid visual images, kaleidoscopic patterns, etc. much more frequently than tactile or auditory sensations.

The exact mechanism of the depressant action of alcohol is not known, but it has been found to impede transmission across synaptic junctions. Under its influence individual neurons become less excitable, repolarise more slowly after excitation, and their spontaneous electrical activity is reduced.

In terms of a crude analogy, psychoactive drugs have access to the switchboard of the nervous system and are capable of opening some switches and closing others (hence, for instance, their usefulness as analgesics). The mystery is, why the victim finds such interference pleasant enough to seek its repetition, why the use of the drug becomes addictive in some people but not in others, and how withdrawal symptoms arise after prolonged use.

Another form of addiction may be relevant to the problem. Animal experiments with electrodes implanted in various parts of the brain show that electric impulses applied to the electrodes are perceived as pleasant in some parts of the brain, unpleasant in other parts, while the major part of the brain is insensitive. If the animal itself can operate the contact delivering impulses to electrodes implanted in the pleasure areas of its brain, it quickly learns to use it, then proceeds to activate it several thousand times in an hour, in preference to food, and, if separated from it, will brave electric shocks to reach it again. Such behaviour amounts to a form of addiction. Similar electrodes have also been implanted in the brain of human subjects, e.g. in patients in the terminal stage of cancer to relieve intractable pain, or in epileptics in an attempt to prevent or cure epileptic seizures. Such patients report 'relief of tension', 'a quiet, relaxed feeling'. The experience seems only mildly pleasurable.

The presumable natural function of non-specific pain and pleasure areas of the brain is to monitor internal conditions and register needs, like thirst or hunger, by unpleasant sensations, followed by a sense of contentment when the needs are satisfied. Addictive drugs apparently give access to such pleasurable sensations without the fulfilment of needs. The reaction of the body to such interference is apparently a re-balancing of the system so as to resist and counteract the effect of the drug. Due to increased resistance the addict needs greater doses of the drug to achieve the same effect, but in addition to this the reaction of the body seems equivalent to the application of an antagonistic drug. Thus narcotic addicts derive unclouded pleasure only from the first few applications of the drug, after which unpleasant sensations intermix with the pleasant ones. At a still later stage the drug is needed mainly to relieve these unpleasant sensations and restore 'normality'. If drug-taking is discontinued, the body is left, so to speak, under the effect of the antagonist, with symptoms opposite to those of the drug. Narcotics, for instance, contract the pupil, their withdrawal causes pupillary dilation. Barbiturates can stop epileptic convulsions, their withdrawal induces such convulsions. The biological mechanism whereby these antagonistic effects are achieved is not known. In general the reaction to the drug is a bias in the opposite direction. When the use of the drug is discontinued, the bias remains, giving rise to the withdrawal syndrome, until a new re-balancing removes the bias. Some drugs, however, cause permanent brain damage, so that normality may not always be completely restored.

Dental Caries

Caries (from the Latin word meaning decay) is the commonest disease afflicting civilised mankind, affecting 98 per cent of people in England and Wales. Twenty five per cent are totally toothless by the age of 40, and 75 per cent by the age of 60.[12] In contrast, caries in the form that we see it today is virtually never seen in ancient skulls, and the disease is still rare in modern-day primitive communities. It began to be common in Europe in the mid-nineteenth century, at the same time as cheap sugar became abundant.

But the discovery of the link with sugar came originally not from epidemiology but from experiment. The American W.D. Miller, in 1883, began experiments on healthy teeth in the test tube, and observed that typical caries was produced if certain oral bacteria were added, but only in the presence of sugar or bread. In experimental animals, caries is produced when they are fed on a high-sugar diet but not when they are reared in a germ-free environment. So the bacteria are necessary for caries. On the other hand, these organisms are always present in the healthy human mouth to some extent, and cause no damage or trouble unless sugar is consumed. So both factors are critical. Sugar – especially sucrose (cane or beet sugar) – causes the bacteria to multiply abnormally and produce excessive amounts of acid and of a complex carbohydrate slime. The acid can be sufficient to reduce the pH of the mouth from neutral to below 5 within seconds, and the slime ensures that the acid remains for as much as an hour at that level. At this degree of acidity the hard enamel of the teeth begins to dissolve. Eventually the enamel gives way, and bacteria flood into the tooth pulp, there to set up infection, inflammation, and thus toothache, abscesses etc.

Of course, there are many other factors influencing caries, as well as bacteria and sugar. Enamel can be made less soluble by flouride, for example. Different bacteria have different caries-inducing capacity. Simple tooth brushing, if done effectively several times a day with antiseptic toothpaste, would probably be sufficient to keep the bacterial population under control. The age, sex, race and nutrition of the individual all have a bearing. But towering above all these factors is sugar. No amount of tooth brushing and flouride will prevent caries when the sugar consumption is high.

This has been demonstrated so many times, by epidemiological observations and experimental interventions in humans, that the case linking caries with sugar is probably the strongest that has ever been made for a dietary disease. In a scientifically excellent (if ethically dubious) experiment on Swedish mental institution inmates in the 1950s, some patients were denied all sugar while others were encouraged to consume toffee *ad lib* day and night, and other groups were assigned an intermediate intake. The resulting differences in caries incidence were rapid and huge, although it was noted that *some* caries occurred even at zero sugar intake. In contrast to the sugar story is the once fashionable theory that fibrous 'cleansing' foods such as carrots and apples protect against caries by cleaning plaque away from the teeth. This is not true. A high carrot and apple intake does not protect against caries unless sugar intake is reduced at the same time.[12,13]

Coeliac Disease (Idiopathic Steatorrhoea; Non-tropical Sprue[14–21])

Some people can slowly starve in the midst of plenty because they cannot digest the food that they eat. This is a state called malabsorption. To some degrees malabsorption occurs whenever we catch gastroenteritis – a 'tummy bug' – but this is usually over within a few days. But when it continues for months, or years, it becomes a problem and comes to the attention of doctors. The causes are many, including congenital absence of certain digestive enzymes, tropical infections, diseases of the pancreas, surgical removal of lengths of small intestine, and even overenthusiastic use of purgatives. In 1888 Dr Samuel Gee, a physician at St Bartholomew's Hospital, London, described a disease of children that he called 'the coeliac affection', in which malabsorption was the main feature but was not apparently due to any known cause. In retrospect the disease was probably known to Arataeus the Cappadocian in the fifth century, but Gee's was the first, and still the classic, description.

The disease is mainly seen in children, beginning with the first two years of life, often soon after weaning. The picture is essentially of frequent motions – four or more daily. The motions are soft, frothy, having an offensive smell, pale, bulky, and floating on water. There is abdominal distension and wind, though after a while the limbs are noticeably emaciated. The mouth is full of painful ulcers (the synonymous term *sprue* is derived from the Dutch *spruw*, which means mouth ulcers). The child becomes thin and growth is retarded. Although mental ability is unimpaired, the mood is usually miserable and irritable, with excessive crying and occasionally severe loss of appetite. After a few months various vitamins and mineral deficiencies start to become apparent, and may include anaemia (iron, folic acid, vitamin B12, vitamin E), spontaneous bruising (vitamin K), bone pains or sometimes frank rickets (vitamin D, calcium), tingling of the extremities, sore tongue, dermatitis (vitamin B), and muscle weakness (potassium, calcium). If the patient survives childhood he is usually markedly shorter than his siblings and parents. Adults can also suffer from coeliac disease, and here the characteristic bowel looseness may be absent. Instead, the diagnosis is made during the investigation of an unexplained anaemia, weight loss, or bruising tendency.[14–16]

The wall of the intestine is thin, the mucosa lacks the normal finger-like projections called villi, the crypts are increased in size and cellular contents, and there is sometimes considerable inflammation (Figure 1.2). The enzymes of the intestinal wall are reduced. Obviously the gut is deficient both in anatomical and chemical requirements for digesting food, so it is not surprising that much of the dietary fat is not digested for the body's use but excreted in the faeces (steatorrhoea). There was much learned discussion in the medical literature about what the cause might be. Pancreatic failure? Blockage of gut lymph vessels? Primary enzyme failure? Bile deficiency? Intestinal tuberculosis? None of the ideas really fitted well.

As the cause of coeliac disease was unknown, it was often difficult

Figure 1.2: Diagram of Epithelium (Surface) of Small Intestine. Normal on left. The epithelium is arranged in finger-like projections called villi. Food molecules approach from the lumen (above) and are fully digested in passage through the layer of epithelial cells, beneath which is the lamina propria, which normally contains blood vessels, lymph vessels, some muscle and a few lymphocyte and plasma cells. In the coeliac intestine the villi are stunted or absent, whereas the crypts are larger and more densely infiltrated with lymphocytes and plasma cells.

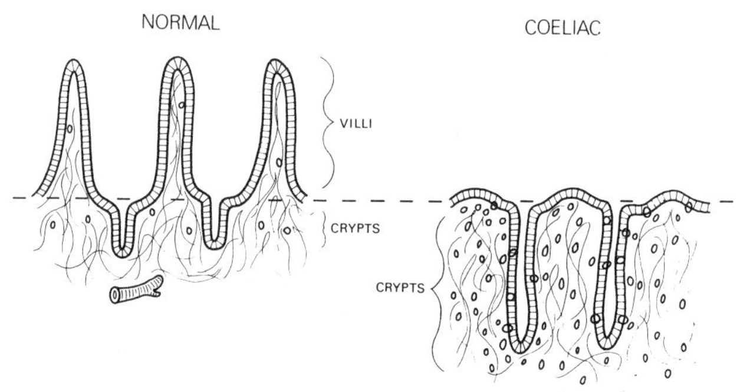

to distinguish it from other kinds of malabsorption syndrome. Apart from supplementing the diet with appropriate vitamins, there was not much that doctors could do. Since a lot of fat was being lost in the faeces, increasing the body's calcium loss, most doctors recommended a low-fat diet. Bananas were found to be beneficial, or at least well tolerated, by the patients, and for a while in the 1940s the 'banana diet' enjoyed a vogue. But doctors were well aware that a diagnosis of coeliac disease was an admission of their own helplessness, and were often reluctant to make the diagnosis. It was an unpopular disease. Gee himself seems not to have appreciated the importance of his observation, since in subsequent years he never alluded to it in his entry in the Medical Directory. Today he is chiefly remembered for Gee's Linctus.

But all this changed in 1945. A Dutch physician, Dr W.K. Dicke, noticed that in the closing stages of the second World War coeliac disease had become rare in Holland. The years 1943–4 had been lean years in Europe, with famine and much hunger, but this was not the reason for the disease's unwonted rarity as in neighbouring European countries it still occurred. And after the War, when food supplies stabilised again, coeliac disease came back to Holland too. So had there been anything different about the Dutch famine? There had. Fondness for bread and grain products had never been a national characteristic of the Dutch, and in 1943-4 hardly any wheat had been consumed in Holland. The stoic Dutch obtained such starch as they could from whatever root or other vegetables they could find. On the other hand in France and Belgium, where bread is a traditional national delicacy, wheat was still to be found during those lean years. Could coeliac disease be caused by some toxic component of wheat?

Within a few years Dicke and his colleagues had found the culprit.[15] The storage protein of wheat grains is called gluten, and gluten contains proteins known as gliadins. Gliadins are generally toxic to human intestinal tissues, though in normal individuals the dose needed to cause trouble is enormous. Coeliac patients are unusually sensitive to the poisonous action of gliadin, perhaps because they do not digest it properly, perhaps because gliadin binds unusually firmly to the surface of their intestinal cells, perhaps because they become immunologically sensitised to the proteins. Remove the gliadin from the coeliac patient's diet and his illness disappears within a few weeks (sometimes more slowly) – and also his deranged intestine becomes normal again and the enzyme levels are restored. Rye, barley and (to some extent) oats also contain gluten-like storage proteins, but the proteins of maize and rice are quite different and are safe for coeliacs. Complete digestion of gliadin to amino acids yields a product that is safe even for coeliacs, but digestion of proteins in the gut is not normally complete until the molecules have passed into the absorptive cells (see Chapter 7).

It must have come as a shock to the physicians of 1945 to realise that good wholesome bread – the staff of life – could sometimes make people ill. Moreover, the poison was not an artificial additive but a perfectly 'natural', nutritive component. One man's bread, if not one man's meat, was quite literally another man's poison. Nevertheless, to its credit, the medical profession accepted the concept quite rapidly and without controversy. To some extent this is because the commercial vested interest of the wheat farmers and bakers was never seriously threatened. Coeliac disease is, after all, mercifully rare, being of the order of one case in several thousand people (though it varies geographically – in western Ireland it rises to about one in three hundred). The vast majority of people find wheat perfectly harmless and beneficial, and Dicke's discovery never threatened to make a big impact on the habits of the general population. On the other hand the medical profession nowadays sometimes shows a perilous tendency to believe that all the problems of coeliac disease have been solved. There remains, alas, a small minority of patients who do not get better on a gluten-free diet; what of them? Beyond suggesting that such patients can't be keeping to their diets, many doctors prefer to disbelieve their existence, or else remark that if they don't get better on a gluten-free diet they can't have coeliac disease (this may bring some comfort to the doctor, but is less than helpful for the luckless sufferer). But there has been a recent suggestion that some of these people might also be sensitive to proteins of soya preparations.[19] There is no *a priori* reason to believe that wheat is intrinsically more dangerous than any other plant food, and it may be that many foods can produce a coeliac-like disease in certain sensitive individuals.

Coeliac disease can occasionally be triggered in a previously healthy adult by taking extra helpings of wheatgerm or bran on the advice of doctors or the 'health food' fraternity. Curiously, the incidence of childhood coeliac disease appears, in recent years, to be falling in at least three centres in Britain – Leeds, Glasgow and Taunton[17] – in spite of increasing awareness and improvements in diagnosis. Perhaps this is due to the recent resurgence of breastfeeding and delayed weaning. The situation will be watched with great interest in coming years.

Failure to Utilise an Essential Nutrient

Acrodermatitis Enteropathica[23–26]

This rare disease is a good example of the interaction between heredity and environment.

The illness begins in infancy and terminates, if untreated, in death in early childhood. Characteristically, it appears first when the baby is weaned from the breast (though earlier in bottle-fed babies). Resumption of breast-feeding causes the illness to retreat, but this obviously cannot be maintained indefinitely. The baby has persistent diarrhoea, which often smells foul. There is a scaly red rash, especially around the anus and on the face. The hair and nails grow slowly and are of unhealthy appearance, with persistent infections around and beneath the nails. The child's growth and development is retarded. He rarely smiles, and avoids eye-to-eye contact. He appears withdrawn, depressed, irritable, even schizoid. Apart from feeding on breastmilk, the only treatment available before 1973 was the drug diodoquin, which is a chelating agent (i.e. it binds on to metal ions).

But this drug was not always effective. Two doctors at the Great

Ormond Street Hospital for Sick Children in London, Moynahan and Barnes, discovered that one of their diodoquin-non-responsive patients was also intolerant of lactose. Lactose is the sugar that provides milk – cow, human or other – with its carbohydrate. It can only be digested if the intestine contains the enzyme lactase. The vast majority of babies have plenty of lactase, of course, but the occasional congenital lactase deficiency means that the unfortunate baby cannot digest milk, and may die unless a lactose-free formula can be provided. Moynahan and Barnes were pleased to see their patient respond well to a lactose-free breast milk (they mixed it with lactase enzyme before giving it), but this highly expensive feed could not be continued for long. On a regular lactose-free formula – one based on modified cow's milk – the symptoms reappeared. Careful analysis of the nutritional composition of this formula indicated that it was deficient in zinc.

Now it had been known for some time that zinc is a minor, but essential, part of human diet.[24] Years earlier Prasad, in Iran, had described a group of hypogonadal dwarfs – adolescents or young adults who failed to grow or develop sexually in the normal way – who were deficient in zinc because of their diet. The local staple food – an unleavened wholemeal bread known as *tanok* (rather like the Asian *chapati*) – contains high levels of phytate, which binds to zinc, calcium and other elements in the diet so that the body cannot utilise them properly. In the Iranian climate, zinc loss would be aggravated as well by excessive sweating. Prasad's dwarfs regained normal growth and development when he fed them supplements of zinc.

So Moynahan and Barnes at Great Ormond Street reasoned that if the low-lactose feed they were giving their patient was zinc deficient as well, this might account for the relapse. They gave her extra zinc sulphate, and were delighted to see her get better and remain well, though she could still not tolerate lactose.

At this stage there was no reason to suppose that zinc deficiency might be directly related to acrodermatitis enteropathica. After all, its symptoms are not very like those of Prasad's Iranian dwarfs, it is clearly an inherited disease (transmitted from parents to children as an autosomal recessive), and in any case most patients with acrodermatitis enteropathica have a perfectly normal zinc content in their diets, and (being babies) do not consume noteworthy amounts of phytate.

But Moynahan could not stop thinking about the gratifying cure he had given his lactose-intolerant patient by zinc supplementation. Response to a supplement, after all, does not prove that the disease was caused by previous deficiency – the supplement might have some unsuspected beneficial effect by itself. Tentatively, Moynahan gave zinc sulphate capsules to his other acrodermatitis enteropathica patients. It was one of the fairy-tales of medical discovery. All the children got better when given extra zinc (in amounts that for normal individuals would be a gross overdose), and no longer needed any drug or other dietary treatment. In a letter to the *Lancet* in 1973 Moynahan described acrodermatitis enteropathica as a 'lethal inherited human zinc deficiency disorder',[22] a verdict that has been confirmed by numerous reports in the world literature since then. Like pernicious anaemia a half-century earlier, a terrible and inexorable killing disease had been vanquished, by a simple dietary supplement.

This story of discovery is noteworthy for the remarkable number of false clues that lay in wait to mislead investigators. Consider the relationship with milk. The disease first appears when the baby is taken off the breast and/or given cow's milk and it retreats if breastfeeding is reintroduced, only to reappear when other foods are given again. With hindsight, investigators soon established that breastmilk has a higher available zinc content than cow's milk. But at the time that sequence could easily have been mistaken for allergy to cow's milk, or at least lactose intolerance. Again, the drug diodoquin was originally prescribed not for its chelating activity but because of its ability to kill the protozoan parasite *Giardia lamblia*, under the mistaken belief that the diarrhoea was caused by this parasite. And then again, acrodermatitis enteropathica is associated with a profound deficiency in immunological functions[25,26] – skin tests to tuberculin remain stubbornly negative in spite of TB vaccination, the lymphocytes refuse to respond to stimulation, the polymorphs fail to migrate in response to the proper stimuli. For a while, indeed, some experts believed that acrodermatitis enteropathica was caused by immunodeficiency. But once Moynahan had shown that the disease gets better on zinc supplementation, it was quickly realised that all of the immunological abnormalities return to normal as well. They are the effects of the disease, not the cause. It is always dangerous, when observing that a certain disease is *associated with* a certain set of abnormal functions or dietary habits, to infer that the disease is *caused by* them. This is a lesson that should be borne in mind when reading Chapter 2.

Food as a Source of Infection

Food Poisoning and Brucellosis[27–29]

Most of us refuse bad meat because we know it would make us ill. The picture of acute food poisoning ('gastric 'flu'; 'tummy bug') is so familiar that it needs little description. What parent has never sat up all night nursing a vomiting toddler, glumly contemplating the probability that within a few days the whole household will be similarly affected? As the infection passes down the alimentary tract the vomiting is replaced by abdominal pains and then by diarrhoea, and with luck the whole miserable episode is over within two or three days. Mind you, the illness can be severe, and is not always so benign. In the tropics, diarrhoea diseases are a major cause of childhood death, and the vicious circle of infection → malnutrition → infection is the scourge of all poor countries. Even in the prosperous USA outbreaks of botulism from home-bottled fruit still occur, causing occasional deaths, and in any country the consumption of a strongly flavoured mackerel or salmon can sometimes lead to a nasty attack of scombrotoxin poisoning from bacterial action on the flesh.

The causative organisms are many, including various bacteria, viruses and protozoa. But one bacterium, *Brucella*, causes such a singular illness that we should consider it in some detail.

Brucellosis (Malta Fever, undulant fever) is the collective name given to illnesses caused by infection with these organisms. *Brucella* is primarily an animal parasite, being spread only incidentally to Man. There are three main species: *Brucella abortus* which infects cattle worldwide and causes infectious abortion in pregnant cows; *Br. melitensis* which mainly infects goats, especially in Mediterranean countries; and *Br. suis*, a swine parasite that is especially endemic in the midwest United States. Among humans brucellosis is a well-known hazard for vets, farmers and abbattoir workers, who have close contact with infected animals in the course of their work. Bacteriologists studying the organism sometimes become its victims. The reason for its inclusion in this book is that brucellae frequently settle in the udder of the infected beast and are thus passed into the milk, usually for the animal's lifetime. Brucellae are killed by pasteurisation but some farmers and whole food enthusiasts prefer the taste or composition of untreated milk and so occasionally fall victim. (From the 1 May 1985 a UK government regulation forbids the sale of untreated milk in shops, restaurants and hospitals, or via wholesalers. It will still be legally available at the farm gate. Several states in the USA and EEC have similar regulations.)

The illness is very varied; atypical variants are commoner than typical cases. Some cases are severe, giving rise to classic undulant fever or even a rare malignant form in which high fevers culminate within a few days in death. But most cases are not life-threatening, and the symptoms are remarkable for being vague and non-specific, though quite severe enough to devastate the sufferer.[27,28] The incubation period after infection can last for weeks or months, and the onset may be insidious. At first the patient merely finds that he is becoming easily tired, especially in the afternoons. Then mild headaches begin, a distaste for food (especially towards evening), spells of chilliness and some insomnia. Fever, when it occurs, is usually mild. Then generalised aches and pains make their appearance, especially in the back, with constipation and gradual loss of weight. As the syndrome slowly builds up, drenching night sweats become a feature. Only now is the doctor consulted, and even at its height the story is vague and hard to recognise. Many patients, not surprisingly, have difficulty in defining their ailments, emphasising perhaps one or two symptoms that they can put into words.

The mental symptoms may be quite prominent, with anxiety, severe depression (suicide by infected vets is not unknown), irritability of temper, tears without cause, shyness or diffidence, a dazed feeling, difficulty in concentrating or in finding the right words, a lack of initiative, confidence and willpower.

There are no characteristic physical findings on examination. The spleen or lymph nodes may be enlarged, or may not be. There is usually some anaemia. Occasionally the testicles become inflamed. Skin tests and blood tests are of arguable reliability, though they are certainly helpful. Antibiotics (tetracycline, streptomycin or cotrimoxazole) are often helpful in limiting the disease, though by no means always.

Given the vagueness of the story it is not surprising that some doctors miss the diagnosis, while others (including, as a rule, vets) tend to suspect brucellosis readily (too readily?) for all manner of ill-defined ailments. Dr H. Rowland,[27] writing in 1978 in the influential *Price's Textbook of the Practice of Medicine*, maintained that the disease is generally overdiagnosed, whereas Dr R.J. Henderson and his colleagues,[29] writing in 1975 in the *British Medical Journal*, took the opposite view. They advised that the best diagnostic accuracy is obtain by disregarding the blood tests and taking a careful history, and applying a high index of suspicion. The controversy is impossible to resolve. Had it not been for the historical accident of the disease becoming rampant among British sailors in Malta at the end of the nineteenth century, making necessary the Royal Society Commission of Enquiry of 1905-1907 and its consequent identification of infected goat's milk and cheese as a source of infection, it is likely that chronic brucellosis would have remained forever undefined, the province of psychiatrists, fringe practitioners and quacks. If we had set out to *invent* a clinical picture designed to confuse doctors and make them suspect hysteria, hypochondriasis or malingering, we could hardly have done better (to make the suspicion even more convincing we should have made the patients female). There are parallels here with the so-called 'total allergy syndrome' (see Chapter 7).

With or without antibiotic treatment, most brucellosis sufferers eventually recover most of their health, though episodes of tiredness and residual illness may conspire to spoil their relish for life for many years afterwards. Since the cause is known, and for most people avoidable (by pasteurisation) it is curious that some folk nevertheless continue to take the risk.

References

For Butter Yellow

1. Kinosita, R. 'Studies on Carcinogenic Chemical Substances', *Transactions of the Pathological Society of Japan* (1937) *27*, 665–725.

For Pink Disease

2. Friberg, L. and Vostal, J. *Mercury in the Environment – a Toxicological and Epidemiological Appraisal* (CRC Press, Cleveland, Ohio, 1972) pp. 99–100.
3. Warkany, J. and Hubbard, D.M. 'Mercury in the Urine of Children with Acrodynia', *Lancet* (1948), *i*, 829.
4. Dathan, J.G. 'Acrodynia Associated with Mercury', *British Medical Journal* (1954), *i*, 247–9.
5. Colver, T. 'Pink Disease and Mercury in Sheffield 1947–1955', *British Medical Journal* (1956), *i*, 897–8.
6. Warkany, J. 'Acrodynia – Postmortem on a Disease', *American Journal of Diseases of Children* (1966), *112*, 147–56.

For Alcohol and Other Addictants

7. Hofmann, F.G. *A Handbook on Drug and Alcohol Abuse, the Biomedical Aspects* (Oxford University Press, New York, 1975).
8. Laurence, D.R. 'Non-medical Use of Drugs, Drug Dependence, Tobacco, Alcohol' in *Clinical Pharmacology*, 4th edn (Churchill Livingstone, Edinburgh, 1973).
9. Wilson, A., Shield, H.O. and Modell, W. 'Pharmacology of Central Nervous System and Local Anaesthetics' in *Applied Pharmacology*, 11th edn (Churchill Livingstone, Edinburgh, 1975).
10. Robinson, T. 'The Evolutionary Ecology of Alkaloids' in G.A. Rosenthal and D.H. Jansen (eds.) *Herbivores, Their Interaction with Secondary Plant Metabolites* (Academic Press, New York, 1979).
11. Jaffe, J.H. 'Drug Addiction and Drug Abuse' in L. Goodman and A. Gilman (eds.) *The Pharmacological Basis of Therapeutics*, 4th edn (Macmillan, New York, 1970).

For Dental Caries

12. Silverstone, L.M., Johnson, N.W., Hardie, J.M. and Williams, R.A.D. *Dental Caries: Aetiology, Pathology and Prevention* (Macmillan, London, 1981).

13. Shieham, A. 'Sugars and Dental Decay', *Lancet* (1983), *i*, 282–4.

For Coeliac Disease

14. Bockus, H.L. *Gastro-enterology*, vol. II (W.B. Saunders, Philadelphia, 1944), pp. 229–47. (Interested readers with access to a medical library may care to compare this chapter with the corresponding chapter in the second edition of the same book, written in 1962.)
15. Dissanayake, A.S. 'Coeliac Disease' in S.C. Truelove and D.P. Jewell (eds.) *Topics in Gastroenterology 1* (Blackwell Scientific Publications, Oxford, 1973), pp. 167–83.
16. Wright, R. 'Coeliac Disease and Gastrointestinal Allergy' in R. Wright (ed.) *Immunology of Gastrointestinal and Liver Disease* (Edward Arnold, London, 1977), pp. 27–38.
17. Littlewood, J.M., Crollick, A.J. and Richards, I.D.G., *also* Challacombe, D.N. and Baylis, J.M. 'Childhood Coeliac Disease is Disappearing' (Letters to the editor.) *Lancet* (1980), *ii*, 1359–60.
18. Dossetor, J.F.B., Gibson, A.A.M. and McNeish, A.S. *Lancet* (1981), *i*, 322–3.
19. Haeney, M.R., Goodwin, B.J.F., Barratt, M.E.J. *et al.* 'Soya Protein Antibodies in Man; Their Occurrence and Possible Relevance in Coeliac Disease', *Journal of Clinical Pathology* (1982), *35*, 319–22.
20. Savilahti, E., Viander, M., Perkkio, M. *et al.* 'IgA Antigliadin Antibodies: a Marker of Mucosal Damage in Childhood Coeliac Disease', *Lancet* (1983), *i*, 320–22.
21. Ashkenazi, A., Levin, S., Idar, D. *et al.* 'Immunologic Assay for the Diagnosis of Coeliac Disease: Interaction Between Purified Gluten Fractions', *Pediatric Research* (1980), *14*, 776–8.
22. Green, F.H.J. and Freed, D.L.J. 'Antibody-facilitated Digestion and the Consequence of its Failure' in W.A. Hemmings (ed.) *Antigen Absorption by the Gut* (MTP Press, Lancaster, 1978), pp. 182–97.

For Acrodermatitis enteropathica

23. Moynahan, A.E. 'Acrodermatitis Enteropathica: a Lethal Inherited Human Zinc-deficiency Disorder', *Lancet* (1973), *i*, 676–7.
24. Editorial, 'Zinc Deficiency in Man', *Lancet* (1973), *i*, 229–30.
25. Chandra, R.K. 'Zinc Levels and Cell-mediated Immunity', *Paediatrics* (1980), *66*, 789–91.
26. Cates, K.L. 'Defects in Neutrophil Chemotaxis' in A.D.B. Webster (ed.) *The Assessment of Immunocompetence* Clinics in Immunology and Allergy 1. (W.B. Saunders, Philadelphia and London, 1981), p. 616.

For Brucellosis

27. Rowland, H.A.K. in R. Bodley Scott (ed.) *Price's Textbook of the Practice of Medicine* (Oxford University Press, Oxford, 1978), p. 52.
28. Huddleston, I.F. *Brucellosis in Man and Animals* (The Commonwealth Fund, New York, 1943).
29. Henderson, R.J., Hill, D.M., Vickers, A.A. *et al.* 'Brucellosis and Veterinary Surgeons', *British Medical Journal* (1975), *2*, 656–9.

2 DISEASES SUSPECTED TO BE CONNECTED WITH THE DIET

S. Seely

The Reasons for Suspicion

As already pointed out, once a disease is known to be caused by some item of diet, society tends to lose interest in it. The offending contaminant or food additive is eliminated and lo, the disease disappears like magic. In some cases the causative agent, for example alcohol, is difficult to banish, but at least the potential victims have been warned and have only themselves and their peculiar body chemistry to blame for their plight.

Of far greater concern are diseases – some of them the most important killing diseases of our time – which are suspected to be caused by the diet, since it is possible that literally millions of deaths would be preventable in Western countries, if we were clever enough to identify the causative agents. The most important diseases thought to be diet-related are two disorders of the circulatory system, coronary heart disease and cerebrovascular disease (strokes), and three cancers, those of the stomach, large intestine (colon and rectum) and of the breast.

The first question that arises in connection with these diseases is that if the causative agents are unknown, how is it possible to know, or at least guess, that the diet is involved in their pathogenesis? The answer is that the diseases in question have peculiarities which suggest a connection with the diet. Food in advanced countries obviously does not contain strongly toxic substances, or even mildly toxic ones if their consumption is followed by immediate ill effects. Dietary toxins which evade detection must be substances with a slow, cumulative effect, like lead, or cause overt disease only after a long latent period, like carcinogens. This gives diet-related diseases their first important characteristic: there is something puzzling about them. There is no apparent cause: no microorganisms, no genetic error, no organ failure. Secondly, human diet is highly variable, changing not only with climate, the availability of various kinds of food and other natural conditions, but also with arbitrarily imposed factors, local customs, traditions and the like. Considerable differences can exist between the diet of neighbouring countries, even if their people are ethnically related. Similarly, the prevalence of suspected diet-related diseases shows such apparently capricious variations from one country to the next. In Central Europe, for example,[1] mortality from coronary disease is high in three neighbouring countries, Austria, Czechoslovakia and Hungary, and low in the three adjacent countries of Poland, Rumania and Yugoslavia. The mortality ratio of the two areas is of the order 3/1. The population of the area belongs to three ethnic groups, the Austrians being Germanic, the Hungarians a mixed group preserving traces of Asiatic origin, and the population of the four remaining countries being Slavs, so the high-risk and low-risk areas cut across ethnic boundaries. The high-risk countries are the successor states of the one-time Austro-Hungarian Monarchy, their cultural links apparently overriding ethnic affinities.

The study of large ethnic groups provides two distinct patterns. In one case the prevalence of the suspected diet-related diseases seems to depend on environmental conditions, and in the other, groups take their diseases with them wherever they go. For instance, coronary disease is virtually non-existent in the poorer parts of Africa, but while African negroes appear immune to the disease, they are certainly not immune to it in the United States (where their coronary mortality is much the same as of American whites). The black population of the West Indies or of South Africa fall between the two extremes. Their mortality rates are between a quarter and a third of that in the United States. On the other hand, the mortality from coronary disease of Israelis of European origin in Israel is similar to that of Jews living in Europe or in the United States. Coronary mortality in all English-speaking countries, including the United States, the United Kingdom, Canada, Australia, New Zealand and Ireland, is similar irrespective of climatic variations. Thus if male mortality in the 45–74 age group in the United States is taken as 100, it varies only between 92 and 104 in the other five countries. These findings are consistent with the assumption that if migrants move from a poor to a prosperous country, or from one prosperous country to another similarly prosperous one, they or their descendants gradually adopt the diet of the host country and their diet-related diseases change accordingly. If they go as colonisers to a sparsely inhabited region, they take their diet, and their diet-related diseases with them. Similarly, migrants from a rich to a poor country are seldom willing to adopt the rice, maize or millet diet of their hosts, so that their diet-related diseases tend to remain unchanged.

Groups of Japanese origin living in the United States have been much studied in respect of diet-related diseases, with the finding that they are gradually assimilated by the host country. Among the five major diseases suspected to be of dietary origin, mortality from coronary disease, cancer of the large intestine and breast is high in the United States and low in Japan, while cerebrovascular disease and gastric cancer mortality is high in Japan and low in the United States. It has been found that mortality from the first three causes begins to increase, and from the last two causes to decrease, in first generation Japanese born in the United States, complete assimilation usually taking two generations. There were similar significant changes in Okinawa island (Japanese population about 1 million), while it was under US administration from 1945 to 1972. Mortality from cancer of the stomach, for example, when the island was returned to Japanese sovereignty in 1972, was about a quarter of that prevailing in Japan, though still about 50 per cent higher than in the United States.[2,3] Since the climate and similar conditions are unlikely to have changed under US administration, it is difficult to conceive any other reason for the recession of gastric cancer than changes in diet.

In general terms, the worldwide distribution pattern of the five diseases follows two patterns. All bear some relation to material prosperity, in that their prevalence is very low or non-existent in the poorest parts of the world and high in advanced countries. However, cerebrovascular disease and cancer of the stomach peak at some moderate state of prosperity and begin to decline in the most advanced countries. Coronary disease, breast cancer and cancer of the colon and rectum continue to advance approximately in direct proportion with prosperity and reach their peak in the technically most advanced countries. Table 2.1 shows mortality from these diseases in 22 countries.[4] These are all member states of the Organisation of Economic Cooperation and Development (OECD), for which both detailed mortality and food consumption statistics are available. The mortality rates shown in the table apply to the latest year for which data were available at the time of writing, ranging from 1975 to 1979. The figures represent mortality from a specified disease as a pecentage of the total mortality from all causes in that country.

As seen from Table 2.1, the five diseases account for over 50 per cent of all deaths in a few Western countries, more than from all other diseases combined. Even in those countries where mortality from these diseases is comparatively low, like Yugoslavia, France, Spain and Belgium, they are responsible from a quarter to a third of all deaths.

Table 2.1: Mortality from Specific Diseases as Percentage of Total Mortality

Country	1 Coronary disease	2 Strokes	3 stomach	4 Cancers of colon, rectum	5 breast	Total of columns 1–5
Sweden	36.15	10.54	1.90	2.92	1.57	53.11
Scotland	30.59	14.66	1.71	2.62	1.79	51.37
Australia	32.08	12.60	1.31	3.09	1.64	50.62
Denmark	33.51	9.10	1.60	3.77	2.01	49.94
US	34.14	9.11	0.75	2.80	1.80	48.60
New Zealand	29.80	12.08	1.49	3.40	1.76	48.53
England and Wales	28.86	12.54	1.91	2.19	2.04	48.14
Norway	27.36	13.72	2.11	2.98	1.62	47.79
Ireland	27.76	13.56	2.12	2.80	1.49	47.73
Canada	31.59	9.27	1.32	3.20	2.01	47.39
Finland	30.24	11.69	2.40	1.70	1.32	47.35
Austria	24.65	14.91	2.90	2.94	1.49	46.91
Germany	21.39	14.08	2.64	3.25	1.64	43.00
Netherlands	23.83	10.76	2.37	3.28	2.40	42.64
Japan	9.52	23.05	7.34	2.06	0.56	42.63
Italy	19.11	14.03	2.87	2.40	1.47	39.89
Portugal	9.81	22.08	3.00	1.66	0.89	37.45
Switzerland	18.19	11.83	2.22	2.92	2.24	37.40
Belgium	15.82	12.85	1.94	2.86	1.59	35.06
Spain	10.28	16.97	2.86	1.68	1.10	32.87
France	10.51	12.82	1.73	2.95	1.57	29.58
Yugoslavia	10.87	10.67	2.10	1.20	0.88	25.72

The five diseases together cause something like 2-3 million deaths in advanced countries in a year.

Apart from geographical variations, diet also changes in time, and diet-related diseases can be expected to change with it. In the last two centuries increasing prosperity has made Western diet more varied and abundant, so that the prevalence of diet-related diseases in the past should be comparable with the poorer countries of our time. Even if reliable mortality and food consumption statistics are not available for the distant past, approximate comparisons can be instructive in some cases. This applies particularly to coronary disease which has a well-documented history. It is a comparatively new disease. Whereas its close relative, cerebrovascular disease, then called apoplexy, was already known to the Hippocratean school and references to it can be found in medieval scripts, there is no mention of coronary disease in ancient documents. Its first recognisable description is found in a letter of William Harvey dated 1648. At the end of the seventeenth century the disease was still a rarity. Thus when five cases of sudden death occurred in Rome at around 1700, presumably due to heart attacks, a papal commission was set up to investigate them. In England coronary disease began to emerge as a major disease only at about the middle of the last century. In 1900 it accounted for about 10 per cent of all deaths, the same as tuberculosis. The rise of mortality from 10 per cent to 30 per cent of all deaths which has made it the first-ranking killing disease of our time, took place only in the present century. Some of this rise is doubtless due to increased expectation of life, but the increase is spectacular even if only the mortality rate of a fixed age group, let us say, 45-64, is considered. The history of the disease is, therefore, compatible with the present absence of the disease in poor countries and its gradually increasing importance in moderately prosperous countries. The inference is that if coronary disease is caused by some pathogenic agent in the diet, the foodstuff containing it was either unknown (or was a luxury) in the past, and is still unknown (or an unobtainable luxury) in poor countries to-day, but available to all in prosperous countries.

Cerebrovascular disease is closely related to coronary disease, one affecting the arteries of the brain, the other the arteries of the heart, but both the history and the geographical distribution of the disease point to significant differences in their aetiology. The origin of cerebrovascular disease is lost in antiquity. Its geographical distribution coincides with that of coronary disease in that both are virtually non-existent in the poorest countries of the world, but cerebrovascular disease appears at a lower level of prosperity and reaches its peak at a still moderate level, e.g. in countries like Portugal, Bulgaria, Singapore, Japan. Its prevalence declines in the technologically most advanced countries. If it is caused by a dietary pathogen, that is likely to be present in a foodstuff which may still be a luxury in the poorest countries, but a more modest luxury than the causative agent of coronary disease. It seems to lose favour and tends to be superseded by greater luxuries in the most prosperous countries. Japan is an interesting example in this respect. About 20 years ago Japan was the world leader in cerebrovascular disease mortality. This was the time of rapid rise in prosperity in the country, and it was followed by a spectacular recession in cerebrovascular mortality. The rate halved in about 15 years from 1964 to 1979, and the process is still in progress at present.

Summarising, epidemiological studies provide a fair amount of evidence, even if not proof, that some of the most important killing diseases of our time could be of dietary origin. As far as I know, there is no contradictory evidence. All we have to do is to find the responsible agents, in the same way as our predecessors identified ergot, butter yellow and mercury as the causative agents of important diseases of their age. Once it is realised that important diseases are probably diet-related, the battle is half won. One might, perhaps, say that the battle is over bar the shooting.

Techniques of Searching for Dietary Pathogens

The failure to identify the causative agents of the five most important diseases of dietary origin is certainly not for the want of trying. Prodigious effort has gone into this research and uncounted millions have been spent on various projects. However, the intrinsic difficulties of the task are so great that results so far are inconclusive.

Human diet, which in the present case must be taken in the widest sense of the word to include contaminants, food additives, bacterial toxins and medicines as well as nutrients – anything that goes in at one end and out at the other – consists of thousands of items, the vast majority of which are obviously harmless. Identifying the few mild toxicants among them inevitably brings the needle in the haystack analogy to mind, and even that is inadequate to express one of the foremost difficulties of the task. It is known in advance how the needle differs from the hay, but the greatest difficulty in the given case is that a mildly noxious substance which does not produce immediate ill effects, is not distinguishable from truly harmless items of diet.

Science is mounting a two-pronged attack on the problem, attempting to dig a tunnel, so to speak, from both ends, ultimately hoping to meet in the middle. One obvious task is to scrutinise the foods we eat, examine their chemical composition, test them on animals for toxicity. More of this will be said in the next section of this chapter. The obvious difficulty of this approach is that a substance mildly toxic to one species may be completely harmless to another, particularly if one is a long-lived, the other a short-lived animal. The other approach is the study of the diseases, trying to understand their pathogenesis and looking for epidemiological clues which might lead to the causative agent. The great advances made by both of these studies must not be underrated, but their meeting in the middle of the tunnel is only distantly in sight.

The simplest and least expensive epidemiological technique is the study of the geographical distribution of a disease, together with the worldwide consumption pattern of various foodstuffs, looking for the matching pattern. The probability that a dietary item found by this method is the cause of a disease depends on the accuracy of the matching.

The method has many shortcomings and limitations. Both death certificates and food consumption statistics contain errors, so that the matching can never be perfect. Detailed statistics are available only for advanced countries, particularly food consumption statistics. The most detailed food consumption statistics available for about 20 countries are those published by the Organisation of Economic Cooperation and Development. These consist of about 60 items. If the pathogen of a given disease is not among them, the search will obviously fail. Other difficulties that may arise can be appreciated by recalling some of the examples from the previous chapter. One of the most important factors in the pathogenesis of dental caries is sugar, but clearly, sugar dissolved in drinks, like tea or coffee, makes much less contact with the teeth than, for instance, in toffee. Apart from the quantity of sugar consumption, therefore, the form of sugar intake is relevant, so that the correlation coefficient found between tooth decay and the quantity of sugar consumption may not be high enough to carry conviction. Similar difficulties would arise if an epidemiological survey attempted to establish the connection between rye consumption and ergot poisoning epidemics. Toxicity, even when associated with a given food, may not be the property of the food itself; it may only be the carrier of a pathogen. Consequently the epidemiological survey, which cannot take cognisance of the complex relation between disease and pathogen, may find only an indifferent correlation between disease and food consumption.

A similar difficulty is that a pathogenic agent may be present in more than one food, so that the correlation between the disease and one of those foodstuffs may not be convincing. Another major difficulty is presented by the many false trails caused by indirect correlations. A prosperity-related disease, like coronary heart disease, may show a degree of positive correlation with virtually any index of material advance, like the gross national product, the number of telephones, washing machines or two-car families in a community. A degree of positive correlation could probably be demonstrated between coronary disease and the consumption of lettuces, chocolate biscuits or raspberry jam. Such indirect correlations play the same role in epidemiology as false clues in a detective story.

It has been thought that some of these difficulties could be overcome by examining the diets of individuals known to suffer from a given disease and compare them with controls not affected by that disease. One method used for this purpose was the retrospective questioning of patients and controls about their diets. But it was found to introduce more errors than it eliminated. The data collected by this method are non-quantitative and of poor quality. Apart from the fact that the dietary information that really matters is not the food consumption of the patient at the time, but at a much earlier period, the errors involved are so great as to invalidate the findings. When data obtained by questioning *controls* in such surveys are compared with national food consumption statistics, there is little resemblance between them. For instance, a survey was conducted by A.B. Miller[5] in 1975 in Canada in an attempt to discover differences between the diet of a group of women suffering from breast cancer and a matched control group. The survey estimated the total daily calorie intake of the controls – all adult women – at 1947 Cal/day, in contrast to the average national daily intake in the same year of 3127 Cal/day. Similarly, the total animal fat intake of the controls, estimated on the basis of their replies, was 86.3 g/day, compared with the national daily intake of 145.1 g/day.

Nothing demonstrates the importance attached to diet-related diseases better than the large-scale, multimillion dollar projects called prospective studies. These consist of the selection of a population group, usually more than a thousand people, who are given a thorough medical examination at the beginning of the study and whose medical history is then followed for many years, possibly decades, until some or all participants die. The records kept of each participant include notes on their diet, the ultimate aim being to have statistical data of the food consumption of people who died of a given disease and of those who died of other diseases. The first of these, the Framingham Heart Study, began in 1948 and ran for 30 years. Since then numerous studies of a similar kind have been started in many countries, ranging from Israel to Russia. Several are running at present in the United Kingdom.

There could have been few medical projects in history which started with greater expectations. At one time it was thought that they could not fail to identify dietary items responsible for some of the major ills of mankind. In fact, those completed so far could, and did, fail. The basic difficulty is that it is not possible to keep records of every mouthful of food a person eats. The participants are periodically interviewed about their diet, usually on a '24 hour recall' basis. As before, the data collected in this manner are non-quantitative and of poor quality. The interviewed person does not know the composition of the food he consumed, let alone its quantity. He is likely to forget some items. The periodic samplings are not accurate representations of the whole period. Lastly it is unlikely that records are kept of hundreds of food items. Those recorded are probably the select few which were the suspects of the day when the trial started. If the true pathogenic agent of the disease under examination is not among them, decades of work and millions of dollars or pounds can be wasted.

In another form of study, the intervention trial, a group of participants are persuaded to abstain from consuming certain foodstuffs, while a control group receives no instructions and is presumed to consume the normal diet of the country. The trial continues until a proportion of both groups die, when it is ascertained whether a certain disease caused fewer deaths among the abstainers than among the controls. This method is not a search for dietary pathogens, but a test on already suspected items. Its cost-effectiveness depends on how well founded the suspicions are which the trial sets out to prove. A large trial of this nature, the Multiple Risk Factor Intervention Trial,[6] investigating the connection between coronary disease and the consumption of saturated fats and smoking ended in the United States in 1982. It cost 115 million dollars and its results were inconclusive. There was no significant difference between the coronary mortality of abstainers and controls.

A variation on the same theme is when a captive population, e.g.

that of a prison or asylum, are given a diet from which some particular food item is missing.

I intend to make only a brief mention of non-epidemiological techniques, like immunological studies. These are based on the hopeful assumption that a toxicant, even if it results in clinical disease only decades after its consumption, may produce immediate effects, or, at least, effects demonstrable at an earlier stage. As the animal body sometimes protects itself against noxious agents by the production of antibodies, a branch of research is aimed at detecting antibodies in patients suffering from a given disease, which then may lead to the identifications of the antigens against which these are directed.[7] Another assumption, applied specifically in coronary research, is that an atherogenic agent immediately increases blood cholesterol level. The assumption is impossible to prove, but is widely held to be an axiomatic truth. Consequently, for example, the cholesterol-lowering effect of a substance called clofibrate received much attention at one time and a trial was organised to test it. The trial was a failure. After some years more clofibrate-treated patients died of coronary disease than controls.[8]

While the tracking down of dietary toxins is immensely difficult, there is nothing easier than naming suspects on the basis of superficial evidence. It is still possible to find statements in medical journals comparing the 'low-fat, low-sugar, high-fibre diet' of the poorest inhabitants of Asia or Africa with the high-fat, high-sugar, low-fibre diet of advanced countries. Such simplistic arguments serve only as thin guises of preconceived ideas. The difference between the diets of poor and prosperous countries are innumerable. The diet of the poorest Africans is low not only in fats and sugar, it is also low in carrots, onions, cabbages, strawberries and oranges, to name only a few. They do not flavour their mealie meal with monosodium glutamate and do not take an aspirin when they have a headache. Such superficial arguments have produced most of the suspects connected, for example, with coronary disease: cholesterol, saturated fats, eggs, meat, sugar, coffee and the like, which serve only to mislead the public. The causative agent of coronary disease is not known and much serious work will be needed to identify it.

The Search for Toxic Substances in Food

As already explained, efforts to identify the unknown, but probably dietary causes of various diseases are like digging a tunnel from both ends. At one end the pathogenesis of the disease is investigated, hoping it will throw light on the agent causing it, at the other the foods we eat are scrutinised for possibly toxic substances. All this is done in the hope that the two branches of research will finally converge, the two half-tunnels will ultimately meet in the middle. Unfortunately, for the time being, the middle where they will meet is barely in sight, the two excavations do not even point in the same direction. On one hand epidemiologists and pathologists insist that their clues point to foods of animal origin: fats, cholesterol, meat, milk, eggs, while plant biologists find new vegetable toxins every day, without any corresponding evidence incriminating animal foods.

It is clear that, no matter what their conclusions are at present, both lines of research have to continue. It can even be predicted that ultimately they will become confluent. If results so far are contradictory, the most likely reason is that wrong conclusions have been drawn from some observations, possibly on both sides. Animal foods may not be as harmful as one side believes, nor as harmless as maintained by the other side, and the same probably applies to plant foods.

This book is intended to give a brief survey of both lines of research. So far we have discussed matters mainly from a medical-epidemiological angle, this section is intended to present a short introduction to research on food toxins.

Diet, in the present sense, must be taken in the widest possible sense to include all human ingesta, nutrients as well as food additives, contaminants, bacterial products, medicines, trace elements and the like, in fact, anything that goes into the digestive tract at one end and comes out at the other. Such ingestibles can be divided into three large groups, namely food of vegetable origin, food of animal origin and a miscellaneous group to include substances like food additives, residues of agrochemicals and the like.

For the general reader who had not taken much interest in the subject before, the most surprising feature of the following chapter, where possible toxins in various types of foods will be discussed, is likely to be the enormous number of toxic substances found in vegetable foods consumed every day, even in staples like wheat, potatoes, cabbages and other common fruit and vegetables. Such toxins, (also called secondary plant metabolites or allelochemicals) are the weaponry used by plants to defend themselves against their innumerable parasites and predators: viruses, bacteria, fungi, insects and large herbivores. We may, of course, be of the opinion that plants have been created by a benevolent providence to provide food for man and beast, but (as far as it is possible to read their thoughts) plants beg to differ. They seem to defend themselves vigorously against all comers, even if they are willing to make concessions to pollinators, seed propagators and possibly to cultivators. To some extent they fight back by mechanical means, using thorns against large herbivores, hairs to impede the movement of small insects or sticky exudates to capture them. The standard method, however, is the synthesis of chemical substances which are toxic to animals and microorganisms.

Some of the defence measures employed by plants are of considerable subtlety. It was mentioned in the first chapter that many substances, produced by a variety of plants, interfere with the nervous system of animals, particularly with nervous conduction across synaptic junctions. Some weapons of this chemical warfare possess the incredible property of being addictive to animals. The victim apparently finds the experience of being poisoned pleasant and seeks its repetition.[12]

Other plant toxins interfere with the sexual activity of animals. Many plants produce substances which simulate female hormones (oestrogens) and there is one, gossypol, present in cotton seed, which is a spermicide and is now under trial as a male contraceptive.[13] The presumable function of such hormone mimics is to regulate hormone-dependent physiological activities of animals in a manner inappropriate to their needs, e.g. by inducing a period of oestrus in immature females or needlessly prolonged oestrus (called nymphomania by animal breeders) in mature ones. A hormone mimic acting in a similar manner on insects delays metamorphosis, others hasten its occurrence.

A large class of plant toxins is directed at the digestive system of animals, including a variety of enzyme inhibitors, antivitamins, goitrogens. Antivitamins counteract the effect of vitamins. Antivitamins A, D, E, K, B_{12} as well as antithiamine, antiniacin, antipyridoxine are produced by various plants.[14] Other toxins interfere with the absorption of trace elements, like iodine, hence act as goitrogens. Some penetrative substances, like tannins (present in tea and coffee) may react with the cellular structure of the intestines.[15]

Plants produce a whole arsenal of substances capable of interfering with the circulatory system. Haemagglutinins which can cause the clumping of blood corpuscles, are produced by literally hundreds of plants. Dicoumarol[14] (or dicumerol, as spelt in American literature) is an antivitamin K present in sweet clover. It is an anticoagulant, capable of causing fatal haemorrhages in animals. (Warfarin, a synthetic chemical used as a rat poison and also as an anticoagulant in medicine, was developed on the model of dicoumarol.) Some fruits (pineapple, banana, avocado) contain serotonin, noradrenaline, dopamine, exactly the same substances, mentioned in the first chapter, which are produced by animals. These have a vasoconstrictor effect and tend to elevate the blood pressure. A substance called aminopropionitrile, present in chick peas and sweet peas, is responsible for the disease named lathyrism. This affects mainly the bones, but also the fibre structure of blood vessels, resulting in loss of elasticity, hence predisposing to rupture (aneurysms). Citral, an antivitamin A present in orange peel, has been observed to cause damage to the endothelium of blood vessels in animals. Gossypol, of male contraceptive fame, also has an effect on the heart, capable of causing death in animals by cardiac irregularity.

Chapter 3 will look at these plant chemicals in greater detail and in a more technical manner. It must be noted, however, that new plant toxins are still discovered every year and not all physiological effects of those already known are understood. For example, the primary function of oestrogen mimics presumably is interference with the reproductive cycle of animals. A synthetic oestrogen, diethylstilboestrol, however, also has an adverse effect on the circulatory system. On this analogy it is possible that phyto-oestrogens, like gossypol, may also cause damage to the arteries.

Another point to note is that while plants evolve substances toxic to animals, the animals, in turn, learn to cope with them. Some birds, for example, can eat the fruit of deadly nightshade, several insects live on tobacco plants, red deer can eat the leaves of rhododendrons. The knowledge of the composition of a substance, therefore, is not enough to reveal whether it is toxic to a given species. A new factor in our case is the invention of cooking, which destroys some (but not all) plant toxins. Other forms of processing, for instance the peeling of plant foods, may also have a similar effect.

Animals seldom defend themselves by making themselves toxic to would-be predators, though there are several known examples among insects, fish, frogs, etc. Captain Cook and the naturalist J.B. Forster were severely poisoned when eating the liver and roe of a puffer fish in New Caledonia in 1774. The puffer poison (tetrodotoxin, TXT) induces neuromuscular paralysis, in severe cases leaving the victim apparently dead. According to new findings[16] zombies in Haiti are not living dead but victims of TXT poisoning. When in the paralysed state, they are buried alive, but quickly disinterred, revived and fed 'zombi cucumber' (the hallucinogen *Datura stramonium*). Under the combined effect of anoxic brain damage and hallucinations the victim may behave as an automaton, wholly subservient to the voodoo doctor.

Among animals consumed in advanced countries only the quail has been accused of toxic properties. The Bible[17] describes a case of mass poisoning of Israelites during the exodus. The quail fell dead from the sky and the Israelites gathered them, 'but while the meat was still between their teeth' the anger of the Lord burned against them and he struck them with a severe plague. Quail poisoning still occurs in some Mediterranean countries but probably only if the quail had eaten certain seeds which are harmless to them but toxic to humans, and then it affects only people with a hereditary abnormality of carbohydrate metabolism.[18]

Less exotic circumstances, under which animal foods may acquire toxic properties, e.g. bacterial action, will be described in the next chapter.

The plants we consider edible are obviously those selected for their non-toxic (or mildly toxic) properties and we breed them to achieve a further reduction of allelochemicals. Unfortunately this process also reduces their resistance to parasites and other animals. Having reduced their ability to defend themselves, we have to take over their defence, and this is done with an arsenal of agrochemicals, fungicides, insecticides and the like. Storing plant products may involve the use of further preservatives. Some of these chemicals inevitably find their way into our food, either directly, with the plants, or indirectly, through animals which have eaten the plants. This subject will also be briefly discussed in the next chapter.

The search for food toxins covers a large field, of which only a sketchy exposition can be given in a single chapter. The interested reader's attention can be drawn to some excellent books on the subject, notably *Toxic Constituents of Plant Foodstuffs*, editor I.E. Liener (Academic Press, New York, 1980); *Herbivores, Their Interaction with Secondary Plant Metabolites*, editors G.A. Rosenthal and D.H. Janzen (Academic Press, New York, 1979); *Handbook of Naturally Occurring Food Toxicants*, editor M. Rechcigl Jr (CRC Press, Florida, 1983), and *Toxic Hazards in Food*, editors D.M. Conning and A.B.G. Lansdown (Croom Helm, London, 1983).

References

1. Seely, D. 'Diet and Atherogenesis', *Medical Hypotheses* (1979), *5*, 1067–70.
2. *Statistical Yearbook of Japan 1972*. Tokyo, 1974.
3. Seely, S. 'The Recession of Gastric Cancer and its Possible Causes', *Medical Hypotheses* (1977), *4*, 50–7.
4. World Health Organisation. World Health Statistics Annuals. Geneva, 1976–81.
5. Miller, A.B. 'Role of Nutrition in the Etiology of Breast Cancer', *Cancer* (1977), *39*, 2704–8.
6. Oliver, M.F. 'Does Control of Risk Factors Prevent Coronary Disease?' *British Medical Journal* (1982), *285*, 1065.
7. Davies, D.F. 'Immunological Aspects of Atherosclerosis', *Proceedings of Nutrition Society* (1976), *35*, 293–5.
8. Oliver, M.F., Heady, J.A., Morris, J.N. and Cooper, J. 'WHO Cooperative Trial on Primary Prevention of Ischaemic Heart Disease using Clofibrate to Lower Serum Cholesterol: Mortality Follow-up', *Lancet* (1980), *ii*, 379.
9. Miettinen, M., Turpeinen, O., Karvonen, M.J. *et al.* 'Effect of Cholesterol-lowering Diet on Mortality from Coronary Disease and Other Causes: a Twelve Year Clinical Trial on Men and Women', *Lancet* (1972), *ii*, 835.
10. Mann, G.V. 'Diet/Heart: End of an Era', *New England Journal of Medicine* (1977), *297*, 644.
11. Walter, J.B. and Israel, M.S. *General Pathology*, 4th edn (Churchill Livingstone, Edinburgh, 1974).
12. Lemberger, L. and Rubin, A. *Physiologic Disposition of Drugs of Abuse* (Spectrum Publications, New York, 1976).
13. Drife, J.O. 'Drugs and Sperm', *British Medical Journal* (1982), *284*, 844.
14. Liener, I.E. (ed.) *Toxic Constituents of Plant Foodstuffs* (Academic Press, New York, 1980).
15. Swain, T. 'Tannins and Lignins' in: G.A. Rosenthal and D.H. Janzen (eds.) *Herbivores, Their Interaction with Secondary Plant Metabolites* (Academic Press, New York, 1979).
16. Editorial article. 'Puffers, Gourmands and Zombification', *Lancet* (1984), *i*, 1220–1.
17. Numbers, *11*, 4–6 and 31–4.
18. Ouzounellis, T. 'Quail Poisoning (Coturnism)' in M. Rechzigl Jr (ed.) *CRC Handbook of Naturally Occurring Food Toxicants* (CRC Press, Boca Raton, Florida, 1983).

3 POSSIBLE SOURCES OF FOOD TOXICANTS: PLANTS, SOME FOODS OF ANIMAL ORIGIN, MICROORGANISMS AND FOOD ADDITIVES

G.A. Silverstone

Poisonous Plants and Edible Plants

Fact and fiction are closely entwined in the matter of poisonous plants. We all know they exist and were brought up on tales where poisonous mushrooms or berries were used with deadly effect, and as children we were all warned against eating strange berries however attractive they might look. Which plants are poisonous and which are not is a less straightforward question than might be thought, because hemlock and deadly nightshade only represent one end of a broad spectrum that shades imperceptibly from those we know to avoid to those like carrots or apples or strawberries that we accept and eat without hesitation. The appearance of a plant is no clue to its character; only generations of experience has led us to select certain species for our food and taught us how they should be prepared. The majority of cases of plant poisoning occur among children or, less often, among adults who have either misidentified a plant (pokeweed for radish, tubers of *gloriosa superba* for yam) or misused it in home medication.

Not all components of common foodstuffs are harmless. There may be anti-nutrition factors or chemicals which in large amounts would be lethal, and it is often only the way the food is prepared or the fact that only low levels of toxin are present that allows us to consume them at all. But not always so, for chronic and serious poisoning may arise from certain foodstuffs and other apparently innocuous plants may be stimulated into producing poisons for their own defence.

To begin with the poisonous plants, K.F. Lampe and R. Fugerström divide the poisons into several main types according to their physiological effect.[5] First there are the gastroenteric irritants which vary in action from those which produce immediate pain and so are rarely swallowed, to those which have a delayed effect before symptoms, often very severe, develop. Then there are those poisons which produce cardiovascular disturbances and others which have a nicotine like action on the central nervous system. Different physiological effects are

Table 3.1: Examples of Poisonous Plants

Plant	Action of Poison	Toxin
Spurge laurel	Gastroenteric irritant	Vesicant resin (Mezereinic acid)
Horse chestnut	Gastroenteric irritant	Saponin
English ivy	Gastroenteric irritant	Saponin
English yew	Gastroenteric irritant	Alkaloid
Rhododendron and azalea	Cardiovascular poison	Resin
Foxglove	Cardiovascular poison	Alkaloid
Lobelia	Nicotine-like poison	Alkaloid
Deadly nightshade	Hallucinatory	Atropine alkaloid
Nux vomica	Convulsant	Alkaloid
Morning glory	Hallucinatory	Lysergic acid monoethylamide
Hydrangea	Cyanogenetic	HCN
Ackee plum	Hepatoxic	Hypoglycin B
Mistletoe	Gastric poison and smooth muscle stimulant	Amines

produced by atropine-containing plants and by those which act as convulsants or hallucinogens. The two other main classes are plants producing hydrocyanic acid and liver-damaging plants, but the authors divide poisonous mushrooms into seven classes of their own. Some produce only mild nausea, others are hallucinatory in effect while the most deadly, such as the death cap (*Amanita phalloides*) almost invariably kill.

The types are illustrated with a few examples, mostly from our gardens, in Table 3.1.

Fatalities have resulted from eating all of the species in Table 3.1 but in discussing the nature of these, or similar, toxins we shall be taking our examples not from the plants listed but from the edible fruit and vegetables consumed every day. Toxicity is a matter of degree – not of kind.

Enzyme Inhibitors

Enzymes

This is not a textbook of biochemistry, nevertheless, in order to appreciate the significance of potentially toxic materials it is desirable to have an elementary knowledge of how they act within a living body. It is also the case that since toxins may act in more ways than one we shall find the need to refer back to enzyme inhibition in later sections.

Firstly, what are enzymes? Enzymes are considered as catalysts which enable chemical reactions to be carried out in the body, these chemical reactions being necessary for almost every manifestation of life including muscular activity, digestion and so on. As with all catalysts they assist the reactions without taking part in them and remain unchanged by the process.

Enzymes are made up of protein molecules produced by living cells and, like all proteins, are assembled as polypeptide chains, i.e. chains of amino acids reacted together to form a polymer. As the number of amino acids is large (over thirty may be isolated from physiological fluids) there are many possible assemblies to be made. The overall shape of an enzyme is determined first by the arrangement of amino acids (primary structure), the way the chain of molecules folds along the molecular axis (secondary structure) and the irregular three dimensional pattern of the folded chain (tertiary structure). Such folded chains may link together to give an even more complex pattern. It is not necessary to do more than appreciate the variety of three dimensional structures which may be formed, each one quite unique.

A common analogy likens enzymes to keys and the substrate (i.e. the material which will be modified by contact with it) to a lock. Different enzymes will match different substrates and each enzyme will assist one type of transformation i.e. each key will fit one lock but with the essential difference that when a key is withdrawn, the lock (though it may have been opened or closed) will be mechanically unchanged. When the enzyme and substrate part, the latter will be transformed in one of six major ways. The enzyme, as catalyst, remains ready to repeat the process on another molecule.

The six principal enzyme types are:

Oxido-reductases	which oxidise or reduce the substrate.
Transferases	which transfer a functional group from one substance to another.
Hydrolases	which hydrolyse ester groups to acid and alcohol.
Lyases	which catalyse non-hydrolytic reactions with formation of a double bond or addition to a double bond to give a single bond.
Isomerases	which isomerise the substance to a different geometrical form.
Ligases	which join two substrates together.

Each of the above groups has many specific types, only a few of which will concern us here. Apart from a few exceptions (like trypsin) the name of an enzyme generally ends in the suffix -ase. They occur throughout the system, in saliva, gastric fluids, plasma, lungs and especially the liver where many are concentrated and function to detoxify harmful substances by, for example, allowing their conversion into less harmful materials or into complexes (conjugates) which are water soluble and may be flushed from the body.

An example may be helpful. Potentially toxic amines are detoxified in the body by the enzyme known as monoamine oxidase (MAO) which binds with the amine, allows oxidation to an aldehyde and then, by another pathway, to an acid, relatively harmless and easily excreted.

$$RCH_2NH_2 \xrightarrow[O_2]{MAO} RCHO + NH_3 \xrightarrow[\text{Aldehyde oxidase}]{O_2} RCOOH$$

Anything which interferes with MAO will allow amine to accumulate in the body, just as dirt in a key will prevent it functioning in a lock. The consequences of this we will discuss in a later section.

It is worth noting that all these enzyme reactions take place at body temperature whereas reactions in a laboratory may require high temperature, high pressure, prolonged time or a combination of these. It is not surprising that laboratory and commercial use is now being made of immobilised enzymes, i.e. enzymes isolated and bound to inert polymer supports so that they may be used to facilitate chemical reactions.

An enzyme inhibitor is therefore anything which prevents its normal action. This may be by binding to the enzyme or to the substrate or even by disrupting the enzyme itself. We shall consider a few important members of this group and how certain foodstuffs may suppress them, always bearing in mind that work carried out in the laboratory with experimental animals or in glassware (*in vitro*) is, at best, a simulation of what may go on in a human body. Though enzymes can be isolated from body fluids or from the organs of animals sacrificed for the purpose and the action of inhibitors can be studied *in vitro*, the results must be recognised as part of a more complex chain of events.

Inhibitors of the Digestive Process

When food enters the intestines, its protein content is broken down into its component amino acids, with the aid of many enzymes. The first, and one of the most important of these, is trypsin, which catalyses

Table 3.2: Plants Containing Trypsin Inhibitors

Soyabeans	Kidney beans
Peanuts	Garden peas
Oats	Rye
Chickpeas	Wheat
Buckwheat	Maize
Barley	Beetroot
Lentils	Turnip
Rice	Sweet Potatoes
Runner beans	White potatoes
Butter beans	Lettuce

the first stage of peptide breakdown. If it fails in its function, proteins pass through the alimentary canal without being digested.

The fact that a number of plants contain substances which can interfere with trypsin, hence are called trypsin inhibitors, was first discovered in 1917, when laboratory rats failed to grow when fed on raw soya beans. This was followed by the discovery that rats were able to digest soya beans, if they were well cooked in advance. Later it was found that several other legumes behaved in a similar way: rats could utilise them only after prolonged cooking. Ultimately it was discovered that soya beans as well as many other plants contained trypsin inhibitors which were destroyed by prolonged cooking.

When we consider some of the plants shown to contain trypsin inhibitors we will find them familiar. Though the inhibitor is often concentrated in the seeds, or in other cases the roots and leaves, it may sometimes be distributed through the whole plant. Plants containing trypsin inhibitors are listed in Table 3.2.[6,7,9] Those (except lettuce) are normally subject to cooking which inactivates the anti-enzyme factor although one has, in fact, been isolated from peanuts which have been roasted. A curious sideline is the observation that the factor in peanuts has blood clotting properties which led to a study of its use for treatment of haemophilic patients.[7]

Needless to say, they have been detected in many other vegetables especially in pulses, though often only in the seed. The quantity present depends often on the stage of the plants' growth and in the case of turnips a seasonal variation in content has been observed with an absence of inhibitor in some months. Egg whites too, have been shown to contain an anti-trypsin factor.

It is now known that the growth-depressing action of trypsin inhibitors is not due to the inactivation of trypsin alone. They also initiate other reactions in which the pancreas becomes over-activated, probably due to the failure in receiving one of its essential amino acids, methionine, with the result that amino acids are lost from the digestive system. In plants the production of such inhibitors is a defence mechanism, produced in response to insect attack or physical damage.

Cholinesterase Inhibitors[8]

Nerve impulses are transmitted from one nerve cell to another at *synapses*, namely junctions at which the axon of one neuron terminates on the body or axon of another. The transmission of nerve impulses through synaptic junctions is a complex process. In simple terms, the electric impulse arriving at the junction initiates a chemical change at the synaptic cleft which, in turn, triggers off an electric impulse in the next neuron. After the passage of the nerve impulse it is essential to restore the conditions that existed before it as quickly as possible, so as to make the system ready to transmit further impulses. A notable feature of the system is that various parts of the nervous system employ different chemical transmitters. Synaptic junctions appear to be the special targets of a multitude of plant and bacterial toxins, the effect of which can vary from mild interference, like that of coffee, to the paralysis of the nervous system caused by toxins like curare, strychnine or tetanus toxin.

One of the most important chemical transmitters at synaptic junctions is acetylcholine. This is the chief mediator in the autonomic nervous system which controls glands, visceral and cardiac muscles, that is, parts of the body which function without conscious control. It is also found at some junctions of the central, sympathetic and parasympathetic nervous systems. Acetylcholine, before the arrival of a nerve impulse, is contained in synaptic vesicles in the terminal buttons of cholinergic neurons. The arrival of an electric impulse increases the permeability of these vesicles to calcium ions, the resulting influx of which liberates acetylcholine into the synaptic cleft. Having crossed the cleft, acetylcholine acts on membrane receptors of the post-synaptic cell to increase their permeability to sodium ions, which then triggers off a nerve impulse in that cell.

After the passage of an impulse acetylcholine must be rapidly removed from the synaptic cleft. This is achieved by its hydrolysis to choline and acetic acid with the aid of the enzyme acetylcholinesterase as shown below:

$$\underset{\text{Acetycholine}}{CH_3OCOCH_2CH_2N(CH_3)_3} \xrightarrow[\text{esterase}]{\text{Acetylcholin-}} \underset{\text{Choline}}{HOCH_2CH_2N(CH_3)_3} + \underset{\text{Acetic acid}}{CH_3COOH}$$

Table 3.3: Edible Plants Containing Cholinesterase Inhibitors in the Parts Normally Eaten

Asparagus	Orange
Broccoli	Pepper
Carrot	Strawberry
Cabbage	Tomato
Celery	Turnip
Radish	Apple
Pumpkin	Aubergine
Raspberry	Potato
Vegetable Marrow	

If inactivation fails, acetylcholine accumulates, overstimulating nerves and the glands or muscles they control. This is the effect which, apart from plant toxins, is made use of in phosphorus and halogen-containing insecticides or in nerve gases used in chemical warfare.

A disturbingly large number of plants produce cholinesterase inhibitors, whereas other plant toxins interfere with other synaptic transmitters, like noradrenaline. (These will be considered in a subsequent section dealing with alkaloids.) Highly poisonous plants either produce a high concentration of cholinesterase inhibitors, or a very potent type. Lower concentrations or less potent types appear in a number of garden plants, such as petunia, boxwood, periwinkle or poppy, as well as in edible plants.

Edible plants in which cholinesterase inhibitors are to be found in the parts generally eaten are listed in Table 3.3.[8] Cholinesterase inhibitors are found in the parts not usually eaten of beet, horseradish, Lima bean and soyabean as well as sugar beet and the leaf of the tobacco plant.

Of the above, the structure of the active substances in potato and in tomato is known and will be described in the following chapter, but in some cases the chemical nature is uncertain.

Tests for inhibitors are usually carried out with aqueous or organic concentrates from the plant using enzyme suspensions under laboratory conditions which are not necessarily the same as obtained in culinary use so it may be that they would be rendered harmless or removed by cooking or attenuated by the digestive process. Nevertheless, it must be remembered that potato toxins have affected humans and other plant toxins have poisoned cattle by their anticholinesterase action.

Miscellaneous Other Enzyme Inhibitors[26]

The inhibition of a number of other important enzymes has been

Table 3.4: Miscellaneous Enzyme Inhibitors

Foodstuff	Enzyme Inhibited
Broad beans	Papain
Haricot beans	Papain
Kidney beans	Plasmin
Lima beans	Plasmin
Beans (unspecified)	Amylase
Soya beans	Papain, plasmin
Garden peas	Papain
Potatoes	Kallikrein, invertase
Wheat (13 varieties)	Amylase
Rye	Amylase
Sorghum	Amylase
Wheat flour	Papain
Wheat bran	Papain
Unripe mango	Amylase
Taro root	Amylase

established using extracts from a variety of foodstuffs. In some cases the factor has been isolated and characterised, in other cases it has only been tentatively described and it must be admitted that the precise significance of some is not completely understood.

In Table 3.4 the enzymes named contribute to the living process in this fashion: amylase hydrolyses starch while invertase breaks down sucrose into D-glucose and D-fructose. Papain behaves in a manner similar to trypsin and will attack most proteins. Plasmin occurs in the blood serum and aids in the hydrolysis and dissolution of fibrin, the polymer which forms blood clots. Finally, kallikrein is an enzyme which has an important role in the chain of reactions leading to the formation of antibodies, these being formed to counteract and neutralise foreign materials (antigens) which have entered the system. The antagonism reported is in addition to any already referred to (e.g. cholinesterase inhibition by potatoes).

As before, in some cases the inhibitor would be lost during cooking, others (e.g. the amylase inhibitors in wheat and rye) are destroyed by the digestive process, however, their presence must be noted in overall consideration of the nutritional value of the foodstuff.

The Alkaloids

It is possible to classify toxicants which occur naturally in plants in a variety of ways. The most usual, and the one which for the most part will be adopted here, is to classify according to physiological action rather than according to chemical type. However there is one chemical class which merits separate attention because of its ubiquity in the plant kingdom and the fact that all members of this class exert, when ingested, a marked effect on animal organisms. The substances in this group are known as alkaloids and it has been suggested that from 7 to 10 per cent of all plants contain some to a greater or lesser degree.

Alkaloids, of which several thousand have now been identified, fall into about twenty main classes according to their chemical structure. They may be loosely defined as: naturally occurring compounds, generally alkaline in nature, which possess one or more nitrogen atoms contained in a heterocyclic ring system, i.e. a ring of five or six atoms in which one or more is nitrogen and the rest usually carbon. It is the nitrogen which confers the basic (alkaline) properties on the molecule. Some common alkaloid structures are illustrated in Figure 3.1.

Though recognised as chemical entities only in the early nineteenth century, man has made use of alkaloids in the form of plant preparations for millenia for medical, religious or social purposes. Since the results of ingesting or inhaling such preparations vary between mild stimulation and hallucinatory effects on the one hand and to soporific states or even death on the other, it is not surprising that the main drugs of abuse turn out to be alkaloids. Quite apart from morphine or cocaine and the like, the stimulation of tea, coffee, or tobacco, the bitter taste of tonic water or the more dramatic effect of hemlock, are all due to the alkaloids they contain. Quinine, long used for treatment of malaria, gives tonic water its flavour; Socrates died by taking hemlock.

The first natural alkaloid to be isolated (by Serturner in 1805) was morphine. The name alkaloid was coined by Meisner in 1819 to classify the alkaline materials which were now being found in increasing numbers. Strychnine was isolated in 1817, caffeine in 1819, but it was not until 1826 that Schiff established the structure of an alkaloid for the first time in the case of coniine (from hemlock) and not until 1889 that the structure was confirmed by Ladenburg's synthesis. Since then alkaloid chemistry has become a separate discipline and scarcely a year passes without identification of new members of the group.[10]

Geographical distribution of alkaloid containing plants is widespread[11] and within the plant itself it is common to find the alkaloids concentrated in bark, roots or active tissues. It is usual also to find many different alkaloids in a single plant. Quite apart from the richer, better-known sources of these chemicals such as aconite, cinchona, ipecacuanha, opium poppy, quebracho, strychnos, tobacco, several

Figure 3.1: Some Alkaloids and Related Compounds

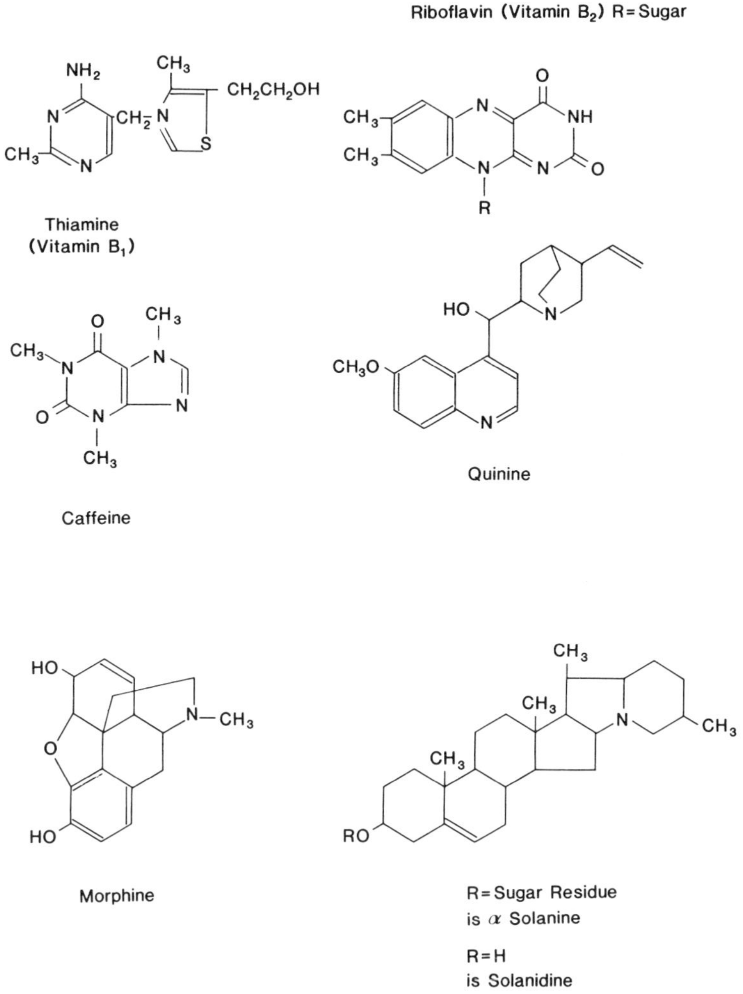

cactus species and a variety of fungi, it is instructive to consider only a few of the more familiar plants in which similar materials are to be found (Table 3.5).

Table 3.5 naturally, does not represent a list of common foodstuffs, although, as we have already pointed out, illness and death have resulted from accidental eating of many of these species. It is important to note that the ingestion of plants containing alkaloids (or other

Table 3.5: Familiar Plants Containing Alkaloids

Autumn crocus	Lupin
Castor plant	Lobelia
Calabar bean	Mandrake
Cola	Pomegranate root bark
Climbing lily	Snowdrop
Deadly nightshade	White hellebore
Delphinium (larkspur)	Veratrum
Hemlock	

toxins) by cattle is a matter of some concern, not only because of the immediate effect, but because some alkaloids are now known to be teratogenic, i.e. they can induce congenital defects in offspring when taken by pregnant animals. Larkspur, lupin and threadleaf have caused cattle poisoning in the USA, as well as the nightshades and similar species.[12]

Although most alkaloids occur in a free state or combined as soluble salts with acidic materials, there are a number which occur in a form where they are linked by way of an oxygen atom, to one, or more, sugar molecules. This is true of several naturally occurring chemical types other than alkaloids. Compounds linked in this fashion are called glycosides (or, in this case, glycoalkaloids). When the sugar molecules have been removed by chemical hydrolysis the resulting material is referred to as the aglycone. There are many forms of naturally occurring sugars and the names glucose, fructose, dextrose and lactose may be as familiar to the reader as the household sucrose. The ability of natural materials to appear in combination with varying groups of sugars means that a single alkaloid (for example) can give rise to several different glycosides all of which will produce the same aglycone.

Mode of Action of Alkaloids[11]

The chemical structure of alkaloids is very close to that of a number of chemicals which are essential to life. One need only name niacin, thiamine (vitamin B_1) and riboflavin (vitamin B_2) as examples (see Figure 3.1). Further, the solubility of alkaloids in water, especially as salts or glycosides, means that transport within organisms may be facilitated even though this might be expected to lead to ready excretion.

Because of their importance as drugs the action of the alkaloids has been intensively studied and many have been found to be quite specific in their action within living organisms. Thus, some will inhibit the production of certain essential materials, others will bind to appropriate sites or break down membrane compartmentation. Yet others will suppress vital enzyme activity as discussed in the section on enzyme inhibitors. Because of the overlapping action of different materials on living systems it is not possible, in a study of this sort, to segregate completely any one chemical class. Earlier we defined enzymes and made reference to cholinesterase and the effects of its inhibition, sufficient then to say that certain alkaloids, by this action, have the same effect as synthetic nerve gases developed for chemical warfare.

It is such quite specific effects as are found in the nervous system of animals and of man when alkaloids are ingested, or injected, that have been most studied. The transmitter substances which pass impulses through nerves and between nerves and the tissues they control, are interfered with. Electrical conductance and transmission are interrupted or the production of chemicals required by the nervous system (e.g. noradrenaline) is slowed down. But naturally, the effect will depend upon the dose, among other complex factors both outside and inside the laboratory.

For many of those who take alkaloids repeatedly the body appears to develop a dependence leading to the phenomenon of addiction, and such becomes the need of the living organism that cessation of the alkaloid supply leads to disturbing physical effects (withdrawal symptoms) only relieved by the same or an alternative drug which may not be addictive.

It is time now to consider our daily diet in relation to possible alkaloid intake. While taking stock we will note that in the plants we eat such alkaloids as may be present are frequently concentrated in portions that are not usually consumed. This is especially true in the case of the first vegetable we will discuss.

Common Foodstuffs Containing Alkaloids[13]

The Potato. With an annual worldwide production approaching 300 million tons it is not surprising to find the common potato a subject of intense study and the alkaloids present in the plant among the most extensively documented. It is over 150 years since the first potato glycoalkaloid, now named α-solanine, was discovered but only about 30 years since a second came to light, named α-chaconine. In fact, if the sugar residue (galactose, glucose and rhamnose in the first case; two rhamnose and one glucose in the second) are removed the identical aglycone, solanidine, is left. In recent years a number of other glycoalkaloids have also been reported.

The flesh of a normal healthy potato tuber contains only 1-5 mg alkaloid per 100 g fresh weight. As there is rather more in the peel and eye (about 30-50 mg per 100 g) the average for a whole tuber is about 7.5 mg per 100 g. One must note that no ill effects have been reported from a normal diet of healthy potatoes. Glycoalkaloid content of sprouts, flower and leaf may rise to 500 mg per 100 g. Bitter tubers have been found to contain from 25 to 80 mg per 100 g. In fact, 25 mg is sufficient to produce a bitter-tasting potato. Neither boiling, roasting nor frying has any effect on the alkaloids which can therefore be found in chips, potato crisps, tinned new potatoes and similar products.[14]

Many well-documented cases of illness, or even death, from consumption of potatoes with a high solanine content have been reported. Among the most recent (1979) 78 boys at a south east London school were affected from 7 to 19 hours after a lunch at which potatoes later shown to contain, when peeled, 33.3 mg glycoalkaloid per 100 g were served. Apart from acute physical discomfort, neurological symptoms ranging from apathy to visual disturbances and hallucinations, were reported. Seventeen of the boys required short periods of hospitalisation.[15]

Different species of potatoes have been found to contain different alkaloid concentrations and so the choice of a strain for cultivation is important. Not only is this so, but bad storage and ill treatment after harvesting can lead to a build up of glycoalkaloids. Exposure to light which causes 'greening' (the actual green colour is due to chlorophyll) or mechanical damage will increase the amount of alkaloid which points to its production being part of a defence mechanism which will be discussed later. Indeed, they do act as a resistance factor against both Colorado beetle and leaf hopper but less effectively, as we shall shortly see, than some other glycoalkaloids.

In tests of a hypothesis that certain birth deformities might be related to consumption of imperfect potatoes, pregnant animals were fed blighted potatoes. Gross abnormalities were found in the offspring but no implication of teratogenicity in humans has been demonstrated.[16]

The Tomato. It was recognised in the 1930s that tomatoes synthesised a defence chemical that has a toxic effect on some microorganisms which are tomato pathogens. This contributed to wilt resistance. The active material was named α-tomatine when isolated in 1948. It proved to be a glycoside having two glucose, one galactose and one xylose molecule attached to a high molecular weight alkaloid belonging to the same chemical class as solanidine. This was named tomatidine.

The amount to be found in red, ripe fruit is about 36 mg per 100 g with higher amounts in green fruit and as much as 200 mg per 100 g in flowers and leaves. It is also found in the juice on pressing. Tomatine has been recognised as a post-infectional inhibitor whose synthesis can occur in response to stress.

The consumption of green tomato plants by pigs has resulted in their illness and death. Toxicity studies in the laboratory have given variable results with evidence of anti-enzyme activity, but it is the anti-fungal action which is most considerable and the possibility of using α-tomatine against certain human fungal infections such as ringworm and thrush has been considered. It is interesting to note that α-tomatine appears to be more effective than α-solanine against Colorado beetle.

The Yam. Although not so widely eaten in the northern hemisphere, the starchy root of the yam is a major food item in many tropical countries where it is widely cultivated. An alkaloid present, dioscorine, is a much smaller molecule than that of those found in the potato or tomato plant, nor does it occur combined with any sugar. It has been shown to be extremely toxic and causes general paralysis of the central nervous system. Extracts from wild yams, which are richer in dioscorine than the cultivated variety, have been used as animal poisons in hunting. In spite of this, the normal cultivated variety appears satisfactory as a staple feedstuff in West Africa and South East Asia. Unfortunately in times of scarcity or of famine the wild yams also get eaten by humans with disagreeable consequences.

Beverages. Infusions made from plant leaves or berries are almost certain to contain alkaloids and so, of course, do the common drinks originating from the far and near east, namely tea and coffee, as well as that first brought from Mexico, namely chocolate (drunk as cocoa). These have been claimed to be both stimulant and soporific. Coffee is widely believed to cause sleeplessness while cocoa, on the other hand, has long been familiar as a bedtime drink and tea is regarded as a particularly soothing beverage. All three contain varying amounts of caffeine while cocoa also contains a related alkaloid, theobromine, and theophylline is present in tea.

Among the cold drinks the well-known cola types contain caffeine found in the Kola nuts used in manufacture but the amount present in a bottle of such drink is less than in the average cup of coffee.

Miscellaneous Other Sources of Alkaloids. Among many other foods containing glycoalkaloids at a level above 10 mg per 100 g, but still regarded as perfectly acceptable, are aubergines and green and red peppers. The burning taste of common black pepper is due to the two compounds piperine and chavicine which are reported to have insecticidal properties. There is no doubt that many other common plants contain minute amounts so it is not surprising that when Hegnauer extracted 100 kg of cabbage in 1963 he was able to isolate 40 mg of narcotine, another alkaloid, i.e. 40 parts per hundred million of cabbage.[11]

Two other important points should be noted. First, many of the active principles shown to be present in fruit and vegetables have not yet been identified. Thus, the cholinesterase inhibitors reported to be present in those plants listed in the section 'Enzyme Inhibitors' may also be alkaloids. Secondly, as the recent work on potato, tomato and yam has shown, choice of cultivar can be made to reduce alkaloid level, although sometimes at the expense of other desirable properties, while cultivation methods may reduce the amount further. It was recently reported that sulphur deficiency in the soil reduced the alkaloid level in the leaf of mustard plants, for example.[17] Lastly, we must remember that post-harvest handling of the fruit and vegetables has to be carried out with care as the plant can still produce defence chemicals in response to attack.

Phytic Acid

Time and time again in the study of plant composition we find that not only are the plants capable of reacting to attack by the production of defensive chemicals but some, which are apparently nourishing due, for example, to high protein content, have somewhere in the matrix a small amount of material which is actively anti-nutritional when ingested. We have seen this already in the case of enzyme inhibitors but can now consider a fairly straightforward chemical which, while not actively toxic, can serve to prevent absorption of essential nutrients.

This is phytic acid, or more properly, *myo*-inositol-hexadihydrogen phosphate.

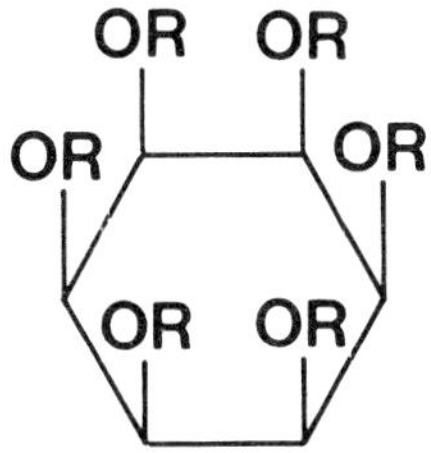

OR OR
OR OR
OR OR

R = H, Myo inositol

R = H_2PO_3, Phytic Acid

Although an alternative structure has been suggested, the above is the most generally accepted form for the molecule.[18] In this, a relatively simple sugar, *myo*-inositol (one of the several isomeric forms of hexahydroxycyclohexane), is combined with six molecules of phosphoric acid. On the face of it, phytic acid ought to be a very rich source of phosphorus, one of the essential elements, but this is not the case.

Before proceeding, let us see the foodstuffs in which it is found. Cereals are one of the principal sources, rye being especially rich in phytic acid, also rice, corn, wheat, nuts, soyabeans, various legumes and root crops. It is present in green beans, carrots, broccoli, potatoes, sweet potatoes, artichokes, blackberries, strawberries, and figs.[20] In cereals it is concentrated in the bran and germ (as much as 6 per cent of the dry matter in corn germ). Much phytic acid goes into the by-products of flour milling and it can become concentrated in high protein flour (it is usually associated with protein in the plant). It is thus a component of much of our daily bread, especially the brown wholemeal varieties, as well as breakfast cereals.

Since so much bread is eaten the content and behaviour of phytic acid in bread of many types has been described. It is established that during bread manufacture some is indeed broken down and may be lost in the form of inorganic phosphorus compounds. Whole grain bread may contain 458–1780 mg phytate/kg, white about 161–381 mg/kg. Breakdown of phytate in the conversion of flour is about 31–46 per cent in the case of whole meal and 88–99 per cent in the case of white. The action of yeast is important in breaking down phytic acid. For example, in rye bread after fermentation only 45 per cent of the original phytate remained, without yeast 64 per cent was present and while a hard wholemeal rye bread was found to contain 89 per cent intact phytate, white was found to have almost none. The unleavened bread of middle eastern countries is thus rich in this material.[18]

Behaviour of Phytic Acid

The main problem with phytic acid with its six acid groups is the fact that it readily forms salts with a variety of metal ions. The resulting salts of calcium, magnesium, zinc or iron, are insoluble in water and tend to pass through the digestive system unabsorbed. There is evidence that some phytic acid can be broken down in the gut and that adaptation may occur enabling the digestive system to deal with it more effectively but this may vary among individuals. A few elements will be considered separately.

Phytic Acid and Calcium Absorption. Calcium is required for teeth and bones and calcium absorption from food is a complex process involving the action of calcium binding protein which is activated by vitamin D. In the absence of vitamin D absorption of calcium will not occur. This leads to osteomalacia, a disease in which bones are decalcified though not deformed. In children deficiency of vitamin D or calcium (or both) will lead to rickets in which bones are deformed.

If calcium in the diet is combined with phytic acid, the resulting phytate will pass into the faeces. Several workers have reported that phytate is a rachitogenic factor in cereals.[27] It has been described as an acute vitamin D factor and if the vitamin D content of the diet is low the phytate effect is much more striking.[21]

Phytic Acid and Iron Absorption. The role of iron in our blood is well known, its deficiency results in anaemia. We normally obtain an adequate supply of iron in our diet, bread being one of the sources, but again we find that it may be present, in some cases, as non-absorbable phytate. Conflicting results have been reported after feeding trials on animals. For example, one report relating to feeding of weanling rats claimed the availability of iron occurring naturally in wheat was not restricted by increasing the phytate level. Yet another study showed that the degree of maturity of soyabeans was important. Although three times as much iron was present in immature beans it was not available for absorption because of its insoluble form.[21]

The case with bread is very similar. Wholemeal bread has more iron than has white. Rats made anaemic by a diet of white bread were, in fact, restored to health by whole cereal, but in the course of prolonged experiments by R.A. McCance and E.M. Widdowson in 1942 the iron content of four men and four women dropped when white bread was replaced by wholemeal of 92 per cent extraction although the brown bread contained 50 per cent more iron. Two of the women went into negative iron balance.[22] It is clear that the rats were able to adapt to the phytate while the humans were not which shows the difficulties involved in relating animal nutrition to our own.

Phytic Acid and Other Trace Elements. Small amounts of many metals are necessary to us. Zinc, for example, is a constituent of several enzymes, copper is required for haemoglobin formation, magnesium and manganese also have a part to play, but all of these metals will combine with phytic acid in an insoluble form, thus, reliance on certain foods (e.g. cereals) to obtain these trace elements could result in deficiencies whereas a more varied diet involving food low in phytates can redress the balance.

Two final points: amylase antagonism has been demonstrated for phytic acid but on the other hand, prolonged trials on monkeys seemed to show a marked reduction in dental caries when a cariogenic diet was supplemented by phytate. It has been described as an inhibitor of tooth plaque and a patent taken for incorporation in dentifrice.[23–25]

Vitamins and Antivitamins

From our food we obtain fuel to supply our immediate energy needs (or to store as depôt fats), the materials for growth and a host of trace components all of which are necessary to regulate our body's many functions; elements such as iodine, zinc, manganese or iron and also the organic compounds we know as vitamins. Deficiency of any of these leads to a characteristic syndrome and each and every one is necessary for health. Long before any vitamin had been isolated and described it was recognised that some ailments could be prevented by the correct diet. In the absence of fresh green vegetables for example, lime juice was once provided for sailors in the British navy to prevent scurvy and it was the vitamin C, ascorbic acid, which was the real requirement. As diseases became recognised as resulting from deficiency the missing factors, vitamins, were identified by letters A, B, C and so on, and in many cases this terminology has been retained even though we now know the chemical structure concerned.

The diseases resulting from absence of any vitamin are well known but it only came to light in modern times that excess of some could also produce serious adverse effects. This knowledge was acquired when pure vitamins, or vitamin concentrates, became available and tended to be used in excess. The danger of consuming too much of any vitamin in a normal diet is almost non-existent, but for an infant fed on fortified milk and cereals, together with such supplements as cod liver oil, it is possible to exceed the average need. Particularly in the case of the oil-soluble vitamins, this should be avoided. Because a small dose of vitamin is good for us it does not follow that a large dose must be better.

Nutritionists have also recognised, in recent years, that antagonists to vitamins may also be present in the diet or that a vitamin may occur in an unavailable form. Its presence in a foodstuff is not enough – it must be able to be absorbed and it must not be degraded while the process is going on. A wealth of data is now available on the effect of both lack of vitamins and excess of vitamins on humans. In the study of antagonists much of the work relates to laboratory or farm animals. No attempt to be comprehensive will be made here, we shall simply outline a number of cases one by one, treating the two classes, oil- and water-soluble vitamins, separately.

Oil-soluble Vitamins

Vitamin A. This familiar vitamin and its precursor, β-carotene, is required for retinal health and one of the first symptoms of deficiency is impairment of night vision. It is present in butter, carrots, spinach and the fish liver oils. Both acute and chronic effects of excessive doses on humans are well-documented. In adults skin disorders and blood clotting disturbances are among the consequences from which recovery can be made, but in the case of children skeletal lesions have occurred which can permanently affect growth. (At one time high dosage of vitamin A was prescribed for acne, this now seems undesirable.)

Vitamin A is the only vitamin where poisoning from a natural food source is known to have occurred. In the 1940s arctic explorers who ate a quantity of polar bear's liver suffered the effects of acute poisoning, because polar bear liver contains a particularly high concentration of vitamin A. (The liver of sharks, seals and whales are also rich sources.) If large amounts of foodstuff containing the vitamin A precursor carotene are consumed a yellow skin pigmentation (carotenaemia) occurs, but this is reversible and does not lead to vitamin A intoxication.[28]

Vitamin A can be destroyed, or its formation *in vivo* inhibited by certain foods. There is some antagonism between unsaturated fatty acids and carotene, especially if only low levels of the latter are present. The lipoxidase enzyme in raw soyabeans can destroy carotene and prevent formation of the vitamin and it has been shown that some factor in yeast destroys vitamin A in the liver of the pig. The unsaturated aldehyde citral, present in orange oil and hence in orange juice made from the whole fruit, in marmalade and in some other fruit juices is also an antagonist of vitamin A.

$$CH_3C{=}CHCH_2CH_2{-}C{=}CHCHO$$

$$CH_3 \qquad\qquad CH_3$$

Citral

Normally we would not be expected to absorb enough citral to cause imbalance but if we did, vitamin supplements can overcome this.[27]

Vitamin D. Vitamin D is found in similar sources to vitamin A and is the vital molecule in whose formation the ultra-violet portion of sunlight plays an important part. The complex rôle of this vitamin in regulating calcium absorption was touched on under the heading of phytic acid and happily the deficiency disease of rickets is now rare as adequate supplies of both vitamin D and calcium are available for children's diet. But too much vitamin D can reverse the process resulting in reabsorption of calcium from the bones with attendant rise in calcium levels in blood and urine. Deposition may then occur in soft tissues, possibly with fatal results. This is reversible if caught in time but effects have been noted in certain hypersensitive individuals on a normal vitamin D dosage. It has been customary to fortify milk with vitamin D and reports show that in the period 1953-5 in the UK when a somewhat high level of fortification was used, an abnormal number of cases of hypercalcaemia of infants occurred (about 100 cases per year). In severe cases of this disease mental retardation, osteosclerosis and other damage – even early death – may result. After 1957 when fortification was reduced the number of cases fell sharply.[28] What is needed is sufficient to prevent rickets and no excess.

Factors which act against vitamin D generally manifest themselves as rachitogenic and once again soyabean meal (or the protein from this) is implicated, as is phytic acid and yeast. Cereals have also been shown to be rachitogenic.

Antagonism between vitamins is also suspected since, in animal feeding trials, heavy doses of vitamin A induced rickets in rats already

Table 3.6: Antagonists of the Oil-soluble Vitamins

Vitamin	Typical deficiency effect*	Effect of excess on humans	Antagonists present in	Nature of antagonist	Ref.
A	Impairment of vision	Toxic	Soyabeans	Enzyme	
			Orange oil etc.	Citral	29
D	Rickets	Toxic (reabsorption of calcium and deposition on tissues)	Soyabeans	Protein	28
			Cereals	Phytic acid	
			Yeast	—	
E	Fertility reduction	Not regarded as toxic	Fish liver oils	Unsaturated fatty acid	28
			Kidney beans		
			Peas, alfalfa, yeast		
K	Haemorrhage	Toxic	Raw soyabean (Anti-coagulant properties not reversed by K)	Enzyme	28
			—	Vitamin A	

* Other than impairment of growth.

being fed a rachitogenic diet and it is possible that a rachitogenic factor shown to be present in grass may be β-carotene.[27]

Vitamin E. Vitamin E, tocopherol, is a naturally occurring anti-oxidant. Green leaves and wheat germ oil are rich sources but it is widely distributed in our food. It serves to control oxidation of unsaturated fatty acids even in our bodies but while doing this is itself consumed. So, in a sense, the fatty acids are antagonists to vitamin E. Highly unsaturated fish oils, such as cod liver oil, are especially destructive and yeast, kidney beans and peas all contain antagonists.[27] Excess of this vitamin, apart from some slight disturbances, seems to do no harm.

Vitamin K. The presence of vitamin K is required to control blood clotting and in its absence haemorrhagic disease can occur. Appearance of this type of disease in children is controlled by vitamin K dosage, but this must be limited to avoid toxic effects.

Anti-vitamin K activity was first observed in animals eating sweet clover which contains dicoumarol, an agent which can block the synthesis of vitamin K and lead to haemorrhage.[20] Studies of this material resulted in the development of the rat poison 'Warfarin' which acts in the same manner.

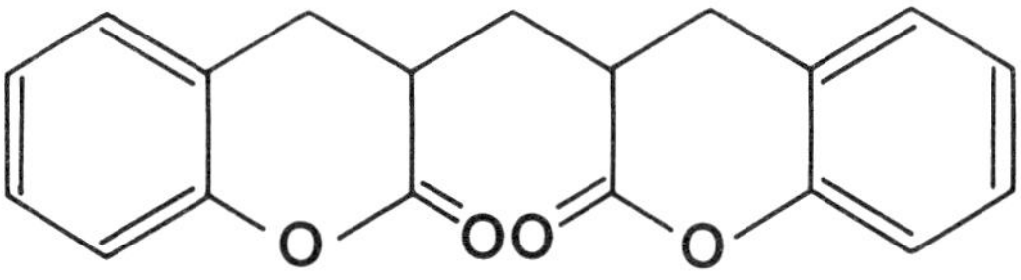

Dicoumarol

Excess vitamin A is antagonistic to vitamin K and the anti-coagulant properties of raw soyabean (attributed to the anti-trypsin factor) on blood are not reversed by vitamin K dosage.[27,28]

The antagonists of oil-soluble vitamins are summarised in Table 3.6.

Water-soluble Vitamins

In Table 3.7 six of the water-soluble vitamins are listed. Apart from some side effects in a few cases large doses seem to do no harm. Their antagonists, some of them enzymes, are also shown in the table. Nicotinic acid, adequate supplies of which we obtain from eggs, milk, liver or yeast, is also present in most cereals, but often in a bound form not available for absorption. This shows itself mainly in the maize-eating areas of some countries where pellagra is endemic (among the unpleasant symptoms of this disease is a form of dermatitis). There is

Table 3.7: Antagonists of the Water-soluble Vitamins

Vitamin	Typical deficiency effect*	Effect of excess on humans	Antagonists present in	Nature of antagonist	Ref.
Thiamine (B_1)	Beriberi	No effect	Blackberries, blueberries, blackcurrants, red beet, water cress, Brussels sprouts, spinach, red cabbage, black cherries, raspberries, mustard seed, crisped cabbage. High carbohydrate diet, raw carp flesh	Enzymes	20, 26, 27
Riboflavin (B_2)	Lesions of lips and mouth	—	Ackee plum	Hypoglycin A	29
Pyridoxine (B_6)	Anaemia	No effect	Flaxseed	Linatine (γ-glutamyl 1-amino-D-proline)	20, 26, 29
B_{12}	Anaemia, spinal cord degeneration	No effect	Raw soya bean, High protein or lard diet	Enzyme	27
Nicotinic acid (Niacin)	Pellagra	Side effects	Maize and other cereals *Sorghum vulgare* (?)	Naicin in bound form Leucine may antagonise niacin	27, 29
Pantothenic acid	?	No effect	Pea seedlings	—	20

* Other than impairment of growth.

a notable exception, however. The nicotinic acid may be released from the grain by treatment with mild alkali and by a happy chance, in Central America, the maize is treated with lime water during preparation. This probably accounts for the low pellagra incidence in these regions.[27]

Goitrogens

The efficient working of the machine we call our body depends on a subtle balance of materials among which trace elements have important roles. Deficiency in any one of these may lead to illness or deformity or incomplete growth. Supplying the deficient element will often cause a complete cure. The condition of goitre which manifests itself by enlargement of the thyroid gland (hyperthyroidism) is due to a deficiency of the one element, iodine, and in most cases a cure is effected by supplying iodine in the appropriate form. Deficiency diseases tend to be endemic in nature and so it can be understood that folklore has long attributed goitre to the eating of certain vegetables. But even so, and now that it has been established that goitrogens do exist in cabbage, turnip and other species it is still uncertain whether they are in fact responsible for endemic goitre in humans.

The uptake of iodine by the thyroid may be readily monitored by feeding humans or laboratory animals with small amounts of radioactive iodine (^{131}I). The iodine taken up by the thyroid may be monitored by a Geiger counter. If the subject is fed goitrogenic material the reduction of radioiodine uptake by the thyroid will be in proportion to the amount fed. Judging by this test many common foodstuffs have shown goitrogenic activity and a variety of organic substances have been isolated and characterised as goitrogens. In a number of other instances the factor responsible remains unknown. Two or three particular chemical types are specifically implicated and one of these, notable for the fact that the molecules contain sulphur, we shall now consider.

Thioglucosides (Glucosinolates)[30]

Many condiments used to add spice to our diet appear to have attracted man because of their pungent nature. Some, like garlic and onion, are inherently pungent; others, such as mustard and horseradish, only develop their pungency when chopped and moistened with water.

The reason here is that the chemicals responsible are aglycones released from their sugar moiety, in this case glucose, by the hydrolytic action of enzymes. These aglycones are capable of rearrangement to give more than one product. In general terms this may be illustrated as follows:

$$RC\begin{matrix} / SC_6H_{11}O_5 \\ \\\\ NOSO_2OK \end{matrix} \xrightarrow[\text{+ enzyme}]{\text{Chopped + water}} [R\begin{matrix} /S^- \\ \\\\ N^- \end{matrix}] + \text{Glucose} + KHSO_4$$

Thioglycoside — Unstable intermediate

$$R{-}N{=}C{=}S \qquad R{-}C{\equiv}N \qquad RS{-}C{\equiv}N$$

Isothiocyanate — Nitrile — Thiocyanate

The nature of the group R varies from plant species to species but one or two are noteworthy.

In kale, turnip, kohlrabi and similar crops R often has the grouping $CH_2{=}CH{\cdot}CHOH{\cdot}CH_2{-}$ and the thioglycoside has the trivial name progoitrin. Because of its –OH group progoitrin can not only form the isothiocyanate as shown above, but can lose water and cyclise to give the potent material known as goitrin, 5-vinyl oxazolidine-2-thione.

$$\begin{matrix} & CH{-}{-}NH \\ & | \qquad | \\ CH_2{=}CH{-}CH & \quad C \\ & \backslash \quad / \\\\ & O \qquad S \end{matrix}$$

Goitrin

Much of the flavour of cabbage, Brussels sprouts, cauliflower and mustard is due to the goitrogen allyl isothiocyanate formed from the precursor sinigrin (R is $CH_2{=}CH{\cdot}CH_2{-}$)

$$CH_2{=}CHCH_2C\begin{matrix} /SC_6H_{11}O_5 \\ \backslash NOSO_2OK \end{matrix} \longrightarrow CH_2{=}CHCH_2N{=}C{=}S + \text{glucose} + KHSO_4$$

Sinigrin — Allyl Isothiocyanate

and goitrin is also present.

The goitrogenic properties of these and many similar compounds have been amply demonstrated and it has also been established that the goitre produced by some of these agents is not alleviated by increase of iodine in the diet. Besides the suppression of iodine uptake by the thyroid, such goitrogens apparently initiate a more complex mechanism than in the simpler reversible goitre type. Two things are reassuring; first, it has been suggested that a daily intake of 10 kg of cauliflower or kale would be necessary to provide enough goitrogen in our blood; secondly, the adverse effects seem to persist only when the iodine content of the diet is already low.[31]

Both isothiocyanate and thiocyanate cause thyroid enlargement. The other possible product of thioglycoside hydrolysis, viz. the nitrile, has other toxic effects.

In addition to the *Brassica* family (cabbage, kale, Brussels sprouts, cauliflower, broccoli, kohlrabi), goitrogenic activity has been found in turnips, garden cress, radish, horseradish, spinach, carrot, peach, pear and strawberry.[26,32]

Other Types of Goitrogen

It is known that certain metallic elements, e.g. cobalt and copper as well as arsenic (powdered arsenic ores have been used in parts of Europe in place of garlic or onion) may cause goitre. So do many other organic chemicals including, for example, certain cyanoglycosides (molecules containing hydrocyanic acid) which are present in the red outer skin covering peanuts and cashew nuts, when tested under laboratory conditions.

Goitrogens which have not yet been identified are present in soya beans and at least one case of human goitre was attributed to a milk substitute made from soyabean.[31] Heating of the beans during processing renders them less goitrogenic but does not remove the offending property. We should note that while the enzyme responsible for hydrolysing the glycoside will be destroyed by heating, the cooking process itself may hydrolyse the inactive glucoside to the active aglycone.

Transfer of Goitrogens in Milk

A notable feature of the chemicals involved in this section is that they may be transferred into milk and passed in their active form to the consumer, whether calf or human. In this manner the components of cruciferous weeds, wild turnip or kale, can be passed to ourselves. Milk taken from cows fed on such diets has been compared with that from animals fed on grass pastures. Uptake of radioiodine by the thyroid was inhibited by the milk from the cows fed on known groitrogenic plants.[32]

A case occurred in Tasmania where children who had been drinking milk from cows fed large amounts of marrow stem kale developed enlarged thyroids (even though the iodine content of the children's diet had been increased).[33] Other studies, although recognising that goitrogens are present in measurable quantities in the milk, have not always confirmed that the amounts consumed would be sufficient to harm humans. On balance, though, it is believed that consumption of large amounts of such milk would cause goitre.

Oestrogens

Among the different classes of chemicals which contribute to the colour, flavour and processing characteristics of food one of the most important is that known as the flavanoids. All plant foods contain some of these in amounts varying from traces to several grams per kilogram of plant. It has been suggested that the average human ingests about one gram of flavanoid material per day. In Figure 3.2 a typical flavanone is shown, variation in the position and number of $-OH$, $-OCH_3$ and $-CH_3$ groups leads to a diversity of structures.

These chemicals have been the subject of very extensive studies and little evidence of toxicity has been shown. In fact, a number of beneficial effects have been suggested for such compounds. For example, many have an inhibiting effect on microbes and viruses. In the wine growing regions around the Mediterranean it has long been the custom to mix wine with water and leave it for some time before drinking the mixture. The weak antibiotic effect of the phenols present in wine renders the water potable. Tea and wine are recommended folk remedies for prevention of certain diseases and while the action is weak compared with modern antibiotics, it is positive.[34]

Thus, while the most commonly occurring flavones are harmless the less common ones exhibit some toxicity. The most potent, tangeretin and nobiletin, are found in the peel and oil sacs of certain citrus fruits. As part of the plant's natural defences they have strong anti-viral and anti-microbial action. But, even these have a low order of mammalian toxicity. Relatively high doses given to adult mice and dogs had little effect though tangeretin caused 83 per cent of the offspring of pregnant female rats to be born dead, or to die within three days, when 10 mg/kg body weight/day was given subcutaneously in carboxymethylcellulose.[34]

A slight modification of the flavanoid skeleton produces the isomeric

Figure 3.2: Flavanoids and Related Oestrogens

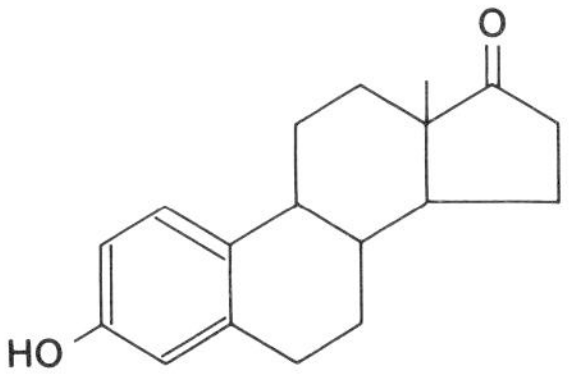

Oestrone

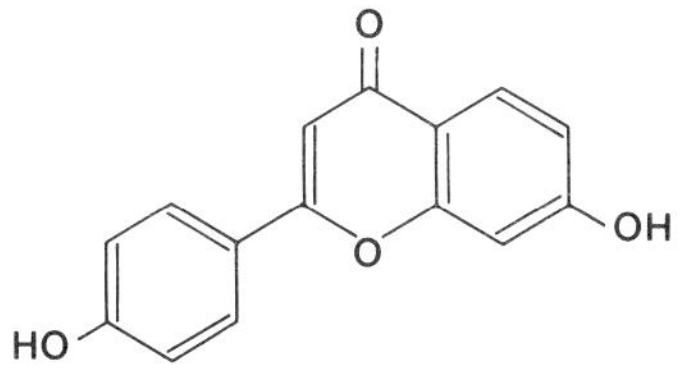

Typical Flavone Structure

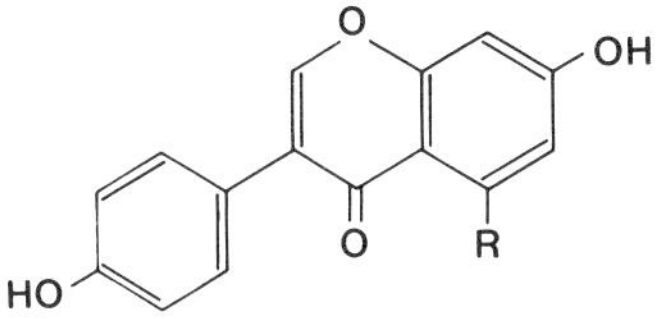

Isoflavone Structure

Genistein	R=OH
Daidzein	R=H
Formononetin	R=H, $-OCH_3$ at 4[1]
Biochanin A	R=OH, $-OCH_3$ at 4[1]

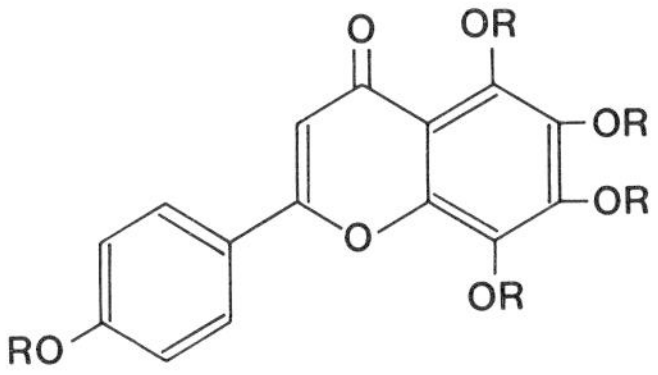

Tangeretin R=CH_3

(Nobiletin = 3[1] methoxy tangeretin)

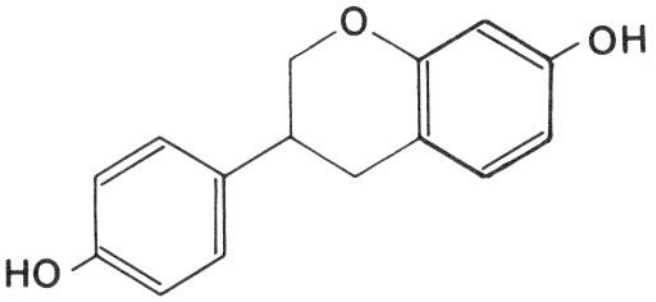

Equol

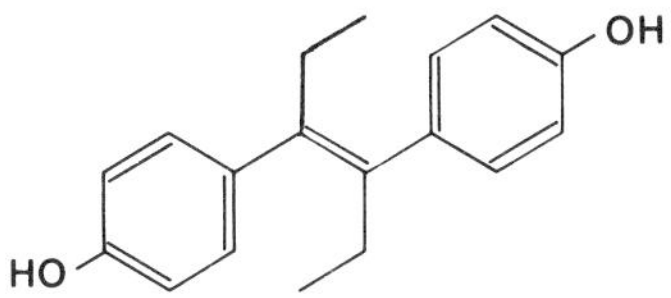

Diethyl Stilboestrol

iso-flavanoids and this has a major effect on the behaviour *in vivo* of these materials. The iso-flavones have been found to exhibit oestrogenic activity. The oestrogens are the steroidal sex hormones which control the development of secondary sexual characteristics and the cycle of oestrus in the female. In Figure 3.2 the structure of the typical hormone oestrone is shown alongside some iso-flavones and the powerfully oestrogenic diethylstilboestrol. (Oestrone is not normally found outside the animal kingdom but, strangely enough, it has been isolated from palm kernel.) It can be seen that the overall shape of the isoflavones together with their aromatic phenolic structure shows distinct similarity to both oestrone and stilboestrol. On this account they are called oestrogen mimics.

This activity first came to light in the 1940s when it was discovered that disturbances in sheep (difficult labour, infertility and lactation in unbred ewes) was leading to severe lambing losses. This was attributed to prolonged periods of grazing in pastures rich in the species known as subterranean clover. Investigation showed this clover to be rich in the isoflavones genistein and formonenetin. Later studies showed that the latter itself was not the responsible factor but was converted, by demethylation and reduction, into the more active equol.[35]

By now all isoflavones tested have been shown to be oestrogenic when given by parenteral injection to animals, but even the most potent (genistein, biochanin A or coumoestrol) have only about 1/50,000 the activity of stilboestrol.

Foods containing isoflavones have been subjected to tests and among those which have given oestrogenic response in the appropriate experimental animal are wheat, rice, soyabeans, oats, barley, carrots, potatoes, apples, cherries, plums, sage leaf, parsley, wheat bran, wheat germ, rice bran and rich polish. In addition, cottonseed, safflower, wheat germ, corn, linseed, peanut, olive, soyabean, coconut and refined and crude rice bran oils have given positive results. The isoflavones genistein and daidzin have been isolated from soyabean and the former has been found in commercial, defatted soyabean at a level of approx. 0.1 per cent. Another isoflavone has been isolated from the fermented soyabean product tempeh. Daidzin has also been found in plums and cherries. These phenolic compounds frequently occur as glycosides.[36,37]

Though livestock losses (particularly of sheep) continue to occur where grazing on different types of clover or other pasture rich in isoflavones cannot be prevented, their relatively weak activity is not expected to produce any physiological effect on humans. Possibly the only case of oestrogenisation in humans are the cases reported during the war in Holland by women who had eaten tulip bulbs to alleviate the food shortage.[38]

One reason for taking note of isoflavones in our diet is based on the observations made relating to diethylstilboestrol. This was at one time used as a palliative in the treatment of prostatic cancer, and was found to cause an increased number of coronary and cerebrovascular deaths. This has led to speculation, whether long-term ingestion of oestrogen mimics (other than diethylstilboestrol) at low levels could have any bearing on coronary disease.[39] But this remains purely hypothetical and degradative pathways may lead to elimination from the system.

Cyanogenetic Glycosides

We have seen how some plant toxins (e.g. alkaloids) may act directly to provide a pathogenic effect, how others (e.g. goitrogens) undergo chemical transformation to form active materials while yet others (e.g. phytic acid) may simply act to deprive us of nutrients. Belonging to the second of these types is a curious class of natural products known as cyanogenetic glycosides. These react to provide a gaseous toxicant which does not occur free in nature. This gas is the notorious hydrogen cyanide (HCN) the inhalation of which, in sufficient quantity, will rapidly cause death due to inhibition of the enzyme cytochrome oxidase required for respiration. Death results, in fact, from cessation of the supply of oxygen.

It seems we are continuously exposed to small amounts of this gas in an industrial environment (it occurs in cigarette smoke, for example) and the taste is not unknown to those who have sampled some of the nut liqueurs of the Mediterranean lands. However several metabolic pathways have been suggested for the detoxification of small amounts in our system one of these involving enzymatic conversion into thiocyanate.

$$\underset{\text{Thiosulphate}}{S_2O_3^{2-}} + \underset{\text{Cyanide}}{CN^-} \xrightarrow{\text{Enzyme}} \underset{\text{Sulphite}}{SO_3^{2-}} + \underset{\text{Thiocyanate}}{SCN^-}$$

Within the plant the hydrogen cyanide is firmly bound into the glycoside structure and as a first stage to liberating the gas enzymatic hydrolysis is required to give a free, but unstable, cyanohydrin together with the sugar. The liberation of HCN from the cyanohydrin may be accomplished with or without the further aid of enzymes. As the required enzymes are usually present in the plant, maceration is all that is needed to initiate the process. Together with the HCN a free aldehyde or ketone is formed.

$$\underset{\text{Glycoside}}{\text{H}-\overset{\displaystyle\text{CN}}{\underset{\displaystyle\text{R}}{\overset{|}{\underset{|}{\text{C}}}}}-\text{O}-\text{Glucose}} \xrightarrow{\text{Enzyme}} \underset{\text{Cyanohydrin}}{\text{H}-\overset{\displaystyle\text{CN}}{\underset{\displaystyle\text{R}}{\overset{|}{\underset{|}{\text{C}}}}}-\text{OH}} + \text{Glucose} \rightarrow \underset{\text{Aldehyde}}{\text{H}-\overset{\displaystyle\text{O}}{\underset{\displaystyle\text{R}}{\overset{\|}{\underset{|}{\text{C}}}}}} + \mathit{HCN}$$

Among the best known of the cyanogenetic glycosides are amygdalin, formed from benzaldehyde, HCN and two molecules of glucose, dhurrin, from *p*-hydroxy benzaldehyde with one molecule each of HCN and glucose, and phaseolunatin which is based on acetone as the carbonyl component. These occur respectively in almonds (and stone fruit kernels), sorghum (or millet) and Lima beans. Though we are focusing our attention on the HCN which may be released, we should not ignore the aldehydes and ketones which may accompany this and add their own complications. We may note as a curiousity at this stage that certain moths and millipedes are known to produce HCN in the same manner.

In addition to the almonds and kernels of lemon, lime, apple, pear, cherry, peach, apricot, plum and prune (acute poisoning from peach and apricot kernels and from choke cherries has been reported) other sources of cyanogenic glycosides are sorghum, millet, maize, Lima beans, immature bamboo shoots and cassava. We can generally avoid eating fruit kernels and most of the other foods are not a major part of our diet in the west, but they are of great importance in other parts of the world. Correct processing of the food can facilitate loss of the HCN before consumption but it is possible that cooking may destroy the enzymes and leave the glycosides intact in which form they may be ingested. It is still uncertain if animal enzymes enable the same chain of reactions to occur or whether digestive acids have a part in the release of toxic material, but the fact is that poisoning from cooked cyanogenic vegetables (Lima beans) has occurred. Another point which cannot be overlooked is that some plants may contain the glycosides but not the enzymes while others, such as lettuce, celery and mushrooms, contain the hydrolytic enzymes but not the glycosides. Mixing of the two will serve to release the HCN.

The quantity of HCN which may be released may vary from 10 mg/100 g plant in the case of American white Lima beans to an astonishing 800 mg/100 g in the case of immature bamboo shoots. The once common bitter almond may contain 250 mg/100 g.[40]

R.D. Montgomery reports that when the toxic nature of a product is known methods are developed to deal with these. Thus it is traditional to wash cassava thoroughly in running water before cooking (it may also be dried in the sun, scraped or smoked in kilns). If it is washed in still water or cooked in a closed vessel the HCN is not removed and, indeed, cases of cassava poisoning have been reported over a 300 year period. Montgomery deals with the subject in detail including advice on how to prevent poisoning by such vegetables.[40]

But what of chronic effects? The same author discusses the possibility at some length, that repeated small doses of HCN may be dangerous. Amblyopia, a form of optic nerve damage, occurs in smokers and among cassava eaters of West Africa (though undernourishment may be another factor) but more significant are the reports, summarised by E.E. Conn,[41] that the ingestion of large amounts of unhydrolysed cyanogenetic glycoside may 'be responsible for a syndrome known as tropical ataxic neuropathy (TAN) encountered in West Africa. Individuals suffering from this condition exhibit lesions of the skin, mucous membranes, optic and auditory nerves, spinal cord and peripheral nerves. The diseases can be correlated with the frequency and quantity of cassava meals'. It has also been shown that patients with TAN have an increased level of plasma thiocyanate, presumably formed during the detoxification process mentioned earlier. An increased tendency to goitre arises from the presence of thiocyanate.

The evidence for chronic HCN poisoning remains circumstantial but the possibility exists that it is involved in the development of ataxic neuropathy.

Amines which Affect the Blood Pressure

In a survey published in 1977, Neurath *et al.* reported the detection of no less than 40 amino compounds in a wide variety of foodstuffs.[42] Amines are organic substances possessing basic nitrogen atoms; primary amines have the group $-NH_2$, i.e. ammonia, NH_3, in which one hydrogen atom is replaced by an organic moiety; secondary amines have two of the hydrogens replaced by organic portions giving the general formula R_2NH. Their appearance in foodstuffs is not surprising in view of the concentration of amino acids (molecules with both an acid and an amine function) in both vegetable and animal systems. It is the primary amines we shall concern ourselves with here, secondary amines will be returned to later.

While primary amines may occur in a free state as normal components of a growing plant they are also produced by bacterial degradation of proteins and amino acids. In fact, such action in food residues in our intestines leads to their further formation. These amino compounds have a characteristic ammoniacal smell which is noticeable in certain cheeses and fish which are no longer fresh. The names putrescine and cadaverine are evocative of the origin of two aliphatic

Figure 3.3: Some Amines Present in Foodstuffs

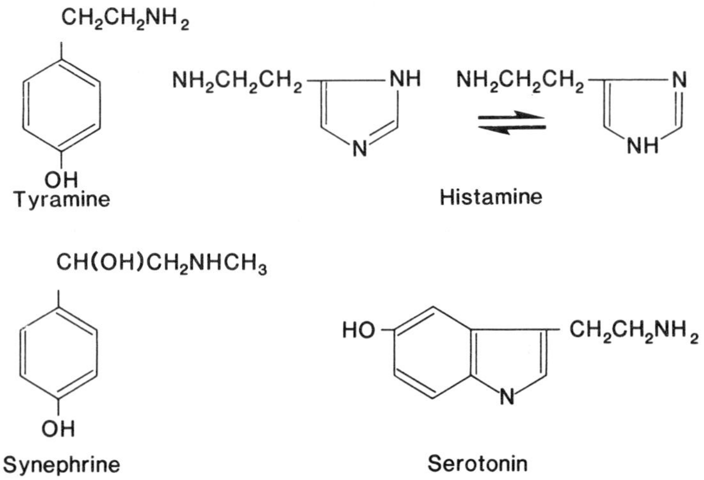

diamino compounds but the majority of amines we are concerned with here are aromatic in the sense that they have benzene rings in their structure (see Figure 3.3).

All such compounds possess, to a greater or lesser degree, the ability to constrict the blood vessels and thereby increase blood pressure. As a result, they have been termed 'pressor amines'. Although every day most of us ingest a quantity of amine which, if injected into the bloodstream, might prove dangerous or even fatal, there is no real hazard in their ingestion. The enzyme monoamine oxidase (MAO) assists in their safe conversion into aldehydes, as we described in the section on Enzyme Inhibitors, and thence to the excretable acids. The reason why some hazard still remains is that some amines may not be well absorbed by the intestines or are passed through our system as conjugates.

One of the major sources of amine is cheese and, not surprisingly, as much as 200 mg of tyramine/100 g has been found in Camembert, while Stilton is another rich source. Fish products and pickled foodstuffs always contain some (e.g. 40 mg histamine/l in sauerkraut juice). Among fruits ripe bananas may have up to 10 mg serotonin/100 g fruit, and amines are to be found in pineapples, passion fruit, paw-paw, plantains (whether raw, boiled or fresh), lemons, plums, grapes, oranges and the tissue of water melons. Broad beans, avocados, potatoes and the beverages wine, beer, tea and chocolate contain detectable quantities. The level in most of these items is only 0.1-3.5 mg/100 g fresh weight which constitutes no problem.[43]

There are two sets of circumstances where risk arises. In cases of excessive consumption of an item rich in amine or if such food is combined with an enzyme inhibitor which prevents its disposal. In certain parts of Africa plantains form a major item of diet and up to 200 mg of serotonin per day may be consumed. A high incidence of a type of heart disease which is accompanied by large amounts of 5-indolylacetic acid in the body is indigenous to these regions. The acid is formed from serotonin by oxidation of the $-CH_2CH_2NH_2$ group to $-CH_2COOH$ by the normal metabolic pathway but, presumably, not fast enough to cancel completely the amine's effect on the vascular system.

Apart from such extreme cases of amine intake, certain drugs are known to be MAO inhibitors and any person under such medication is well advised to avoid amine rich foodstuffs as dangerous levels may accumulate. Complications, and even fatalities, have been reported after consumption of cheese, pickled herring or the yeast extract Marmite.[43,45] Laboratory tests feeding beta-aminopropionitrile (BAPN) and a known MAO inhibitor separately and together to turkey poults revealed little effect when fed separately, but 70-90 per cent of the poults died when the two were fed together and produced the characteristic effect of BAPN poisoning.[43] Thus, when medication is prescribed certain dietary precautions may be necessary, but the normal, healthy human need fear little if overindulgence in amine rich foods is avoided.

Toxins Characterised by Their Action on Blood Cells

Saponins

An interesting example of how we have adapted to cope with apparently toxic components in our foodstuffs and how these components act lethally on other creatures is demonstrated by the compounds we call saponins. The name saponin derives from the soap-like foam producing properties these substances exhibit in water and they may be regarded as naturally occurring detergents.

Detergents depend for their action on the presence within one molecule of a water-soluble and of an oil-soluble (water-insoluble) portion. In synthetic detergents these may be tailored to give greater or lesser degrees of water or oil solubility and the power to drag insoluble material into water or conversely to drag water globules into an oily medium to form emulsions in either case. The ubiquitous

Figure 3.4: Saponin Structures

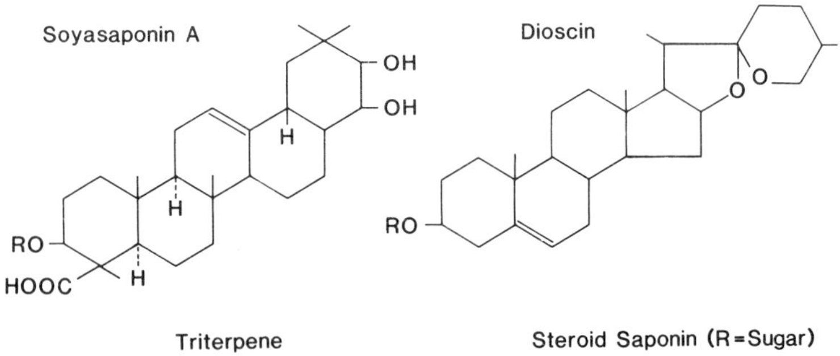

Soyasaponin A — OH, OH, H, H, H, RO, HOOC

Triterpene

Dioscin — O, O, RO

Steroid Saponin (R = Sugar)

naturally occurring sugars provide the water-soluble portions while two classes of large chemical molecules, steroids and triterpenes, provide the water-insoluble parts. When the two are combined saponins are the result. The aglycones, i.e. saponins from which the sugars have been removed by chemical action, are termed sapogenins and the two main sapogenin types are illustrated in Figure 3.4. Sugars are attached via an ether link to the hydroxyl group.

Most known saponins are of the triterpene type but the steroid sapogenins are of especial interest, as they resemble sterols found in the animal kingdom and can be used as starting material for the manufacture of synthetic hormones such as cortisone.

The soap-like properties of saponins cause them to lower surface tension in aqueous liquids and in the bloodstream they have the power of disrupting (haemolysing) red blood cells. They are easily leached from plants by water and such extracts have been used by certain tribes to kill fish since the saponins are extremely toxic to both fish and amphibians. Fish killed in this manner may, however, be eaten without harm. Generally saponins appear to be harmless to warm-blooded animals, though they have been accused of causing bloat in ruminants and certain vegetable materials poisonous to humans, such as horse chestnuts, are certainly rich in saponins.

The presence of saponins in spinach, asparagus, beetroot, yams, soyabeans, sugarbeet, peanuts, tea leaves and in root beer has been reported. They also occur in plants extracts like sarsaparilla and liquorice and have been used as additives in soft drinks, beer and confectionery (as well as fire extinguishers, photographic emulsions and lightweight concrete). Antimycotic and bacteriostatic properties have also been demonstrated in some of these materials.[45,46]

Major studies of the alfalfa and soyabean saponins have been published and from the latter five triterpene sapogenins and six different sugar moieties have been isolated. Each sapogenin appears to be combined with an average of three carbohydrate molecules. The average saponin content of soyabean is only about 0.5 per cent and some, but not all, activity appears to be lost on heating the beans. Though some anti-enzyme activity has been demonstrated *in vitro* this is not regarded as very significant. In fact, nutritional studies with chicks, rats and mice show soyabean saponin to be harmless. Some of the reasons are the destruction of some saponins by intestinal micro-flora, the fact that they are not absorbed into the bloodstream and, most important, blood plasma fully inhibits haemolytic activity on red blood cells.[46] So we see here a clear case of significant difference between *in vitro* activity and *in vivo* behaviour. If this is true of other saponins in normal diet, we are probably well able to cope with them.

Lectins

Of the two groups of compounds characterised by their effect on blood *in vitro* the most ubiquitous, the most complex and the most interesting is that known as lectins. These materials form part of the protein content of many plants (concentrated particularly in the seeds) and, as their alternative name, haemagglutinins (sometimes phytohaemagglutinins) implies they possess the property of agglutinating red blood cells. Since their first discovery in 1889 they have excited interest among workers in several disciplines: indeed, Paul Ehrlich chose these plant components to raise antibodies in animals in his early studies on immunisation.[48]

First isolated from the toxic seeds of the castor oil plant, it was subsequently shown that many edible leguminous plants (beans of all types, for example) contained lectins and as these are important protein sources for much of the world's population, the significance will be obvious. Isolation is carried out by leaching the crushed plant with water or saline solution and purification may be carried out by the technique of affinity chromatography. Those which have been studied show fundamental differences from one another in that some contain several sugar residues, some only a few sugar residues and some, such as concanavalin A from the jack bean, none at all. They have molecular weights around 100,000 and the polypeptide chains, folded into sheet like assemblies, occur as dimers or tetramers. Concanavalin A consists, for example, of four subunits each with 237 amino acids in a sequence which is now known.[49] The agglutinating properties of the lectins arise because each protein subunit contains sites which are capable of binding sugar molecules. (These properties are independent of whether sugars are or are not contained in the structure itself.) Thus a lectin with two subunits each with one binding site can attach itself to two separate blood cells; one with four subunits can attach itself to four cells and so on, in a chain reaction to form polymer clumps and hence agglutination. Metal-binding sites also occur, concanavalin having sites specific for calcium as well as sites for manganese (though this may be substituted by other metal ions).

An important, and unique, feature of the group is specificity for the sugars which may be bound. Lectins from different sources may often bind only with different sugars. For example, barley lectin will bind only with *N*-acetylglucosamine while that from the lentil will bind with glucose or mannose and no other sugars. The specificity extends to blood agglutinating properties since, though some lectins are non-specific (like the highly toxic ricin from the castor oil plant), others will clump cells only of specific human blood types or from some animals, but not others. Scarlet runner bean lectin will agglutinate human blood groups A, B and O (and blood from chicken, goat, rabbit and sheep), that from soyabeans affects human blood groups A and O only (and rabbit blood only of the above). We must note, however, that agglutinating properties and toxicity are not related, i.e. a lectin may agglutinate blood but not exhibit toxicity. The specific binding properties have encouraged biochemists to use lectins in a variety of other fields from insecticides to inhibitors for tumours[50] and those who wish to pursue these matters further will find a list for further reading in I.E. Liener's review.[49]

Injection of lectin concentrates subcutaneously or directly into the bloodstream of laboratory animals, may have fatal consequences but our concern here is only with the possible effects when lectin-containing foods are consumed. Dietary studies are complicated by the fact that a particular item of diet may contain more than one anti-nutrition factor, such as trypsin inhibitors, but there is no doubt that growth inhibition, or even death, may result from excessive consumption of foods with a high lectin content in raw or partially cooked form. Outbreaks of poisoning of humans from partially cooked bean flakes and from runner beans have been reported,[51] though not due to agglutination of the blood. Jaffe[52] suggests that the affinity properties of lectins would allow them to bind to the surface of the intestine and so prevent absorption of nutrients and although alternative suggestions have also been made, other studies seem to confirm this hypothesis.

We have spoken already of the necessity of cooking, preferably in the presence of water, to reduce or destroy the effects of trypsin inhibitors or cyanogenetic glycosides. This applies equally to phyto-haemagglutinins many of which have their activity lowered or removed entirely by moist heating and again we find that most of the foods concerned are those we do not eat raw, viz., kidney, French, black, white, broad, jack of Lima beans, lentils, peas, rice, potatoes or wheat germ. The exceptions to the cooking are bananas and mangoes and peanuts which we sometimes eat unroasted. Once again the soyabean is prominent since the defatted bean may contain up to 3 per cent of a haemagglutinin which has been shown to be toxic. Attention has been drawn to hazards which might arise if legumes are subject to dry heating rather than the normal mode of preparation.[51] Again, the best safeguard is adequate moist cooking and avoidance of overindulgence in lectin-containing foods.

Three Serious Diseases Related to Single Plant Species

In a well-nourished community many items of food may be eaten which if taken by the less privileged, especially over long periods, can cause real and lasting harm. It is necessary for us now to consider three such foods which, while intriguing from the point of view of biochemistry and nutrition, raise profoundly disturbing moral issues.

Lathyrogens

Vetch, the cultured variety of which is said to have come from the Caucasus, is described in culinary works as being prepared and eaten like peas. The most familiar form will be chick peas (or chickling vetch, *Lathyrus sativus*) the basis of cous-cous. No harm appears to come to those who eat it occasionally and it is not a major food item in Europe or North America. However, in times of shortage in Spain, North Africa, India and parts of Asia, it has been more widely used and then disturbing neurological symptoms begin to manifest themselves in humans, in horses and in cattle.

Vetch belongs to the genus *Lathyrus* which includes a fairly large number of species only a few of which are eaten by man. Others provide fodder for animals and yet others are cultivated for their decorative value. Among the last group are the sweet peas, both *L. odoratus* and the perennial *L. latifolia*. The species is scattered world wide but the problem of lathyrism as an epidemic appears to be confined to India where *L. sativus* (chickling vetch) formed 4 per cent of the total pulse crop (this gave 0.5 million tons in the 1950s). Chapaties form one of the staple foods made from it. Being cheap and easy to grow, if other foods become short, more and more will be consumed. If *L. sativus* constitutes more than about one-third of the diet for periods of from three to six months symptoms of muscular weakness, irreversible paralysis of the lower leg and, in some cases, death occur. Young men in the age group 20–29 are said to be especially prone to attack. In 1958 in one district of India alone, there were an estimated 25,000 cases – about 1 in 25 of the population.[53]

This type of disease has been associated with *Lathyrus* for millenia and reference is made to it in classical texts from both East and West, but a serious effort of finding the causative agent became possible only in the present century. It is now recognised that two types of lathyrism occur:[54] neurolathyrism – in which there is damage to the central nervous system, lesions occur together with partial degeneration of the motor tract of the spinal cord; and osteolathyrism – in which the bones and connective tissues are weakened, perhaps by collagen being softened and retained in a soluble form.

A complete explanation of the causes of the disease is blocked by two major obstacles. First, though the plants which produce human lathyrism (which is largely neurolathyrism) are easily identifiable, it is well nigh impossible to induce neurolathyrism in laboratory animals using these plants. Secondly, although active osteolathyrogenic materials have been identified and used successfully in laboratory studies these chemicals do not occur in the *Lathyrus* species used for human consumption. Although a further toxin capable of producing neurotoxic symptoms in the rat has been isolated this again is not found in *L. sativus* or allied species.

The chemical, first isolated from sweet peas in 1954, which is a potent osteolathyrogen, proved to be β-aminopropionitrile which occurs in the plant as β-*N*-(γ-glutamyl)amino propionitrile.

$H_2NCH_2CH_2CN$ $\qquad$ β-aminopropionitrile

This simple naturally occurring chemical (and a variety of similar compounds made synthetically including a number of aminonitriles, hydrazine and some hydrazides) induces osteolathyrism in laboratory animals with great ease. Its discovery was soon followed by the isolation of another similar material from the perennial sweet pea, the flat pea and other plants. This was L-α,γ-diaminobutyric acid

$H_2NCH_2CH_2CH(NH_2)COOH$ L-α,γ-diaminobutyric acid

A neurotoxin has been isolated from the common vetch which often contaminates *L. sativus* but the first neurotoxin to be isolated from the plant itself was found by two groups of workers between 1963 and 1965 and shown to be β-*N*-oxalyl α,β-diamopropionic acid.[55]

$HOOC{\cdot}CO{\cdot}NHCH_2CH(NH_2)COOH$ β-*N*-oxalylα,β-diaminoprionic acid

Although this material does give neurotoxic symptoms in animals the extent to which it is responsible for human lathyrism and the mode of action still remain a matter for speculation. An excellent review (taking the subject up to 1969) by Sarma and Padmanaban is to be found in Reference 2, pp. 267-91. As these authors indicate, in view of the importance of the crop in India it will be necessary to find a suitable substitute, to develop methods for easy removal of the toxins or, best of all, improve the general diet of the population.

Favism

Many people react adversely to certain foodstuffs which are harmless to others, but favism represents a unique and serious case of allergy to one particular plant, the fava bean (broad bean, *Vicia faba*). Those subject to the disease have a hereditary defect which prevents them from metabolising a substance produced by the plant. The illness is a sudden and severe destruction of red blood cells (haemolytic anaemia) after eating fava beans, or even after inhalation of pollen from the plant.

The raw fava beans prove more toxic than those which have been cooked and symptoms appear within 48 hours, sometimes in under 6 hours, but pollen inhalation may lead to distress within minutes. Recovery is usually rapid but children under 6 years of age have been known to die.

The disease is distributed mainly round the Mediterranean littoral and islands with the highest incidence in Sardinia (ca. 0.5 per cent of the population). Elsewhere it is very rare. While considering the occurrence of the disease in Sardinia, Crosby realised that it resembled a similar acute anaemia produced in some patients treated with certain drugs such as primaquine. He suggested that an enzyme deficiency

Figure 3.5: Compounds Suspected of Causing Favism

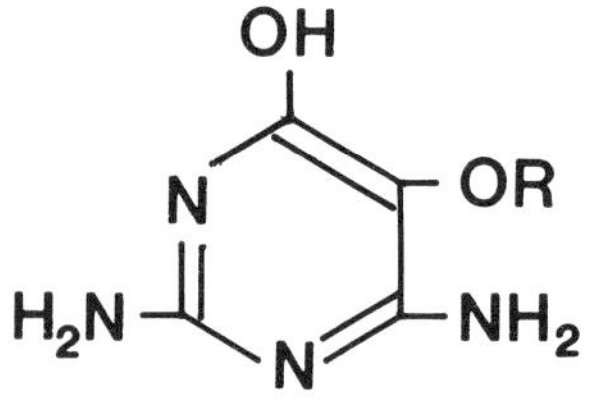

is the underlying cause and further studies revealed that persons susceptible to favism were deficient in an enzyme known as glucose 6-phosphate dehydrogenase (G6PD) the absence of which left the red blood cells unable to cope with the demands created by the presence either of the particular drugs or the fava toxin.[56]

It is now known that G6PD deficiency is hereditary. The incidence differs considerably between ethnic groups. It can be as high as 50 per cent among some Oriental communities and below 1 per cent in Western populations. But in spite of the fact that both the deficiency and the consumption of broad beans are widespread the occurrence of favism remains limited. Many factors must, therefore, be involved and while the defect is hereditary the degree of susceptibility to the effect of the beans will depend upon these unknown factors.[57]

As in the case of neurolathyrism it has not been possible to induce the disease in animals experimentally and the chemical cause of favism has not been definitely established. It is possible to isolate from the beans a glycoside known as vicine which on removal of the glucose gives the pyrimidine divicine (Figure 3.5).

This material has been isolated by several groups of workers and from other plants including one variety of vetch. (It was at one time believed to be the cause of neurolathyrism in humans but this is no longer considered to be so.) The Formosan workers Lin and Ling induced mild effects in the blood of puppies and believed that vicine was therefore the causative agent,[58] but despite this and the *in vitro* studies by other workers the matter remains unresolved.

Cycads

Having noted food-induced diseases in India and around the basin of the Mediterranean we now move to the southwest Pacific where another devastating illness is associated with the consumption of yet one more foodstuff. The disease is amytrophic lateral sclerosis (ALS) and humans suffering from this develop paralysis of the arms and legs with death following in about five years. Animals too are poisoned. The location where this seems to be most prevalent is the island of Guam where there were approximately 100 times as many cases of ALS as in the USA.[60] In this case it is believed that the causative agent has been identified.

The food responsible for this ailment comes from extremely hardy palm-like trees known as cycads. Though also called sago palms they are not the source of the sago familiar to ourselves. This comes from a different species of plant. Cycads grow in the tropics and subtropics and have been found elsewhere though not in Europe. In some regions of the Pacific (e.g. the Philippines) the leaves are eaten like vegetables, but mainly they are used as a source of starch which may be combined with vegetables, used to thicken soups or to make bread and cakes. Sometimes it is fermented. The starch is extracted from the crushed seeds, stem or tuberous portions of the plant, by water and, as with the cyanogenetic cassava, those who prepare the food know that it is toxic if not correctly treated, e.g. by soaking, washing or drying in various fashions. In fact, in Guam, the quartered seeds are soaked for as long as 10 days with several water changes, yet, in spite of this apparent knowledge regarding preparation of the starch, the Guamians also chew the fresh outer coatings of the seeds as a confection.

Of rats fed over a two year period on a diet containing a proportion of washed cycad starch a large number became poor in health. Rats fed dried outer husk of the cycad nuts developed malignant liver and kidney tumours within six months.

The search for the toxic principle in water extracts of cycads produced a number of glycosides with a common aglycone, methyl azoxymethanol.

$$CH_3-\overset{\overset{\displaystyle O}{\uparrow}}{N}=NCH_2OR$$

Cycasin, R= Glucose
Methyl azoxymethanol (MAM)
R=H

$$MAM \rightarrow CH_3OH + CH_2O + N_2$$

Though cycasin is toxic to animals when eaten, it is non-toxic when injected into the bloodstream. It can also be eaten by germ-free rats. The reason is that only intestinal bacteria can split the glycoside into its aglycone and a sugar molecule. Only the aglycone is toxic. Several modes of action of the toxin have been suggested and it can be seen to decompose readily to give methanol, formaldehyde and nitrogen. There is no doubt that MAM is extremely poisonous even though the symptoms produced in rats are not the same as in the human disease. Carcinogenesis will be discussed in the next section, but the problems of the continuing use of cycads as food for humans remains.[61,62]

Carcinogens

Few topics have been of so much concern or controversy than that of possible carcinogenicity of organic compounds. Since the first discovery that cancer could be caused by particular chemicals, gradually the systematic testing of foodstuffs and food additives was put into practice. Since then an ever increasing number of materials have been shown to be capable of inducing tumours and this fact together with the knowledge that particular forms of cancer appear to be particularly prevalent in specific localities, suggests that life styles and diet must be important contributory factors. As examples we can cite the high incidence of stomach cancer in Japan (known to have been prevalent even 100 years ago)[63] or the incidence of oesophageal cancer in other regions of the same country[34] and parts of the Transkei.[26] Tropical Africa shows the highest incidence of liver cancer in the world,[64] but this disease also occurs among Jamaican children,[65] while stomach cancer again ravaged parts of Iceland. In most of these cases a possible link with food has been postulated.

Tests for Carcinogens

Industrial experience demonstrated beyond doubt that many compounds, such as β-naphthylamine used as a rubber additive, promoted cancer in those who had had prolonged contact with them. Even more alarming was the possibility that certain food additives might have the same insidious property. Hence the need became urgent to test all such additives – preservatives, colourants, artificial sweeteners – not to mention cosmetic substances, or indeed all new organic chemicals, for carcinogenic properties – a more difficult undertaking than first realised. Quite apart from any moral issue raised by animal experimentation, such tests are lengthy and expensive; nor do all animals respond equally. Painting substances on mouse skin to see if skin tumours develop may have relevance to human skin contact, but how are we to equate the effects of intravenous, subcutaneous or intraperitoneal injection, implants in organs or prolonged feeding trials (often of unrealistic doses of chosen substance) on rats, mice or hamsters, with the possible effect on ourselves?

During the 1970s B.N. Ames and his co-workers developed a test to detect carcinogens. This involved the use, not of animals, but of the microorganism *Salmonella typhimurium* under carefully regulated conditions, to establish whether mutation (i.e. an inheritable change in the organism) was induced by the substance under test. Over the years the technique has been modified and improved in sensitivity, but the question remains whether mutation in the Ames Test means that the substance is carcinogenic to animals? In practise it often does – but not always. Sugimura[63] in comparing the overlap of Ames Test results with animal tests, found that some types of compound (chlorinated hydrocarbons) gave almost no overlap, whereas other types (alkylating agents) gave almost 100 per cent. Of more than 1,000 compounds tested in his laboratories there was 70–80 per cent overlap. We must conclude then that a positive Ames Test means a high probability of carcinogenicity and, in many cases, an urgent need for corroboration by other methods.

A further complication is the possibility that carcinogenesis takes place in two stages. In the first, initiation, changes in DNA (i.e. deoxyribonucleic acid, the nucleic acid which transmits genetic material and alteration of which results in an inheritable change, or mutation) takes place. In the second stage, promotion, no mutagenic activity need occur. Some of the difficulties are discussed by Sugimura[63] but our concern here is with the possible presence of carcinogens in what we eat. Apart from additives, deliberate or adventitious, we have three potential sources of carcinogen: (1) naturally occurring materials; (2) materials produced by microorganisms and (3) materials produced during food processing.

Naturally Occurring Carcinogens

Poisonous plants – even when the poisons have been shown to be carcinogens – may act on man in several ways. If large amounts are consumed over a short period, the acute effects take precedence over all others, but, as we have seen in the case of amytrophic lateral sclerosis believed to arise from eating cycads, the chronic effect may not be cancer. Plants containing the cancer-promoting pyrrolizidine alkaloids (the species *Senecio*, *Crotalaria* and *Heliotropium*) are very widespread but they are seldom eaten by humans. Some are believed to be used as food in tropical Africa and some are used to

Figure 3.6: Three Natural Carcinogens

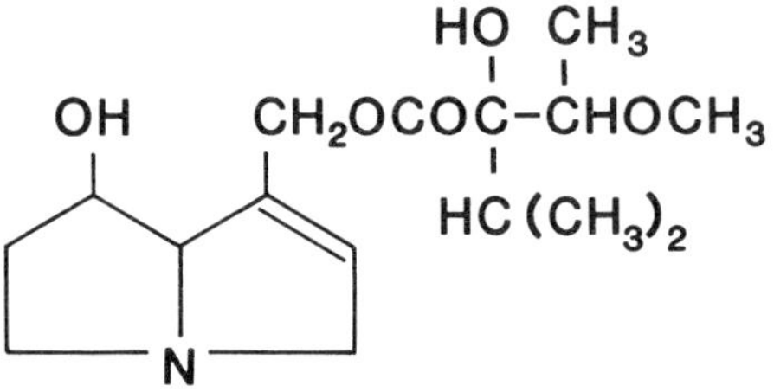

Heliotrine

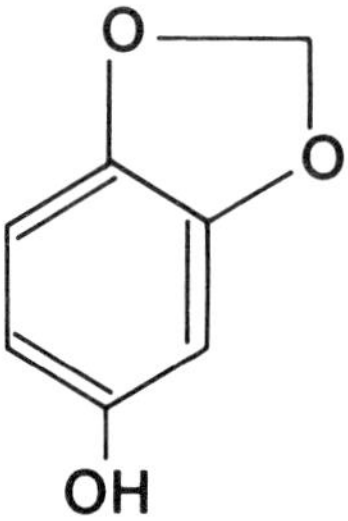

Safrole

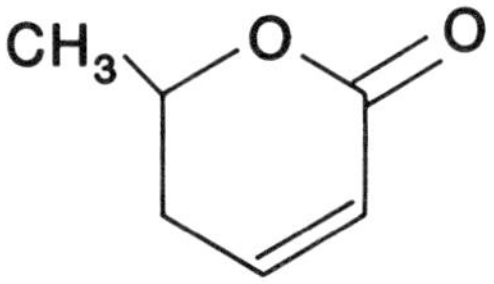

Parasorbic Acid

prepare 'bush teas' in Jamaica, which may account for the high incidence of liver cancer in these places, but the main danger from them lies in accidental contamination of other foodstuffs. More than one such occurrence has been noted. The most recent was probably in Afghanistan in 1976 when wheat was contaminated by seeds containing the alkaloid heliotrine[64] (see Figure 3.6) and acute effects were produced.

Since cattle eat plants of these groups, such as ragwort, there is the possibility of indirect transmission of pyrrolizidine alkaloids to man in milk or in meat. Though the risk is thought to be small we shall have occasion to return to this subject.

Yet another hazard is deliberate adulteration of foodstuffs. In India cooking oil has been adulterated by addition of argemone oil containing the possible carcinogen sanguinarine.[66]

Table 3.8 lists these and other known, or suspected, carcinogens.

Table 3.8: Carcinogens Occurring in Foodstuffs

Toxin	Plant source	Food use	Conjectural effect
Pyrrolizidine alkaloids	*Senecio* *Crotalaria* *Heliotropium*	Some plants may be eaten in Africa. 'Bush teas'	High incidence of liver cancer in tropical Africa.[64] Danger from contamination of grain[66]
	Comfrey	Herbal teas	Hazard exists but no evidence of effect[66]
Methyl azoxymethanol	Cycads	Source of edible starch	Amyotrophic lateral sclerosis in Guam[62]
Sanguinarine	'Prickly poppy'	Argemone oil used to adulterate cooking oil in India[66]	Hazard exists but no evidence of effect
Safrole	Sassafras	Oil of sassafras	
	Nutmeg,* mace,* cinnamon leaf*	Flavourings[67]	Hazard exists but no evidence of effect
Parasorbic acid	Mountain ash berries and cranberries	Syrups, flavourings,[68] medicaments	Hazard exists but no evidence of effect
Nitrosamines	*Solanum incanum*	Juice used to curdle milk	Oesophageal cancer in Transkei[66]
Tannin	Betal nuts	Chewed in East	High incidence buccal cancer[26]
	Sorghum	Bantu beer, porridge	Oesophageal cancer in Transkei[26]
Unknown	Bracken	Eaten in Japan[63]	Direct effect not proven

* Traces only present.

Safrole comprises nearly 90 per cent of the essential oil of sassafras but is only a minor component of nutmeg and other spices. Since its tumourigenic properties were demonstrated its use as a flavouring has been discontinued. Parasorbic acid represents yet another chemical type. This is the α,β-unsaturated δ-lactone of hexenoic acid, but there is yet no evidence that occasional contact with mountain ash berries carries any danger. In fact, though it has shown mutagenicity, feeding trials of parasorbic acid on rats showed no adverse effects.[69]

The inclusion of bracken in Table 3.8 may come as a surprise but it is still eaten in Japan (and to a very small extent elsewhere) although the danger has been widely publicised.

As well as the primary amines known to be present in cheese, a number of secondary amines have been identified. They occur at a low level also in radishes and some other vegetables and can be regarded as possible precursors of the carcinogenic *N*-nitroso compounds. The formation of these chemicals can arise through enzymatic reduction of nitrate (present in fertilisers as well as certain vegetables) to nitrite which can then react with the amines,[42] but their presence in vegetables is unusual.[66]

$$\begin{array}{lcccl} R_1 & & & & R_1 \\ \quad\backslash & & & & \quad\backslash \\ \quad\quad NH & + & {}^{-}NO_2 & \longrightarrow & \quad\quad N{-}NO \; + \; {}^{-}OH \\ \quad / & & \uparrow & & \quad / \\ R_2 & & \text{Enzymes} & & R_2 \\ & & | & & \\ & & {}^{-}NO_3 & & \end{array}$$

From the foregoing it will appear that the danger of direct consumption of known carcinogens is not great. Many other food chemicals have been tested but even when mutagenicity has been demonstrated results are not always reproducible and so remain inconclusive. The lack of certainty is best illustrated with reference to tannins.

Tannins. Extracts from bark, wood, leaves and other plant parts have served for centuries to transform animal skins into durable leather. This comes about because the extracts contain complex polyphenolic substances we know as tannins and these bind in polymeric form the protein present in the skins to give the tough, familiar material with so many uses.

Tannins are complex and occur in several forms and in varying molecular weight. Binding to protein begins at a molecular weight of about 350 and ceases at about 5,000. The two principal types are known as hydrolysable and condensed tannins. The suggestion has been made that they evolved in plants as protection againt microbial and fungal attack, but they also impart an astringent taste which deters animals from feeding on those of high tannin content. In our foodstuffs they are present in fruit, nuts, certain grains (sorghum), cider, cocoa, tea, red wine, spinach, persimmon, bananas and vine leaves. In the case of drink stored in barrels tannin is leached from the wood.

The binding ability of tannin may well extend to dietary protein. This can be regarded in two ways: either the tannin is preventing absorption or else the protein is aiding removal of tannin from the system.[34] Contradictory laboratory results have been reported. Growth of ducklings has been suppressed by a high tannin diet and liver cancer has been induced in rats by injection of tannin,[34] but no adverse effects were reported in similar experiments in other laboratories.[26] Cattle losses from eating acorns are known but it is very difficult to establish a definite effect on humans. Buccal cancer among betel nut chewers and oesophageal cancer in the Transkei where high tannin sorghum is used for Bantu beer and porridge are alleged to be due to tannins.[26] In certain parts of Japan where the rice is cooked in tea – and consumed while scalding hot – the same type of cancer has a high incidence,[34] but in spite of this Singleton concludes that the role of tannins in human cancer remains uncertain though they may be responsible for cellular damage because of repeated irritation and not DNA mutagenesis.[34] This may mean that tannins act as promoters of the second stage of the disease and not as direct initiators. It is worth recording, though, that according to the same author tannins at the appropriate level can apparently suppress detrimental microflora in the alimentary tract and stimulate growth and good health.[34]

Carcinogens Produced by Microorganisms

In Chapter 1 the havoc which may be wrought by such fungi as ergot has been described. The poisonous metabolites of mould origin are given the name mycotoxins, and many of these promote cancer of the liver in poultry, fish or laboratory animals. The most notorious are the group of aflatoxins produced by *Aspergillus flavus* and first detected in mouldy peanut meal responsible for the death of turkey poults and ducklings in 1960. Austwick and Mattocks describe aflatoxins as the greatest known carcinogenic hazard to man.[66,70] The results of mycotoxicosis may be neither acute, as with ergot poisoning, nor the slow development of tumours. For example, a crippling form of osteo-arthritis endemic in Eastern Siberia and adjoining regions, and known as Kashin-Beck disease, has been shown to be caused by eating grain infected by the fungus *Fusaria spirotrichielia*. Incidence of the disease was reduced by importing grain to the region.[71]

The danger from mycotoxins is especially great because the fungi may appear in almost any foodstuff and the metabolites may also be transmitted in milk or in meat. Dairy cattle fed aflatoxin-containing fodder gave milk containing aflatoxin or aflatoxin metabolites, and the same toxin has been detected in meat from cattle fed infected grain. The fact that they can be found in man is illustrated by the aflatoxins shown to be present in the blood and urine of Sudanese children who had eaten infected groundnuts and chickpeas. These children were suffering from the disease of kwashiorkor, which may derive from the effects of the aflatoxins.[72] A relationship has been suggested between primary liver cancer in Africa and South East Asia and the ingestion of aflatoxin B_1 (Figure 3.7) but the precise degree of risk is difficult to assess.[66] As sensitive detection methods have shown the presence of mycotoxins, albeit in minute amounts, in a wide variety of foodstuffs, and as the conditions which favour fungal development are known, active steps are being taken to eliminate this type of hazard where possible.

It is important to realise that only a restricted number of micro-organisms have been shown to produce carcinogenic toxins and that none are produced for instance by the organism used to make blue cheese (*Penicillium roquefortii*) or soya sauce (*Aspergillus oryzae*). Food which shows signs of mould growth where they should not be any (normal hard cheese, preserves, meat or fruit) should be rejected.

The field of mycotoxins is well documented and we shall restrict ourselves here to a few examples only. The aflatoxins (of which there are several) are produced by *Aspergillus flavus*, an exceedingly common fungus; several species of *Penicillium* give patulin, a compound which has been found in apple and grape juice, cider and mouldy fruit such as apples, plums and peaches.[26] Under conditions of dampness and warmth rice is attacked by *Penicillium islandicum* with the production of the toxin luteoskyrin.[73] All these materials are carcinogenic.

Though a watch is now being kept on vulnerable products such as grain during harvesting and storage, it is obviously difficult to obtain representative samples from the huge quantities involved. Even if the toxins are well within acceptable limits, moulds may still develop

Figure 3.7: Two Mycotoxins

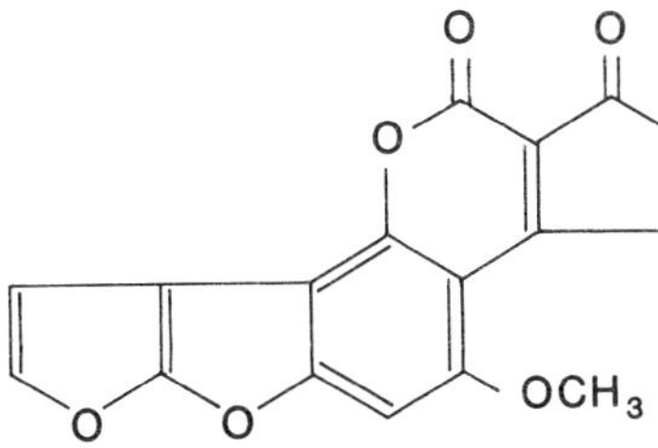

Aflatoxin B_1

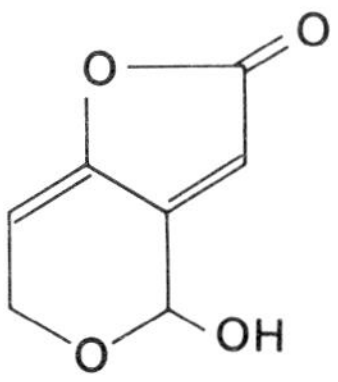

Patulin

at a later stage, after processing, for example. Imported foodstuffs require the same scrutiny. It is hoped that with our present knowledge and continuous vigilance risk can be kept to a minimum.

Evidence for one more, and unexpected, type of carcinogen in crops was reported by Petrun who claimed to have found a high level of the carcinogenic hydrocarbon, benzo(α)pyrene, in crops and soil in sites free of intensive contamination. He suggested the origin lay in synthesis by vegetable or soil micro-organisms,[74] but the danger of benzo(α)-pyrene is greater from industrial pollution than from that source.

Mutagens Produced During Food Processing

Polycyclic hydrocarbons may sometimes arise during the process of smoking of food using burning wood for the purpose of preservation, but danger exists only when the diet consists almost exclusively of smoked products and the high incidence of stomach cancer in parts of Iceland was believed to be from this cause.

Changes in food chemicals may be induced by the action of heat as in frying, roasting or braising. Boiling seems to be instrumental in removing toxins rather than producing any. The effects of deep fat frying have been studied mainly to determine what happens to the cooking oils used but more recently attention has been turned to grilled beef and fish – especially to the charred parts – and fairly strong mutagenic activity was observed (see Figure 3.8). Similar activity was found in heated beef and beef extracts and later mutagens were isolated from broiled sardines, beef or squid. These mutagens were formed from the pyrolysis of amino acids in the proteinous foods, and a whole range of alkaloid like materials were isolated and characterised. These new

Figure 3.8: Trp-p-I Mutagen Isolated from Cooked Beef

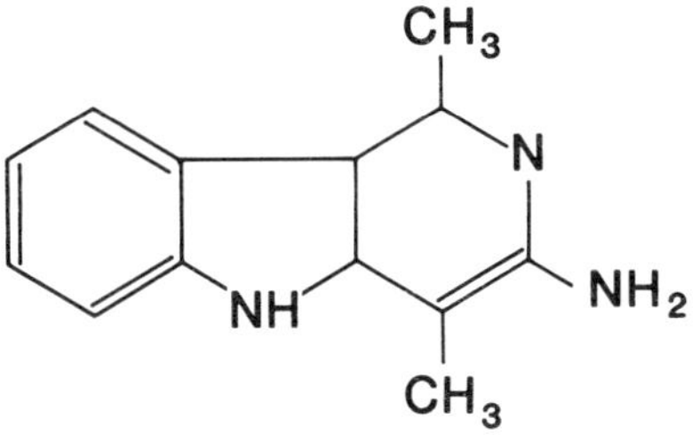

materials were found in food at a very low level and the effect on human beings is not known.[63,70]

General Remarks on Carcinogens

We must recall that the presence of a mutagen does not prove the presence of a carcinogen in our food. Mutagens have been found in a number of spices, alcoholic spirits and other beverages, but no proof of cancer promoting activity has been demonstrated. Also, there is evidence that suppression of certain steps in the process of carcinogenesis may be induced by other items in our diet. (Sugimura cites the fact that the oxidation of amines to nitrosamines may be inhibited by vitamin C.)[63] With a varied diet, care in food preparation and its storage the risk of carcinogens is greatly reduced.

Non-nutritive or Toxic Lipids

The fats and oils in animals and plants are made up of triglycerides. These are esters of the trihydric alochol glycerine with three molecules of long chain fatty acid. The biosynthetic route favours even numbers of carbon atoms in the chain and those with 12, 14, 16 or 18 members are the most widely occurring. The 18 carbons are commonest, viz. the fully saturated stearic acid, the unsaturated oleic (stearic less two hydrogen atoms), the diunsaturated linoleic (stearic less four hydrogen atoms) and the triunsaturated linolenic acid (stearic less six hydrogen atoms) which is the major acid in linseed oil. The fully saturated acids tend to be solids at ambient temperature while the unsaturated acids have lower melting points and remain liquids. Nature also prefers *cis* configuration around the double bond rather than the *trans* isomers which also generally have higher melting points. The question of saturation is significant in living systems as it is desirable to deposit fluid oils rather than hard waxes in the body. Fish swimming in cold waters have a high proportion of polyunsaturated oils, those in tropical waters can support a higher proportion of saturated fats.

The triglycerides we consume and store in our bodies as concentrated sources of energy come from anything that contains fats and oils. We have been advised in the last two decades or so to avoid animal fats with their associated cholesterol in favour of vegetable fats, and the battle continues between those who say saturated fats may be harmful and those who say otherwise. Some of the dangers attributed to animal fats, and the virtues attributed to unsaturated fats have been greatly exaggerated. The subject will be discussed in the next chapter.

It has been claimed that in those countries where a large quantity of fish oils with omega-3 unsaturation are consumed there is much less incidence of multiple sclerosis than elsewhere. Of course, such correlation does not prove that fish oil is responsible but it would certainly warrant further study.[75]

Unfortunately the unsaturated fats are themselves not above suspicion. The problem is that the unsaturation which leads to the desireable low melting points also produces centres capable of chemical reaction – in particular oxidation, with the formation of hydroperoxides. Oxidation may occur at ambient temperature and is accelerated by light or traces of metal. Rancidity is the result of such oxidation and the formation of breakdown products. At higher temperatures the hydroperoxides decompose more rapidly to form radicals which are now capable of a variety of reactions.

Unsaturated fats ⟶ Hydroperoxides
↓
Scission ⟵ Free radicals ⟶ Carbonyl / Hydroxyl / Epoxy / Carboxylic } Compounds
↙ ↘
Polymerisation Cyclisation

Quite apart from this the peroxidised fats are themselves toxic so it is usual to add antioxidants to protect polyunsaturated oils. When heated above 100°C or so reactions which occur include dimerisation or further polymerisation, and cyclisation. Even unoxidised cells may polymerise or cyclise but temperatures in excess of 250°C are needed. (These dimerisation reactions of fatty acids are carried out commercially, usually with clay catalysts, to produce intermediates for the manufacture of polyamide resins used in printing inks for packaging.)

There is strong evidence that some of these reaction products are toxic and the question arises as to what extent they may be formed in cooking oils, particularly in deep fat frying. The answer appears to be that small amounts are indeed formed, but even in fats which have been drastically overused the amounts do not seem significant. Since it has been reported that some of the by-products of heated fats resulted in tumours when fed to rats together with 2-acetylaminofluorene (AAF), whereas the control group fed AAF with fresh corn oil were not affected, a further and more serious question as to what degree they may act as co-carcinogens remains unresolved. Care in the handling of cooking oils used for frying and regular replacement before serious deterioration has occurred should minimise dangers.[67]

It was mentioned above that unsaturated acids having *trans* configuration around the double bonds have higher melting points than those with *cis* configurations and that most naturally occurring olefines are *cis*. In the hydrogenated fats produced for margarine manufacture, e.g. partially hydrogenated soyabean oil (PHSBO), small amounts of *trans* olefines and also of conjugated dienoic acids are formed. The dietary significance of this has given rise to much discussion but the opinion seems to be that *trans* isomers formed are innocuous.[76]

Less Common Fatty Acids

We have adapted to the normal glycerides we find in fish, meat and vegetables, but many modifications of fatty acid structure are known in nature and our bodies do not always react favourably to these. As the length of the fatty acid carbon chain increases so the melting point rises further. An example is the C_{22} unsaturated erucic acid which is a major component of cruciferae such as rapeseed. Rats fed as little as 15 per cent of this acid in an otherwise normal diet suffered accumulation of lipids in the heart leading to myocardial fibrosis. New varieties of rapeseed with only low levels of erucic acid (and higher levels of oleic acid) are being developed for margarine production.[77]

Acids with additional groupings in the chain are not always well absorbed. The powerful laxative effect of castor oil is due to the presence of ricinoleic acid, oleic acid with an added hydroxyl group at the twelfth carbon atom. Other hydroxy acids occur widely in nature and although it has been shown that they can be absorbed as part of a normal diet their laxative effect makes them unsuitable for nutrition.

Several plants contain epoxy fatty acids such as vernolic acid (*cis*-12,13-epoxy oleic acid) which occurs in the diet of inhabitants of the

Figure 3.9: Wyerone

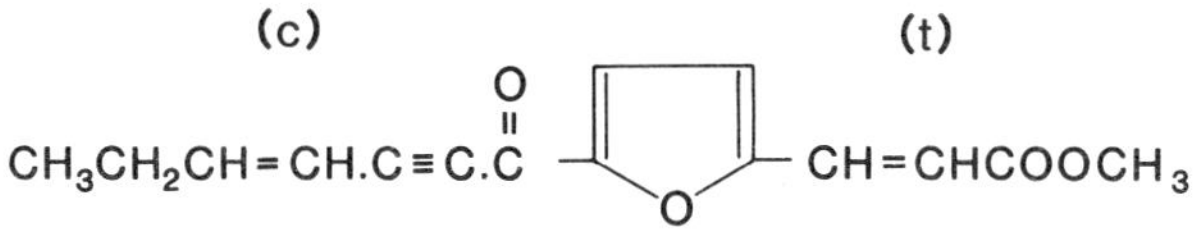

$$\underset{(c)}{CH_3CH_2CH{=}CH.C{\equiv}C.\overset{O}{\overset{\|}{C}}}-\text{(furan ring)}-\underset{(t)}{CH{=}CHCOOCH_3} \qquad \text{Wyerone}$$

West Sudan. Another type, the cyclopropane or cyclopropene containing acids, can be toxic. It is known that animals and birds which feed on plants containing cyclopropenoid fatty acids store them in their bodies and eggs so that they can be transmitted through the food chain. The only significant edible oil which contains such acids is cottonseed oil, sometimes incorporated in salad oils. During the refining process, and especially during deodorisation, most of the cyclopropenoid acids are destroyed, but small amounts may remain (0.1-0.5 per cent).[77]

Yet another group of fatty acids contain the triply unsaturated acetylene grouping and these have, on occasion, proved lethal to both livestock and to man. The broad bean (*Vicia faba* L.) contains an unusual furanoid acetylenic ester, wyerone (Figure 3.9), which has antifungal properties.

Though not an acid, a toxic acetylene compound has also been isolated from carrot and from celery, but the concentration of this material, carotatoxin, is low.[78]

$$(C_9H_{17})-C{\equiv}C-C{\equiv}C-CH_2\overset{OH}{\overset{|}{C}}HCH{=}CH_2 \qquad \text{Carotatoxin}$$

A number of other toxic lipids, such as ω-fluoro-oleic acid (the only known naturally occurring fatty acid containing a halogen) in a West African plant, or cyanolipids which are found only in Sapindaceae species, are known but none of these are components of our normal diet. A number of oils are, of course, produced purely for industrial purposes. Castor oil is one (its pharmaceutical use is minimal). Another is tung oil. Cattle grazing in tung groves have been poisoned as have humans who ate the attractive nuts from these plants. The toxic components have again proved to be acids and esters of unusual structure (unsaturated keto compounds).

In summary we can say that the wide range of cooking oils and salad oils available are desirable adjuncts to our diet and that unsaturated oils are preferable provided they are protected from oxidation and not abused by overheating. Oils from unusual plants should be treated with caution and on no account should industrial oils be used for food purposes.

Phytoalexins

It is now generally recognised that in the course of time plants have evolved defence mechanisms of several types. Beyond the first line of defence, the woody texture, the prickles or spikes, we have the production of defence chemicals, secondary metabolites, which deter by irritation, or taste or even poisoning of any herbivore incautious enough to feed from such plants. Some of the cheaper forms of defence are tannins or resinous materials rendering plants unpalatable. A more costly and more interesting form of defence is the production of metabolites in direct response to attack, as when invaded by pathogenic organisms. Such chemicals are known as phytoalexins and all plants seem able to produce them when required. These phytoalexins must not be confused with the mycotoxins. The latter are actually produced by the microorganisms (as the aflatoxins of *Aspergillus flavus*), the former are produced by the plant with the purpose, one presumes, of destroying, or inhibiting, the attacker.

Not only micro-organisms stimulate this response but almost any stress such as physical damage, light or, in other cases, frost, drought or high temperatures which result in the synthesis of flavanoid or cyanogenetic compounds or alkaloids. The production of solanine and tomatine by potatoes and tomatoes has been described under the appropriate heading. A slightly different, but interesting, illustration of chemical production is afforded by the observation that when caterpillars attack plants an almost even distribution of holes throughout the plant results. When the leaf is chewed proteinase inhibitor begins to accumulate and this probably causes caterpillars to chose fresh leaves rather than one already bitten.[79]

A problem of a different sort has resulted in California from infestation of the celery crop by a particular mould or virus to which the plant reacts by production of furanocoumarins (psoralenes). These coumarins are responsible for producing dermatitis among the crop pickers. When such an attack has occurred in temperate climates, the attackers die in winter, but in the warm climate of California they persist throughout the year and have proved difficult to eradicate.

Poisoning, we know, has resulted from potatoes with a high solanine

Figure 3.10: Structure of Some Phytoalexins Referred to in the Text

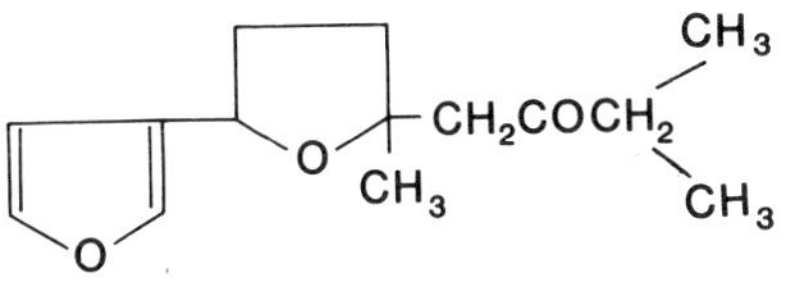

Ipomeamarone

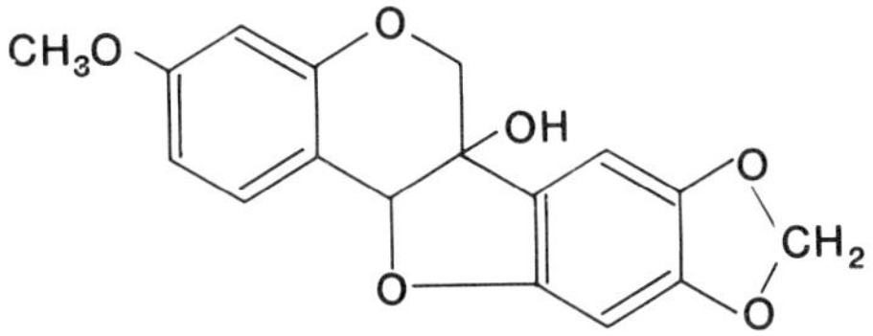

Pisatin

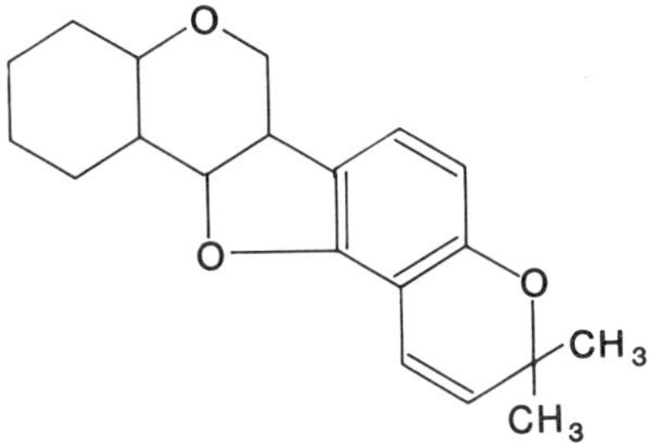

Phaseollin

content. The sweet potato also produces stress metabolites when infested or treated with heavy metal salts, for example. Mouldy sweet potatoes have poisoned farm animals and though the most abundant metabolite, ipomeamarone (a furano sesquiterpene, see Figure 3.10), has been shown to be hepatotoxic, infected animals develop lung oedema and die from asphyxiation. The toxins have been detected in sweet potatoes offered for sale and it should be noted that they are not eliminated by boiling or baking.[26]

Carrots held for prolonged periods in cold storage have developed a bitter taste due to the production of 6-methoxy mellein and, strangely, this material may be produced if carrots are stored near apples as the

Table 3.9: Phytoalexins Produced by Food Plants

Beans (*Phaseolus vulgaris*)	Medicarpin, phaseollin, phaseollidin, phasellinisoflavone, kievitone
Broad bean (*Vicia faba*)	Wyerone, wyerone acid
Pea	Pisatin, maackiain
Beetroot	2,5-dimethoxy-6,7-dimethyl dioxyflavanone 2-hydroxy-5-methoxy 6,7-dimethyl dioxyflavanone

ethylene evolved from apples causes the carrots to react. The garden pea synthesises the phytoalexins pisatin and dimethyl pterocarpin and beans produce phaseollin. The former compounds result from anything that produces cellular damage including ultra-violet light, and the materials have been shown to be toxic to higher animals.

Notable features of phytoalexins are that they are produced throughout the plant but are concentrated in tissues containing the parasites or directly adjacent to the point of infection or attack. They are, furthermore, non-specific to attackers, some of which are susceptible, some not. Potatoes grazed by Colorado beetles produce solanine which has no effect on the beetle whereas if beetroot is infested by beet fly from 29 to 100 per cent of the fly have been observed to be killed by the flavanones synthesised as a result.[80] The type of phytoalexin is determined by the genotype of the plant and plants of the same family synthesise chemicals of similar structure. Many of the defence chemicals of non-edible plants such as orchids have been identified. In addition to the carrot, sweet potato and beetroot mentioned above, phytoalexins have been isolated from barley, turnip, broad bean, green pepper, soyabeans, rice and maize.

Some of the materials synthesised and some typical formulae are shown in Table 3.9.[81]

The nature of the plant reaction serves to emphasise the need to store our crops with care.

Foods of Animal Origin

Unlike plants, animals rarely defend themselves by making themselves unpalatable or toxic to other animals. A few examples exist among insects, but among vertebrates only some frogs and fish are toxic to their predators. No suspicion of toxicity has ever arisen against animals used for human consumption. Yet diet-related diseases produce numerous examples of strong correlation with prosperity, and the main difference between the diets of poor and prosperous countries is the comparatively high proportion of animal foods in the latter. This is the presumable origin of the belief that vegetarian foods are wholesome, while it is animal foods that give rise to diseases of the affluent society. Cholesterol and animal fats, for example, were prominent among suspected causes of coronary disease, cow's milk is notable among foods causing allergies, high meat consumption may be associated with cancer of the colon. The question is that if animal foods are non-toxic, what is the explanation of their connection with diet-related diseases. Probably there are several reasons.

(1) While the animal does not defend itself by making itself toxic to predators, its aim in building its body is not to make itself good food for other animals. Some foods of animal origin, notably fats, pack a large number of calories, so their consumption can lead to obesity. Although they are unlikely to be toxic, they are hydrophobic substances, so that their transport in a waterbased system, (the bloodstream) can pose difficulties. They are normally transported in the blood by carrier proteins, acting, in effect, as packing cases. Normally large quantities of lipids are transported in the body by this means without trouble, but the system is not absolutely foolproof. Gallstones, so to speak, are the result of traffic jams.

Milk and the nutritive content of eggs have been designed for the needs of rapidly proliferating cells in a growing organism. Proliferating cells need a comparatively large quantity of cholesterol for the construction of cell membranes, growing bones need calcium. Hence milk and eggs contain too much cholesterol and calcium for the needs of an animal which has already reached its adult size and for which food is primarily a source of energy.

Some animals can store large quantities of certain vitamins. The liver of animals living in the arctic regions (polar bears, whales, seals) carries a large store of vitamin A, an excess intake of which can be toxic to the human consumer. The case of the arctic explorers who suffered vitamin A intoxication after eating polar bear livers, has already been mentioned in this chapter.

(2) Foods of animal origin can become toxic on account of their vulnerability to invasion by micro-organisms. Some of these may be present in the live animal and passed on to the human consumer, for example, in its milk. Before the introduction of pasteurisation cow's milk was a notable vehicle for the spreading of diseases like bovine

tuberculosis or brucellosis. A multitude of micro-organisms invade the carcass of dead animals. Some of these, like salmonella and botulism bacillus, are sufficiently heat resistant to survive light cooking, as found, for instance, in the inside of a large piece of meat or in the inside of a frozen chicken without adequate thawing.

Even if the food, as consumed, is sterile, the large intestine in the human body supports an enormous bacterial flora, the composition of which depends on the diet. A largely vegetarian diet favours a different population of micro-organisms than one containing a significant proportion of animal products. Some bacteria may produce metabolites which could be carcinogenic or otherwise toxic to their host. This point will be raised again later in this book in Chapter 5.

(3) The eggs of parasitic worms passed on to humans in animal foods are a hazard virtually eliminated under conditions of advanced civilisation.

(4) Natural or artificial toxins, originating in poisonous plants or in weed-killers, pesticides, etc. consumed by an animal can be transmitted to the human consumer in the meat, milk and eggs of that animal. Some examples will be given in the subsequent sections of this chapter.

(5) Metabolic disorders (lactose intolerance, phenylketonuria, familial hypercholesterolaemia, etc.) can make normal nutrients harmful for some people.

(6) Dietary proteins are mostly broken down into their component amino acids before they are absorbed into the bloodstream, but small amounts of partly digested protein molecules do reach the circulation. This happens to a greater extent after acute intestinal infections and other disorders (see Chapter 6). These foreign proteins entering the circulation provoke the formation of antibodies. As will be mentioned in the next chapter, cow's milk antibodies have been demonstrated in patients suffering from coronary disease and may have a bearing on their condition. Allergic symptoms can also arise from the antigen-antibody reaction following the ingestion of foreign proteins.

(7) Animal hormones ingested with meat or milk, like testosterone or oestrogens, may be absorbed by the human consumer. Such hormones may not be appropriate to the consumer's needs.

(8) Allowance must be made for the possibility that some foods of animal origin may contain toxic or noxious agents, the exact effect of which is not yet understood. In Chapter 4, for example, it will be pointed out that a strong correlation exists between coronary disease and the consumption of milk. What exactly in milk could be responsible for its apparent pathogenic effect on the arteries is still a subject of debate.

Transfer of Toxins into Milk, Meat and Fish

There are many well-documented examples of the absorption of natural toxins by animals which then may transmit them through several links of the food chain. One example is poisonous honey from bees which have gathered nectar from poisonous plants like oleander. The milk of cows which have eaten poisonous plants, may contain toxic substances. Probably the most toxic of such substances are fish poisons, like ciguatera. These are thought to arise from blue-green algae and may be passed through several links of the food chain without causing harm to the carrier. A paralysing poison which can be transferred by clams and mussels, probably originates in dinoflagellates on which they feed.[82] More often, however, the transferred toxins are artificial. Fish and shellfish are notorious accumulators of industrial toxins, such as organomercurials. Many cases of human poisoning from this cause are known.

Minamata Disease[83] (see also Chapter 8, p. 244)

Possibly the most extensively documented and publicised cases of industrial poisoning occurred at Minamata Bay and on the Agano River in Japan. From about 1950 onward abnormal behaviour of marine animals and of birds had been observed in Minamata Bay in the south of Japan. Dead fish were found floating in the water, octopus floated to the top and could be caught by hand. Crows were falling out of the sky, domestic animals, especially cats, had convulsions, jumped into the sea and died in madness. In April 1956 a six-year-old girl was found to have unusual nervous symptoms. In the following months more and more patients were admitted to hospital with an unclassified disease to which the name Minamata was given.

Symptoms included sensory disturbances, constriction of the field of vision, impairment of hearing and sometimes of speech. Dizziness, loss of coordination and muscular weakness and, in a small number of cases, convulsions were reported. It was three years before a theory of mercury poisoning was submitted and another two before it was proved. By 1971 there were 658 cases with 78 deaths in the Minamata region alone. A second outbreak on the Agano River on the western Japanese coast had occurred in 1964–5.

Most of the sufferers were fishermen and their families, and warnings had been given against eating fish in the polluted areas. In all, by late 1975, 899 cases were recognised and there were 143 deaths. A further 3,454 patients were appealing for official recognition.

The combined effort of a number of scientific groups eventually identified the causative agent as methyl mercury, generally occurring in the form of salts, arising from mercury losses in factories producing acetaldehyde, where inorganic mercury was used as a catalyst. It was estimated that in the period 1932–68, 81 tons of mercury had been discharged into the bay with the waste. It has been shown that one of the sources of organic methyl mercury compounds was bacterial action. In both major outbreaks water downstream from acetaldehyde plants was contaminated. Fish accumulated the poison and became the immediate source of the ingested mercury.

Draconian measures were required to eliminate the cause of the disease, including the removal of 3.6 million cubic metres of sediment, containing about 25 μg of mercury/g dry weight, from the bay. In some Swedish lakes fish with even higher levels of mercury than those in Japan have been found, but as the consumption of fish in Sweden was low, no epidemic occurred.[84]

Meat and Milk: The Hazards of Free-range Cattle

Meat and milk are also potential vehicles for the transfer of toxins which domestic animals ingest accidentally or which are administered to them deliberately. In the latter category belong growth promoters for poultry and meat-producing animals, as well as milk yield enhancers for dairy cattle. Thus organo-arsenicals are often incorporated into poultry feed to control disease and enhance growth, and oestrogens were used in the rearing of calves for veal. The latter practice had a great deal of publicity and the use of oestrogen-based drugs is now banned in many countries, though still employed in some. In Puerto Rico, for example, it is suspected that the synthetic oestrogen diethylstilboestrol used for fattening cattle and reaching the human consumer in meat, may be responsible for precocious puberty in girls as young as five or six, and of feminisation of boys.[85] As will be pointed out in subsequent chapters, stilboestrol also increases the risk of artery disease and possibly of cancer.

Free-range animals are also exposed to various hazards from natural and synthetic sources. A variety of poisonous plants in pastures constitute the natural hazards. Grazing animals normally avoid these, but they may be unable to separate some of them from the plants they eat. The disease called milk sickness (or the trembles), for instance, of which Abraham Lincoln's mother is thought to have died, is caused by the milk of cows which have eaten the poisonous plant snake root, containing an unsaturated alcohol, tremetol. Such plants are also

Figure 3.11: Anagyrine

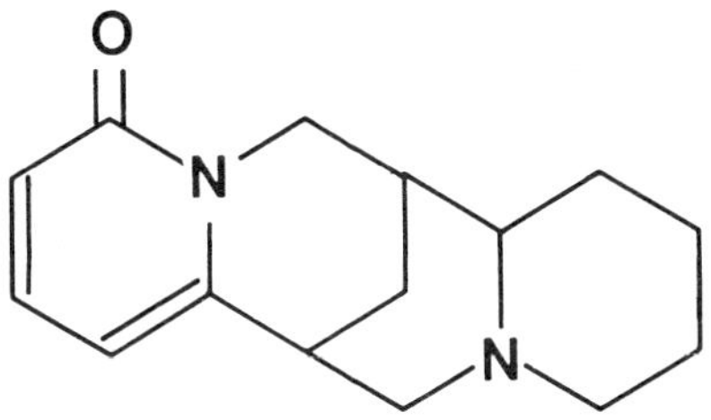

Anagyrine

poisonous to the cows.[86] A more subtle case is the transfer of bracken fern toxicity which passes from the cows to their offspring in the milk.[87] The transfer of goitrogens in milk from cows eating cruciferous plants, marrow stem kale and the like, has already been mentioned. Ragwort is a source of carcinogenic pyrrolizidine alkaloids. Cows fed dried tansy ragwort for two weeks at a level of 10 g/kg of body weight/day produced milk containing 9-17 μg/100 ml.[88] Generally, cattle grazing on alkaloid-containing plants are likely to excrete some of the alkaloid in their milk and some may accumulate in meat. Though the amounts are small, there is circumstantial evidence of teratogenic effect in humans.

The presence of the alkaloid anagyrine (Figure 3.11) in lupin plants eaten as forage has been linked with crooked calf disease, a condition in which calves are born with deformed limbs, spine and skull. In a distressing case in north west California a child was found to have hands and arms deformed in the same manner and it is known that the mother had drunk goat's milk throughout pregnancy from goats foraging where lupins grew. (The woman herself believed that the herbicide 2,4-D was responsible, but while this has shown teratogenicity on laboratory rodents, there was no evidence linking it with this particular case.) This case has led to the recommendation that expectant mothers should avoid milk from foraging goats during the first three months of pregnancy, and drink only commercial milk, which appears to be quite safe.[89]

Milk as a Model of the Environment

No commonly available foodstuff better reflects the environment in which it has been produced than milk. The cow stands between this environment and ourselves, absorbing through its food supply, breath and skin everything that is present there and excreting some of it, either directly or as metabolites, into its milk. Some of the natural contaminants have been mentioned in the previous section, this section will consider the following sources:

(1) Veterinary materials;
(2) Inhalation or skin absorption (after the spraying of barns, etc.);
(3) Contamination from the milking process;
(4) Through the food and water supply.

The milk of cows undergoing medication is not permitted to be sold. When, for example, penicillin or other antibiotics have been used for the treatment of bovine mastitis, the animal must be segregated until the milk is free of their residues. Nevertheless, a small number of milk samples containing penicillin or sulphonamides continue to be reported. The dairy industry in this country penalises producers in an attempt to reduce such cases, not only to protect the public, but because the presence of antibiotics in milk can prevent 'starter' reactions in cheese-making or the manufacture of other fermented dairy produce.

Contamination that can arise during the milking process is from the detergents and bactericides used on the cow before milking. Guidelines issued to dairy farmers require the removal of such substances by warm water rinses, but the inadequate observation of these instructions can result in traces of quaternary ammonium, chloro- or iodo-compounds in milk.

The speed with which pesticides are absorbed by the cow after spraying of barns is quite remarkable. In a case where malathion and ronnel were used, the milk contained traces of these materials on the evening immediately following the spraying and persisted for several weeks afterwards. But these materials also find their way into milk through the cow's food supply, since this is subject to exactly the same hazards as our own (except that it will be free of added colourants and flavourings). The transfer of the herbicide maleic hydrazide to milk will be mentioned later. In another case dairy cows grazing on endive which had been treated with pentachlorointrobenzene were found to have pentachloroaniline in the milk (ca 0.09 mg/kg of fat) together with hexachlorobenzene which is a contaminant of the nitro compound.[90]

Among pesticide residues usually found in milk are polychlorinated biphenyls. Levels vary from country to country but are usually well below the acceptable maximum. Tuinstra *et al.*[91] published the curious finding that milk contained more chlorinated biphenyls than could be accounted for by residues in their food supply, but it is still not known where the rest came from.

Bacteria can find their way into milk from the cow. Before the introduction of pasteurisation this made milk the most important vehicle for the transfer of bovine tuberculosis and brucellosis to humans. Fortunately most pathogenic micro-organisms are heat sensitive and the comparatively simple expedient of heating milk to about 70°C destroys them. Pasteurisation does not destroy all bacteria in milk, but those left are harmless. Occasional slips with the pasteurisation process, or the sale of unpasteurised milk can still result in sporadic cases of brucellosis, or salmonella or campylobacter infection. Bacteria can also invade milk after pasteurisation and contaminate it with bacterial toxins, like aflatoxin.

Human milk is also subject to contamination. Most important among its contaminants are drugs and medicines taken by the mother. Infants breast-fed by a drug addict mother have withdrawal symptoms after weaning and have to be 'dried out' as if they had been drug addicts themselves. Generally, mothers who regularly take medicine for some condition, e.g. epilepsy, would probably do better if they did not breast-feed their infants.

Milk is a complex biological fluid and we have not attempted to list all the chemicals which have been found in it from time to time. We want to make a brief mention of phenols which are probably the degradation products of lignins,[92] the woody parts of plants. Natural steroid hormones, mainly oestrogens, are present in milk originating in the cow (see Chapter 4) and oestrogen mimics could be present originating in plants eaten by the cow or in micro-organisms invading milk. The quantities are unlikely to be significant.

Control of Adventitious Additives

A recent review[93] considers infant food with particular regard to milk. The authors point out that methods of analysis have now become so sensitive that the concept of 'zero value' can no longer have meaning. A pragmatic approach, in which practical residue limits are proposed, together with the tightening of controls and still better analytical procedures, seems to lead to slow but measurable improvements in quality.

Some countries still have no legal ruling on pesticide contamination, but one hopes that the example of those who do, combined with continual activity in the field of prevention of contamination (particularly microbial) will lead to a world-wide improvement.

Food Contaminants and Food Additives

The production and distribution of food in industrialised communities is a massive and complex operation involving the handling and protection of vast quantities of perishable materials. Many separate stages are involved and at each one the probability of contamination exists. Consider agriculture. Even before the crops are planted, the soil must be prepared by eradication of weed and by chemical fertilisation. The seeds may be dressed with fungicide; herbicides are used in the soil; predators are discouraged by the periodic spraying of crops throughout growth. The harvest may be fumigated for its further protection. Certain crops require chemical processing, and before some goods are packaged, perservatives, colourings or flavourings, as well as traces arising from the packaging, may be added. In spite of all precautions, unfavourable combinations of temperature and humidity can conspire to bring about degradation and spoilage. Most food which finally comes to our table is pleasing to the eye, acceptable to the palate and nourishing to the body, but it contains residues indicating every stage of preparation through which it has passed – tiny residues, invisible, tasteless and probably in most cases innocuous. Let us consider these stages and see of what these traces consist.

Chemicals Present Prior to Sowing or Planting

Even before cultivation is begun, conditions may prevail which influence the composition of future crops. Certain soils contain abnormal levels of trace elements, like selenium or tin, which may become concentrated in plants. Cabbages, for example, accumulate selenium, and while we need some for health, an excess is undesirable. Pollution may arise from industrial waste and excess lead, mercury or cadmium may be present. In the neighbourhood of nuclear power plants or after atmospheric testing of nuclear weapons radioactive fallout will occur at very low but measurable levels, and natural radioactivity makes its own contribution both to soil and water.

The next step is the preparation of the soil with fertilisers and herbicides. Nitrate fertilisers have low inherent toxicity, but enzymatic reduction within plants can give nitrite which is more toxic and which may react with amines to form carcinogenic nitrosamines.

The mercurials used for many years to control seed-borne disease are not regarded as serious sources of pollution, since the main source of mercurial pollution is from industrial applications. Nevertheless, cases have occurred when such dressed seed has been eaten with outbreaks of poisoning as the result.

Chemicals Used During Growth

At all stages of cultivation herbicides may be used to control the weeds. The number and variety employed is legion, some being specific in action, some general. Examples are the notorious 2,4,5-T (2,4,5-trichlorophenoxyacetic acid, Figure 3.13), notorious because of the traces of dioxin which may be present, used to kill broad-leaved or woody plants and 2,4-D (2,4-dichlorophenoxyacetic acid) which attacks both annual and perennial weeds. Growth inhibitors such as maleic hydrazide are used and have been found, not only in plants, but in milk from dairy cows grazing on them.[94]

During growth, at fixed intervals, crops are sprayed to prevent disease and control pests. These pesticides have received much publicity and detailed study. They fall into five major types according to use, viz., insecticides, acaricides, nematocides, molluscocides and rodentocides for the control respectively of insects, spiders, nematodes, snails and rodents. The names aldrin, dieldrin, malathion and DDT will be familiar – but there are many more in use, usually containing chlorine or phosphorus. The technical literature is replete with figures for individual pesticides in specific fruit, cereals or vegetables but it is pertinent here to consider only whether any interaction may take place with the food and how much pesticide or metabolite will reach our tables.

With regard to the first point, studies have shown that both herbicides and pesticides may influence the concentration of nutrients in foods into which they are absorbed. The level of carbohydrates may, for example, be affected by herbicide while the phosphorus insecticide dimethoate is known to reduce the level of vitamin C in blackcurrants by over 30 per cent.[95] Interactions of this type require detailed examination. On the second point, many countries now monitor pesticide residues not only in food and drinking water but in human tissues, blood and milk. Particular attention is given to chlorinated hydrocarbons for two reasons. First, they persist in the environment, secondly, they can be detected at very low levels (below 1 part in 10^9) by modern instrumental methods of analysis. International organisations such as the WHO recommend methods and suggest tolerance levels in terms of ADI (Acceptable Daily Intake) but residues vary from country to country and some materials persist for years after use has been banned.

Typical of the systematic approach is the monitoring of pesticides in the environment by the US Food and Drug Administration. A recent report describes the purchase of 20 market baskets in 20 different cities with the food obtained being divided into 12 categories each of which was analysed for 6 metals and 41 different organic substances. Of all the composite samples 52 per cent contained traces of organochlorine pesticides, though the levels were frequently below 0.01 p.p.m. and within the ADI, so no suggestion was made that harm would accrue from this.[96]

Post-harvest Treatment

Infestation of fruit and other crops is commonly eradicated by the practice of fumigation. Methyl bromide, ethylene dibromide, ethylene oxide and even hydrocyanic acid may be used. Low residues of bound bromine have resulted from the first two. Ethylene oxide may be converted by naturally occurring inorganic chlorides in foodstuffs into the toxic chlorohydrin while HCN can form cyanohydrins with fructose. The amount of such by-products, all of which can be measured, depends very much on the type of fruit or vegetable being treated and evaluation of this problem is continuing.[26,67]

Processing of Foods

When chemicals are chosen for use in food processing several factors must be considered; the toxicity of the chemical, its ease of removal, the stability under processing conditions and the possibility of reaction with food components such as amino acids. This is best illustrated by some examples. Oil is extracted from soyabean meal by use of solvents. At one time trichloroethylene was used for this purpose as it is non-inflammable, a powerful solvent for oils and is also sufficiently volatile to be readily removed and recovered for reuse. However, it was found that in meal extracted with trichloroethylene a toxin was produced which led to aplastic anaemia in cattle and its use had to be abandoned. In 1957 severe losses of poultry occurred to contamination of oleic acid used in poultry feed by a chlorinated aromatic compound referred to as chick oedema factor. This substance must have been produced artificially during the treatment of the fats, although how it had arisen is not known. Much of the flour we consume is bleached and conditioned by chemical means. The use of nitrogen trichloride for this purpose had to be dropped because flour so treated if used in the diet of dogs produced symptoms of hysteria.

Such adverse effects led to many studies of the toxicity of the reagents. The conditioners and bleaches now used, chlorine dioxide and benzoyl peroxide, are believed to be quite safe and not to give rise to harmful by-products.

Traces of white mineral oil may appear in bakery products since in some countries it is used as a release agent or lubricant and small amounts are also added to dried fruit such as raisins and sultanas during handling.

Food Additives

It is in the nature of foodstuffs (unless refrigerated) to deteriorate and the need to store supplies from one season to the next and then throughout barren winters must have been the spur which prompted man, throughout the ages, to devise ways of preserving his stocks. The discoveries that dried foods, smoked foods or salted foods would last were major developments, pickling and fermenting must have followed later, but each of these methods, each in its own unique way, modified the taste of the food being preserved and so it is hardly surprising that attempts are now being made to maintain food in a state of freshness by the use of newer materials and methods.

Two of the principal mechanisms which degrade the food are bacterial attack and oxidation. For control of the former anti-microbials are used chief among which are sodium benzoate, sorbic acid and sulphur dioxide. Some concern has been expressed regarding the last named which is used in beverages, and it would be possible to absorb more sulphur dioxide through drinking than through industrial pollution. In some countries antibiotics have been used on fruit but this practice is to be discouraged as resistant strains of organisms might be produced. Oxidative degradation is suppressed by use of antioxidants, typically butylated hydroxy toluene (BHT) or butylated hydroxy anisole (BHA).

The extreme caution required in choosing preservatives may be illustrated by the case of AF-2 (2-(2-furyl)-3-(5-nitrofuryl) acrylamide) used in Japan to preserve meat and fish products. This functioned successfully and was used from 1965 until in 1974 it was proved in animal experiments to be a carcinogen when it was promptly banned.[63]

Colourants are widely used, perhaps too widely, to heighten existing colours, to give food a deceptive appearance of freshness, to identify fruit cordials or simply to make the product more attractive. They come in two types, natural and synthetic and typical of the former are cochineal, turmeric, carotene, caramel, chlorophyll, grape skin extracts and so on, while the latter are in fact dyestuffs. In the last few decades these have been subjected to intensive screening and a whole spectrum of colours has been withdrawn after toxicity, usually carcinogenicity, was demonstrated. Colours now used are generally subject to certification and maximum levels are given. Thus, Citrus Red No. 2 is used up to 2 p.p.m. by weight to colour oranges, Orange B up to 150 p.p.m. by weight for sausage casings and so on.[97] A high degree of safety is believed to exist now but as testing continues it is likely that the number of acceptable colours will continue to be restricted.

Artificial sweeteners are under the same scrutiny and the promotion and banning of cyclamates will be recalled by all who take an interest in this subject. Even though saccharine has been used for so many years its use is reviewed from time to time and investigation of new materials is taking place all the time. Some are unlikely to be acceptable because of slight taste delay or after taste. One of the more useless would seem to be a natural glycoprotein called Miraculin which, if chewed for 10 minutes before a meal, makes all sour tasting substances taste sweet for 1 to 2 hours afterwards.[98]

Among the unnecessary additives one can include monosodium glutamate which is used in a wide variety of foods as an alleged flavour enhancer. This compound, which is present in soy sauce, is said to result in a minor ailment known as Kwok's syndrome if taken in excess by certain sensitive individuals, but this may be an allergic response rather than one from toxicity.

Texture in many processed foods is modified by the use of surface active agents. Some of these are modified natural glycerides and are made from natural materials, e.g. sugar esters. Other agents may be produced by the use of ethylene oxide and as there is evidence that higher molecular weight poly(oxyethylene) compounds may not be well absorbed, control of manufacture and use of such emulsifiers is important.

The last class we shall consider are artificial flavourings. These may be used to replace natural flavours or, like colourants, to enhance those already present. Many are added in the form of essential oils which are, so to speak, the concentrated flavours or aromas of plants. Most such oils are non-toxic but some citrus oils have demonstrated weak tumour promoting activity when applied to mouse skin, and sesame oil gave some incidence of tumours when fed to rats.[99] Among flavouring materials we may include wormwood of which the major component thujone produces convulsions. This was the toxin in the once widely drunk absinthe.

Figure 3.12: Myristicin

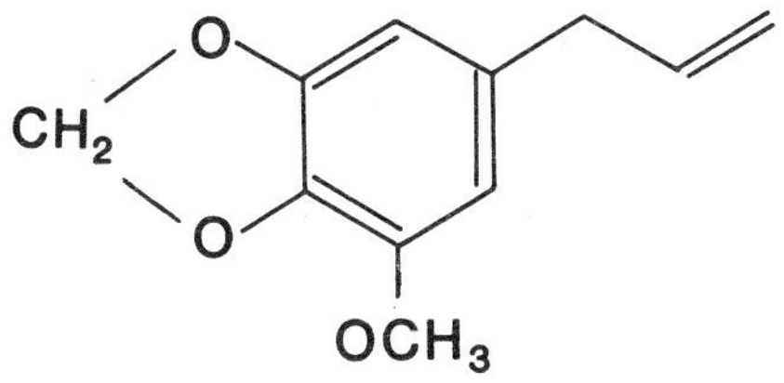

Most essential oils are unlikely to cause harm if used in small amounts at reasonable dilution. We use dill, celery, parsley, mint or nutmeg safely even though myristicin (Figure 3.12), which can produce profound psychological effects on animals, is present in each, but large quantities of nutmeg or mace if consumed produce narcotic effects rather like alcohol intoxication.

In addition to the essential oils individual constituents of such oils, viz. esters, alcohols, aldehydes or acids, may be used alone or in mixtures. Not only has the toxicity of such materials been studied but generally the metabolic pathways by which small amounts are rendered innocuous in our bodies are known.

Packaging Materials

Even the last step before distribution when the food is packaged for its protection, in plastic film or paper or metal foil or even in glassware, can be a further source of taint. Improperly washed glassware may contain detergent or germicide, paper contains size and coating materials, plastic has antioxidants, plasticisers and release agents, cartons may use adhesives and printing inks are ubiquitous. The extent such toxins are transferred to food will depend upon temperature, humidity and the food being packaged. Fatty foods are more prone to extract impurities – but all these matters are well known and it is the duty of the manufacturer, who knows what material he is using and its properties, to ensure that the goods packaged will be as free from taint as possible.

Miscellaneous Factors

Not all poisons fall tidily into the categories we have used, nor do the effects which may be produced in man. In this section we will consider some other possibilities.

Figure 3.13: Chemical Structures of Some Materials Referred to in the Text

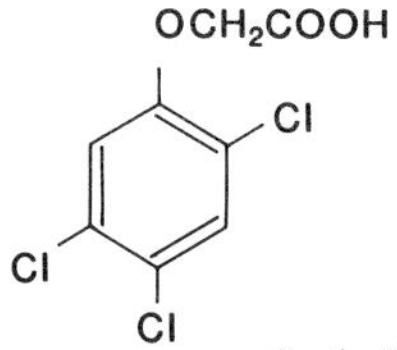

2, 4, 5-T

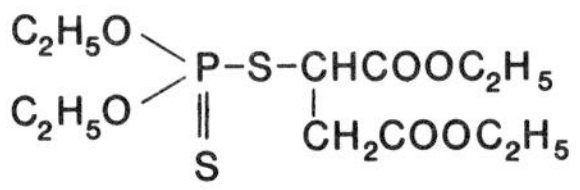

Malathion

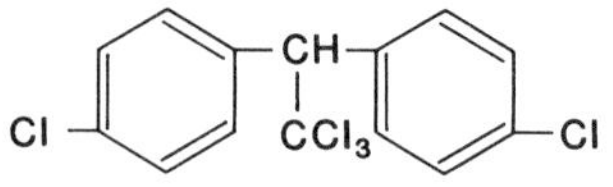

DDT

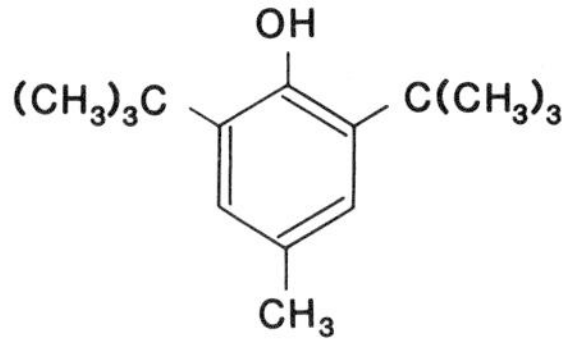

BHT

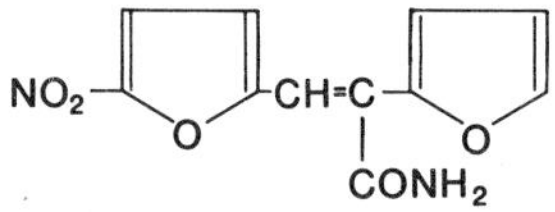

AF-2

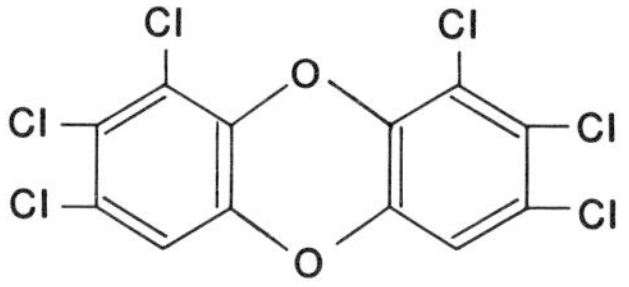

Chick Oedema Factor

Photosensitisation

Certain plant components may sensitise individuals to produce contact dermatitis (as with poison ivy). Others will produce a condition where damage from light may occur. Two types of photosensitiser have been postulated: primary sensitisers which directly cause skin damage where light is present and hepatogenous sensitisers, i.e. substances which can inflict a degree of liver damage. This prevents detoxification of some materials, such as chlorophyll breakdown produces. If these products accumulate in the blood, photosensitisation will develop.[100]

Prominent among such toxins, and often present in essential oils, are the furanocoumarins derived from psoralene and angelicin (Figure 3.14). Some sensitisers have been detected in citrus fruits such as the rinds of orange, lime or bergamot (candied bergamot peel is used in confectionery), in figs, carrots, parsnips, celery and fennel, in angelica and also in dill, rue, mustard and coriander.[101] Only sensitive individuals are likely to be harmed by normal contact with these foods, herbs

Figure 3.14: Common Phytoalexins

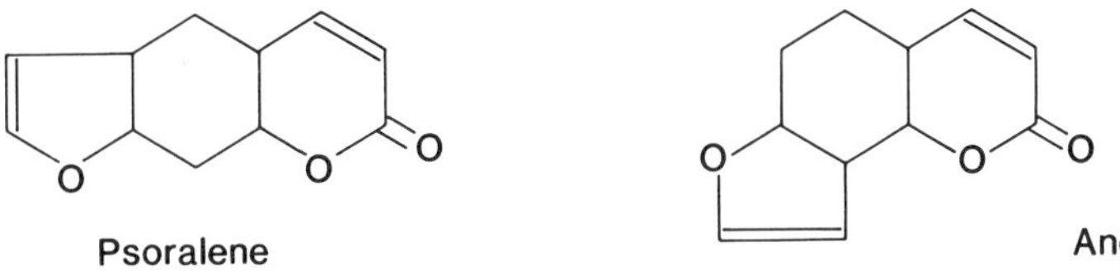

or spices, but clearly excessive contact with the essential oils would carry certain dangers and the use of bergamot oil in sunscreen preparations is under attack.

Oxalates and Anthraquinones

Many green plants such as lettuce, cauliflower, carrots and turnips contain oxalic acid in the form of calcium or potassium salts. but by far the highest concentration is in rhubarb and spinach. From time to time reports of fatalities from the eating of raw rhubarb or rhubarb leaves appear. Though the symptoms recorded usually include 'corrosive' effects as well as severe gastrointestinal irritation, some doubt exists since the oxalate is bound as a neutral salt. Though the cases of poisoning are well documented it is uncertain whether it was the oxalate in the rhubarb or toxic anthraquinone compounds also known to be present, which were responsible.[102] It is likely that a very large quantity of rhubarb would have to be eaten to provide toxic quantities of oxalate. Generally this acid merely serves as an anti-nutrition factor preventing the absorption of calcium.

The anthraquinone glycosides present in rhubarb stalks and leaves vary in quantity during the season and may be as high as 1 per cent in early summer, leaves and uncooked stalks should be avoided for this reason.

Gossypol

Among the vegetable oils cottonseed oil has a relatively unique place since it is a by-product of the cotton industry with a little over one-quarter of the world production coming from the cotton-producing states of North America. It is used in salad oil, margarine and shortening and the meal from the crushed seed is a rich protein source for swine and poultry. Cottonseed flour has also been made for human consumption. One aspect of the oil's uniqueness arises from the presence of pigment glands in the cottonseed which contain the reactive phenolic pigment gossypol (1,1^1,6,6^1,7,7^1-hexahydroxy-5,5^1-di-isopropyl-3,3^1-dimethyl(2,2^1-binaphthalene)-8,8^1-dicarboxaldehyde) which has been shown to have definite chronic toxicity effects in a variety of animals. It has spermicidal properties and has been tried as a male contraceptive. The gossypol may be present in a free, biologically active, state or in the less active combined form. Commercial processing methods are designed to reduce the free gossypol to a very low level. Commercial products containing cottonseed flour have been tested for human consumption over many years. Though there are no recorded cases of gossypol poisoning of humans, the knowledge that this pigment is definitely harmful prompts continual research and the future for cottonseed oil and meal will lie in the development of the glandless varieties which have (at least in the American variety) gossypol-free seed.[103]

Overindulgence, Combination Effects and Afterthoughts

Over-reliance on many plants may create problems. Carotenaemia from excessive absorption of carotene merely results in a yellow skin pigmentation, but excessively large amounts of tomato juice can cause illness by accumulation of an aliphatic hydrocardon, lycopene in the liver; but this serves merely to warn that most foods *taken in excess* might produce some harmful effect.[19]

The greatest imponderable in food toxicology must be the possibility of combination or synergistic effects. That is, the possibly harmful results arising from interaction of components to produce a toxin or the enhancement of toxic effects by the presence of what we may term a co-toxin. Tissue damage from over exposure to tannins might lead to weakening of resistance to mutagens, similar damage from large quantities of saponins might allow alkaloids to penetrate protective barriers and the inhibition of enzymes can prevent detoxification of amines, cyanides or other poisonous species. Other more complex or bizarre effects are known, as when alcohol is taken after eating certain mushrooms such as the 'inky cap' (*Coprinus atrimentarius*). Some hours after eating such fungi sensitivity to alcohol intake reaches a peak and severe physical distress may result from even one alcoholic drink. Fortunately the symptoms are short lived and not reported to cause permanent injury.[5,100]

It is not the purpose of this discourse to promote anxiety regarding what foods we may combine (should nitrate-containing spinach be eaten with amine-containing cheese?). Nutritionists should take these matters into consideration with special regard to synergistic or anti-nutritional effects from adventitious additives. The food industry and the various protection agencies are well aware of acute hazards and their estimates for permissible daily intake of individual materials over a lifetime may be accurate – but what of the effect of the pesticide in combination with the natural toxins? More work is needed here.

In the meantime what shall we do? Plenty of variety in our diet, avoidance of fadism (we have shown that free-range cattle or poultry may be a greater source of danger than the factory fed; that even vitamins in excess may be harmful), care in storage of all foodstuffs and in their preparation and cooking. When experimenting with exotic foods it is best to follow the method of preparation customary in the countries of origin.

References

1. Food Protection Committee (eds.) *Toxicants Occurring Naturally in Foods* (National Academy of Sciences, Washington, 1967).
2. Liener, I.E. (ed.) *Toxic Constituents of Plant Foodstuffs* (Academic Press, New York and London, 1969).
3. Rosenthal, G.A. and Janzen, D.H. (eds.) *Herbivores: Their Interaction with Secondary Plant Metabolites* (Academic Press, New York and London, 1979).
4. Eurotox Symposium: The Chronic Toxicity of Naturally Occurring Substances, *Food and Cosmetics Toxicology* (1964), *2* (6).
5. Lampe, K.F. and Fugerström, R. *Plant Toxicity and Dermatitis* (Williams and Wilkins, Baltimore, 1968).
6. Ambrose, A.M. 'Naturally Occurring Antienzymes (Inhibitors)' in Food Protection Committee (eds.) *Toxicants Occurring Naturally in Foods* (National Academy of Sciences, Washington, 1967), pp. 105–11.
7. Liener, K.F. and Kakade, M.L. 'Protease Inhibitors' in I.E. Liener (ed.) *Toxic Constituents of Plant Foodstuffs* (Academic Press, New York and London, 1969), pp. 6–68.
8. Crosby, D.G. 'Natural Cholinesterase Inhibitors in Food' in Food Protection Committee (eds.) *Toxicants Occurring Naturally in Foods* (National Academy of Sciences, Washington, 1967), pp. 112–16.
9. Ryan, C.A. Proteinase Inhibitors' in G.A. Rosenthal and D.H. Janzen (eds.) *Herbivores: Their Interaction with Secondary Plant Metabolites* (Academic Press, New York and London, 1979), pp. 599–618.
10. Cordell, G.A. 'Alkaloids' in R.E. Kirk and D.F. Othmer (eds.) *Encyclopedia of Chemical Technology*, 3rd edn (Interscience, New York, 1978), vol. 1, pp. 883-943.
11. Robinson, T. 'The Evolutionary Ecology of Alkaloids' in G.A. Rosenthal and D.H. Janzlo (eds.) *Herbivores: Their Interaction with Secondary Plant Metabolites* (Academic Press, New York and London, 1979), pp. 413–18.
12. Keeler, R.F. 'Alkaloid Teratogens from L. Lupinus, Conium, Veratrum and Related Genera' in R.F. Keeler, K.R. Van Kampen and L.F. James (eds.) *The*

Effects of Poisonous Plants on Livestock (Academic Press, New York and London, 1978).
13. Jadhav, S.J., Sharma, R.P. and Salunkhe, D.K. 'Naturally Occurring Toxic Alkaloids in Foods', *CRC Critical Revues in Toxicology* (1981), *9*, 21–104.
14. Jones, P.G. and Fenwick, R.G. 'Glycoalkaloid Content of Some Edible Solanaceous Fruits and Potato Products', *Journal of the Science of Food and Agriculture* (1981), *32*, 419–21.
15. McMillan, M. and Thompson, J.G. 'An Outbreak of Suspected Solanine Poisoning in Schoolboys. Examination of Criteria of Solanine Poisoning', *Quarterly Journal of Medicine* (1979), *48*, 227–43.
16. Poswillo, D.E., Sopher, D. and Mitchell, S. 'Experimental Induction of Foetal Malformation with "Blighted" Potatoes', *Nature* (1972), *239*, 462–4.
17. Singh, O. 'Sulphur Deficiency and Alkaloid Content in Mustard Plants', *Indian Journal of Plant Physiology* (1979), *22*, 78–80.
18. Cheryan, M. 'Phytic Acid Interaction in Food Systems', *CRC Critical Revues in Food Science and Nutrition* (1980), *13*, 297–336.
19. Coon, J.M. 'Discussion' in Food Protection Committee (eds.) *Toxicants Occurring Naturally in Foods* (National Academy of Sciences, Washington, 1967), pp. 281.
20. Reese, J.C. 'Antivitamins' in G.A. Rosenthal and D.H. Janzen (eds.) *Herbivores: Their Interaction with Secondary Plant Metabolites*, (Academic Press, New York and London, 1979), p. 316; 'Compounds that Block Utilisation of Nutrients' Ibid., p. 321.
21. Sinclair, H.M. and Hollingworth, D.F. (eds.) *Hutchinson's Food and the Principles of Human Nutrition*, 12th edn. (Edward Arnold, London, 1969), pp. 111 and 300.
22. McCance, R.A. and Widdowson, E.M. 'Iron Exchange of Adults on White and Brown Bread Diets', *Lancet* (1942), *1*, 588–90.
23. Cole, M.F., Eastoe, J.E., Curtis, M.A., Korts, D.C. and Bowen, W.H. 'Effects of Pyridoxine, Phytate and Invert Sugar on Plaque Composition and Caries Activity in the Monkey', *Caries Research* (1980), *14*, 1–15.
24. Harth, H., Raaf, H. and Wagner, H. 'Two Phase Dentifrices' German Offenlegensschrifft 2 313 914 (25 Oct. 1973). British Patent Application 4848/72 (2 Feb. 1972).
25. Nordbo, H. and Rolla, G. 'Plaque Inhibiting Capacity of Glycophosphate and Phytic Acid', *Microbiologia Espanola* (1971), *24*, 507–9.
26. Salunkhe, D.K. and Wu, M.T. 'Toxicants in Plants and Plant Products' *CRC Critical Reviews in Food Science and Nutrition* (1977), Sept. 265–324.
27. Lepkovsky, S. 'Antivitamins in Foods' in Food Protection Committee (eds.) *Toxicants Occurring Naturally in Foods* (National Academy of Sciences, Washington, 1967), pp. 98–104.
28. Ostwald, R. and Briggs, G.M. 'Toxicity of the Vitamins' in Food Protection Committee (eds.) *Toxicants Occurring Naturally in Foods* (National Academy of Sciences, Washington, 1967), pp. 183–220.
29. Liener, I.E. 'Antivitamins' in I.E. Liener (ed.) *Toxic Constituents of Plant Foodstuffs* (Academic Press, New York and London, 1969), p. 423.
30. Van Etten, C.H. and Tookey, H.L. 'Chemistry and Biological Effects of Glucosinolates' in G.A. Rosenthal and D.H. Janzen (eds.) *Herbivores: Their Interaction with Secondary Plant Metabolites* (Academic Press, New York and London, 1979), pp. 471–501.
31. Wills, J.H. Jr. 'Goitrogens in Foods' in Food Protection Committee (eds.) *Toxicants Occurring Naturally in Foods* (National Academy of Sciences, Washington, 1967), pp. 3–17.
32. Van Etten, C.H. 'Goitrogens' in I.E. Liener (ed.) *Toxic Constituents of Plant*

Foodstuffs (Academic Press, New York and London, 1969), pp. 103–42.
33. Clements, F.W. and Wishart, J.W. 'Thyroid Blocking Agents in the Etiology of Endemic Goiter', *Metabolism, Clinical and Experimental*, (1956), *5*, 623–39.
34. Singleton, V.L. 'Naturally Occurring Food Toxicants: Phenolic Substances of Plant Origin Common in Foods', *Advances in Food Research* (1981), *27*, 149–242.
35. Harborne, J.B. 'Flavanoid Pigments' in G.A. Rosenthal and D.H. Janzen (eds.) *Herbivores: Their Interaction with Secondary Plant Metabolites* (Academic Press, New York and London, 1979), pp. 619–56.
36. Liener, I.E. 'Estrogenic Factors' in I.E. Liener (ed.) *Toxic Constituents of Plant Foodstuffs* (Academic Press, New York and London, 1969), pp. 410–11.
37. Stob, M. 'Estrogens in Foods' in Food Protection Committee (eds.) *Toxicants Occurring Naturally in Foods* (National Academy of Sciences, Washington, 1967), pp. 18–23.
38. Boyland, E. 'Estrogens' in Eurotox Symposium, *Food and Cosmetics Toxicology* (1964), *2*, 666.
39. Seely, S. 'The Possible Connection Between Phytooestrogens, Milk and Coronary Heart Disease', *Medical Hypotheses* (1982), *8*, 349–54.
40. Montgomery, R.D. 'Cyanogens' in I.E. Liener (ed.) *Toxic Constituents of Plant Foodstuffs* (Academic Press, New York and London, 1969), pp. 143–67.
41. Conn, R.E. 'Cyanide and Cyanogenic Glycosides' in G.A. Rosenthal and D.H. Janzen (eds.) *Herbivores: Their Interaction with Secondary Metabolites* (Academic Press, New York and London, 1979), pp. 387–412.
42. Neurath, G.B. and Schreiber, O. 'Primary and Secondary Amines in the Human Environment', *Food and Cosmetics Toxicology* (1976), *15*, 387–98.
43. Strong, F.M. 'Pressor Amines' in Food Protection Committee (eds.) *Toxicants Occurring Naturally in Foods* (National Academy of Sciences, Washington, 1967), pp. 94–7.
44. Liener, I.E. 'Stimulants and Depressants (Pressor Amines)' in I.E. Liener (ed.) *Toxic Constituents of Plant Foodstuffs* (Academic Press, New York and London, 1969), pp. 413–14.
45. Parke, D.V. *The Biochemistry of Foreign Compounds* (Pergamon, Amsterdam, 1968), p. 144.
46. Birk, Y. 'Saponins' in I.E. Liener (ed.) *Toxic Constituents of Plant Foodstuffs* (Academic Press, New York and London, 1969), pp. 169–210.
47. Applebaum, S.W. and Birk, Y. 'Saponins' in G.A. Rosenthal and D.H. Janzen (eds.) *Herbivores: Their Interaction with Secondary Plant Metabolites* (Academic Press, New York and London, 1979), pp. 539–66.
48. Stillmark, H. 'Ueber Ricin', *Archiv fuer Pharmakologie*, Institut Dorpat (1889), *3*, 59.
49. Liener, I.E. 'Phytohemagglutinins' in G.A. Rosenthal and D.H. Janzen (eds.) *Herbivores: Their Interaction with Secondary Plant Metabolites* (Academic Press, New York and London, 1979), pp. 567–98.
50. Aub, J.C., Tieslau, C. and Lankester, A. 'Reaction of Normal and Tumor Cell Surfaces to Enzymes (I). Wheat Germ Lipase and Associated Mucopolysaccharides', *Proceedings of the National Academy of Science, USA* (1963), *50*, 613–16.
51. Jaffe, W.G. 'Hemagglutinins' in I.E. Liener (ed.) *Toxic Constituents of Plant Foodstuffs* (Academic Press, New York and London, 1969), pp. 69–101.
52. Jaffe, W.G. 'Ueber Phytotoxins aus Bohen', *Arzneimittel-Forschung* (1960), *10*, 1012–16.

53. Sarma, P.S. and Padmanaban, G. 'Lathyrogens' in I.E. Liener (ed.) *Toxic Constituents of Plant Foodstuffs* (Academic Press, New York and London, 1969), pp. 267–93.
54. Selye, H. 'Lathyrism', *Revue Canadiene de Biologie* (1957), *16*, 1–82.
55. Liener, I.E. 'Lathyrogens in Food' in Food Protection Committee (eds.) *Toxicants Occurring Naturally in Foods* (National Academy of Sciences, Washington, 1967), pp. 40–6.
56. Crosby, W.H. 'Favism in Sardinia', *Blood* (1956), *11*, 91.
57. Mager, J., Razin, A. and Hershko, A. 'Favism' in I.E. Liener (ed.) *Toxic Constituents of Plant Foodstuffs* (Academic Press, New York and London, 1969), pp. 293–318.
58. Lin, J.Y. and Ling, K.H. 'Favism II. The Physiological Activities of Vicine *in vivo*', *Journal of the Formosan Medical Association* (1962), *61*, 490; 579.
59. Liener, I.E. 'Favism' in Food Protection Committee (eds.) *Toxicants Occurring Naturally in Foods* (National Academy of Sciences, Washington, 1967), pp. 47–50.
60. Whiting, M.G. 'Toxicity of Cycads', *Economic Botany* (1963), *17*, 271–302.
61. Miller, J.A. 'Cycads and Cycasin' in Food Protection Committee (eds.) *Toxicants Occurring Naturally in Foods* (National Academy of Sciences, Washington, 1967), pp. 30–2.
62. Yang, M.G. and Mickelson, O. 'Cycads' in I.E. Liener (ed.) *Toxic Constituents of Plant Foodstuffs* (Academic Press, New York and London, 1969), pp. 159–68.
63. Sugimura, T. 'Mutagens, Carcinogens and Tumor Promoters in our Daily Food', *Cancer* (1978), *49*, 1970–84.
64. Robins, D.J. 'Pyrrolizidine Alkaloids – Pharmacological and Biological Studies', *Royal Society of Chemistry Specialist Periodical Report. The Alkaloids* (1981), vol. 10, p. 60.
65. Liener, I.E. 'Senecio Plants' in I.E. Liener (ed.) *Toxic Constituents of Plant Foodstuffs* (Academic Press, New York and London, 1969), pp. 417–18.
66. Austwick, P. and Mattocks, R. 'Naturally Occurring Carcinogens in Foods', *Chemistry and Industry* (1979), Feb., 76–83.
67. Friedman, L. and Shibko, S.I. 'Adventitious Toxic Factors in Processed Foods' in I.E. Liener (ed.) *Toxic Constituents of Plant Foodstuffs* (Academic Press, New York and London, 1969), pp. 349–409.
68. Dickens, F. 'Lactones' in Eurotox Symposium, *Food and Cosmetics Toxicology* (1964), *2*, 668.
69. Gaunt, I.F., Hardy, J., Kiss, I.S., Butterworth, K.R. and Gangolli, S.D. 'Long Term Toxicity of Parasorbic Acid in Rats', *Food and Cosmetics Toxicology* (1976), *14*, 387–98.
70. Grasso, P. 'Carcinogens in Food' in D.M. Conning and A.B.G. Lansdown (eds.) *Toxic Hazards in Food* (Croom Helm, London, 1983), pp. 122–44.
71. Eurotox Symposium: The Chronic Toxicity of Naturally Occurring Substances, *Food and Cosmetics Toxicology* (1964), *2*, 677.
72. Hendrickse, R.G., Coulter, J.B., Lamplagh, S.M., Macfarlane, S.B.J., Williams, T.E., Omer, M.I.A. and Suliman, G.I. 'Aflatoxins and Kwashiorkor. A Study of Sudanese Children', *British Medical Journal* (1982), *285*, 843–9.
73. Tatsuono, T. 'Metabolites of *Penicillium islandicum*, Supp.' in Eurotox Symposium: The Chronic Toxicity of Naturally Occurring Substances, *Food and Cosmetics Toxicology* (1964), *2*, 678.
74. Petrun, A.S. 'Levels of Carcinogenic Polycyclic Hydrocarbons in Cultivated Plants', *Ratsional'noe Pitanie* (1977), *12*, 71–5.

75. Stansby, M.E. 'Development of the Fish Oil Industry in the United States', *Journal of the American Oil Chemists Society* (1978), *55*, 238-43.
76. Applewhite, T.H. 'Nutritional Aspects of Hydrogenated Soya Oil', *Journal of the American Oil Chemists Society* (1981), *58*, 260-9.
77. Seigler, D.S. 'Toxic Seed Lipids' in G.A. Rosenthal and D.H. Janzen (eds.) *Herbivores: Their Interaction with Secondary Plant Metabolites* (Academic Press, New York and London, 1979), pp. 449-470.
78. Liener, I.E. 'Carrots' in I.E. Liener (ed.) *Toxic Constituents of Plant Foodstuffs* (Academic Press, New York and London, 1969), p. 437.
79. Janzen, D.H. 'New Horizons in the Biology of Plant Defences' in G.A. Rosenthal and D.H. Janzen (eds.) *Herbivores: Their Interaction with Secondary Plant Metabolites* (Academic Press, New York and London, 1979), pp. 331-50.
80. Rhoades, D.F. 'Evolution of Plant Chemical Defence Against Herbivores' in G.A. Rosenthal and D.H. Janzen (eds.) *Herbivores: Their Interaction with Secondary Plant Metabolites* (Academic Press, New York and London, 1979), pp. 1-55.
81. Deverall, B.J. *Defence Mechanisms of Plants* (Cambridge University Press, 1977).
82. Wills, J.H. Jr 'Seafood Toxins' in Food Protection Committee (eds.) *Toxicants Occurring Naturally in Foods* (National Academy of Sciences, Washington, 1967), pp. 147-63.
83. Tsubaki, T. and Irukayama, K. (eds.) *Minamata Disease* (Elsevier, Amsterdam, 1977).
84. Mariani, A., Santaroni, G.P. and Clements, G.F. 'Mercury in the Environment', *Bibliotheca Nutritio et Dieta* (1980), *29*, 32-8.
85. Ferriman, A. *Observer*, 29 May 1983, 3.
86. Couch, J.F. 'The Compound that Produces "Trembles" (Milk Sickness)', *Journal of the American Chemical Society* (1929), *51*, 3617-19.
87. Evans, I., Jones, R.S. and Mainwaring-Burton, R. 'Passage of Bracken Fern Toxicity into Milk', *Nature* (1972), *237*, 107-8.
88. Dickenson, J.O., Cooke, M.P., King, R.R. and Mohamed, P.A. 'Milk Transfer of Pyrrolizidine Alkaloids in Cattle', *Journal of the American Veterinary Medical Association* (1976), *169*, 1192-6.
89. Crosby, D.G. Quoted in *Chemical Engineering News*, 11 April 1983, 37.
90. Goursaud, J., Luquet, F.M. and Casalis, J. 'Hexachlorobenzene and Pentachloroaniline Contamination of Milk Produced in an Endive Area', *Industrie Alimentaire et Agricole* (1977), *94*, 1291-4.
91. Tuinstra, L.G.M.T., Traag, W.A. and Van Munsteren, A.J. 'Determination of Individual Chlorinated Biphenyls in Agricultural Products by Automated Capillary Gas Chromatography. Determination in Cattle Feed and its Relation to Milk Residues', *Journal of Chromatographic Science* (1981), *204*, 413-19.
92. Brewington, C.R., Parks, O.W. and Scwarz, D.P. 'Conjugate Compounds in Milk, II', *Journal of Agriculture and Food Chemistry* (1974), *22*, 293-4.
93. Mueller, H.R., Secrtetin, M.-C. and Blanc, E. 'New Aspects of Preventing Contamination of Infant Foods', *Bibliotheca Nutritio et Dieta* (1980), *29*, 89-105.
94. Kashsfutdzinov, G.A. and Tsarev, S.G. 'Effect of Silage Obtained from Beet Tops and Treated with Maleic Hydrazide in the form of its Sodium Salt', *Gidrazid Maleinovoi Kistloty kak Regulyator Rosta Rastenii* (1973), pp. 340-3
95. Berger, S., Pardo, B. and Skorkowska-Zielenieska, J. 'Nutritional Implications of Pesticides in Foods', *Bibliotheca Nitritio et Dieta* (1980), *29*, 1-10.

96. Johnson, R.D., Manske, D.D., New, D.J. and Podberac, D.S. 'Pesticides, Metals and Other Chemical Residues in Adult Total Diet Samples (XII), August 1975–July 1976', *Pesticide Monitoring Journal* (1981), *15*, 54–69; 'In Infant and Toddler Foods', *Pesticide Monitoring Journal* (1981), *15*, 39–50.
97. Klaui, H. 'Present Problems of Food Colours', *Bibliotheca Nutritio et Dieta* (1980), *29*, 75–81.
98. Lindner, K. 'Non-nutritive Sweetening Agents', *Bibliotheca Nutritio et Dieta* (1980), *29*, 92–88.
99. Bryson, G. and Berschoff, F. 'Tumours in Evans Rats Fed Vegetable Oils', *Proceedings of the American Association for Cancer Research* (1964), *5*, 8.
100. Tampion, J. *Dangerous Plants* (David and Charles, Newton Abbot, 1977), p. 129.
101. Lewis, W.H. and Elvin-Lewis, M.P. *Medical Botany* (Wiley, New York and London, 1977), pp. 79–81.
102. Fassett, D.W. 'Oxalates' in Food Protection Committee (eds.) *Toxicants Occurring Naturally in Foods* (National Academy of Sciences, Washington, 1967), pp. 257–66.
103. Berardi, L.C. and Goldblatt, L.A. 'Gossypol', in I.L. Liener (ed.) *Toxic Constituents of Plant Foodstuffs* (Academic Press, New York and London, 1969), pp. 212–66.

4 DIET-RELATED DISEASES OF THE ARTERIES

S. Seely

The circulation of animals is essentially a transport system in which nutrients and other essentials of life obtained from the outside world are delivered, in some cases after suitable processing, to the cell population which utilise them, while the waste products of the cells are transported by the same system to organs which can remove them from the blood and return them to the outside world. The system is waterborne, but a very small quantity of water carries a comparatively large quantity of nutrients and other cargo. The volume of the water content of the plasma, and that of the substances dissolved or floating in it are, in fact, approximately equal.

The most easily transported of these substances are nutrients or waste products which are water-soluble, like glucose or most salts. Among those most difficult to transport in an aqueous medium are gases, like oxygen and carbon dioxide. Both are soluble in water, but if the respiratory system had to rely on gases dissolved in the plasma, a very large amount of water would be needed. The addition of haemoglobin to blood increases its oxygen carrying capacity 70 times. On the other hand, the system is not of high efficiency: venous blood carries a large quantity of oxygen and arterial blood a moderate amount of carbon dioxide. The transport of gases accounts for about 40 per cent of the total blood volume, if only the red blood cells performing the actual transport are considered. Assuming an equal quantity of water needed to float them, 80 per cent of the total capacity of the circulatory system is engaged in supplying oxygen to tissue cells and removing carbon dioxide from them.

Another class of substances transported with difficulty in a water-based system are lipids. Fatty substances discharged into water-filled vessels would tend to stick to the vessel walls and ultimately result in blockages. There are two solutions to the problem. One is the conjugation of an individual water-insoluble molecule with one or more other molecules, forming a water-soluble complex. The usual expedient in the case of lipids is transport by means of carrier proteins. These are large molecules in comparison with the lipids they carry and can serve, in effect, as packing cases for them. The protein molecule turns a hydrophilic outer surface to the watery medium in which it floats, but can have a large collection of hydrophobic molecules, shielded from contact with water, inside. The protein carrier together with its lipid cargo constitutes a lipoprotein. Since lipids are lighter than water and proteins heavier, the specific weight (or density) of the combination depends on the proportion of lipids and proteins. Transport proteins collecting lipids in the liver after a fatty meal contain a large proportion of lipids, hence they are comparatively light and are called very low density lipoproteins (VLDL). As they deliver parts of their cargo to various destinations, they gradually become heavier. When the cargo is mainly cholesterol, they are called low density lipoproteins (LDL). Carrier proteins are needed not only to deliver lipids to cells, but in some cases to transport them in the opposite direction. Cholesterol in particular is a highly stable substance which cannot be digested or degraded by tissue cells or macrophages. Hence cholesterol residues, usually the remains of dead cells, have to be carried from tissues to the liver for re-use or excretion. The proteins serving this purpose carry comparatively small loads, hence form high density lipoproteins (HDL).

The fluid portion of the blood, the plasma, carries an enormous number of organic and inorganic substances. Among them are three kinds of proteins, albumin, globulin and fibrinogen, serving various purposes. The blood also carries the chemical messengers – hormones – from the organs which produce them to receptors in other parts of the body. The hormones can be free, conjugated, or attached to carrier proteins. Enzymes, drugs, metallic ions, bilirubin, arising from the breakdown of haemoglobin, etc. are among the many substances always in transit in the blood.

The circulatory system is also the highway which invading micro-organisms attempt to utilise for spreading in the body. Tumours also attempt to spread by blood-borne fragments. The circulatory system is also one of the main targets of various secondary metabolites (or allelochemicals) which plants produce to ward off, or kill, animals feeding on them. To cope with these hazards, the circulation is defended by an immune system and by several types of white blood cells (polymorphonuclear leukocytes, lymphocytes and monocytes) which play specialised parts in seeking out, ingesting and killing bacteria, invade areas of infection, phagocytose foreign material, dead cells and the like. All these add to the heavy traffic the circulatory system has to carry.

In the case of injuries, blood from the circulatory system leaks into tissue spaces or the outside world and it is essential that such leaks are quickly stopped. A temporary plug is formed by platelets adhering to injured tissues and subsequently converted into a solid plug by clotting agents. The potential adhesiveness of platelets and the existence of clotting factors is an essential defence mechanism, but an error which might activate this mechanism in the absence of injuries can convert it into a weapon of self-destruction. A blood clot can obstruct an artery with possibly fatal results.

Similarly, the regulation of blood pressure has to steer a middle course between opposing demands. The best example to show the risks and problems is that of Dr Barney Clark who,[1] in the terminal stage of chronic congestive heart failure, was the first recipient of an artificial heart which kept him alive for about four months. When the artificial heart was set at 70 beats per minute, to provide a moderate output, renal function was unsatisfactory. Setting it at a high output of 110 beats per minute improved diuresis, but caused seizures due to hyperperfusion of the brain. Similarly, treatment with anticoagulants ensured that no blood clots were formed, but it was found at autopsy that the patient had several small haemorrhages.

Blood clotting and the regulation of blood pressure are also those points of weakness where plant metabolites try to attack animals. Plants produce a whole array of haemagglutinins as well as some anticoagulants. Other plant metabolites contain hypertensive agents.

Like any other organ, the circulatory system is subject to congenital abnormalities, deficiencies and neoplastic changes. In leukaemia the custodians themselves, the white blood cells, proliferate uncontrollably.

It is easy to realise that the complex and multitudinous tasks falling on the circulatory system make it highly vulnerable to pathogenic influences. It is, in fact, the most vulnerable organ system in the body, its disorders accounting for as many deaths in Western countries as all other diseases combined. The surprising fact about the circulatory system is that its disorders are prominent *only in advanced countries*. In other mammals, as well as in humans living more nearly under natural conditions, the circulatory system performs its duties without apparent difficulties. It seems that the system is well able to cope with its natural hazards. Civilisation seems to have added something to its difficulties which must have made all the difference between a trouble-free, and a highly disease-prone organ system. As already hinted, the transformation is likely to have something to do with Western diet, but, in spite of claims to the contrary, the identification of dietary pathogens still awaits future developments.

In view of the fact that artery disease is the most important medical problem of our day, it is intended to examine the relevant facts, hypotheses and speculations in some detail.

Construction of the Artery Wall

Figure 4.1 is a schematic diagram of a segment of the wall of a small artery. It is a three-layered structure, with a tough, white layer of connective tissue, the adventitia, on the outside. The medium layer, the media, forms the bulk of the artery wall. This consists mainly of muscle. By far the most important structure from the present point of view is the inside layer of the wall, the intima, of which more will be said later. In small arteries the layer of muscle is between two sheets of elastic tissue which form its boundaries both with the intima and the adventitia and are called the internal and external elastic laminae. In larger arteries layers of muscle alternate with such elastic sheets. Generally, the larger the artery, the more elastic tissue it contains. In the aorta the greater part of the middle layer consists of thick elastic laminae.

The function of the muscular layer is the regulation of blood flow through the artery. When the muscles contract, they constrict the lumen of the artery, when they relax, the bore of the artery is enlarged. Half of the animal body consists of muscle, and muscles in particular need several times as much blood to supply them with oxygen and nutrients when they are working to the limit of their capacity than when they are at rest. Hence blood flow to various organs, but particularly to muscles, has to be regulated in accordance with needs. This regulation is the task of the muscular layer of the artery wall, acting, in effect, as taps in a man-made water supply system.

The function of the elastic laminae in the arteries is to even out, to some extent, the pulsating pressure applied to the circulatory system by the heart. During systole, when the heart actively pumps blood into the system, these elastic sheets expand, storing energy in elastic tension, during diastole they contract, returing stored energy and tending to maintain pressure in the arterial system. The importance of these elastic sheets can be best appreciated from the fact that the heart in its active phase compresses its own arteries, so that it is not supplied with blood during systole. It receives its blood supply during diastole, elastic tissues providing the motive force. In old age the artery wall tends to lose some of its elasticity. If it lost it completely, the heart would be in difficulty in supplying itself with blood.

Figure 4.1: Segment of the Artery Wall. Abbreviations: E = endothelium, IEL = internal elastic lamina, EEL = external elastic lamina, I = intima, M = media, A = adventitia, SM = smooth muscle. Note. In large elastic arteries elastic laminae are interposed between layers of smooth muscle in the media.

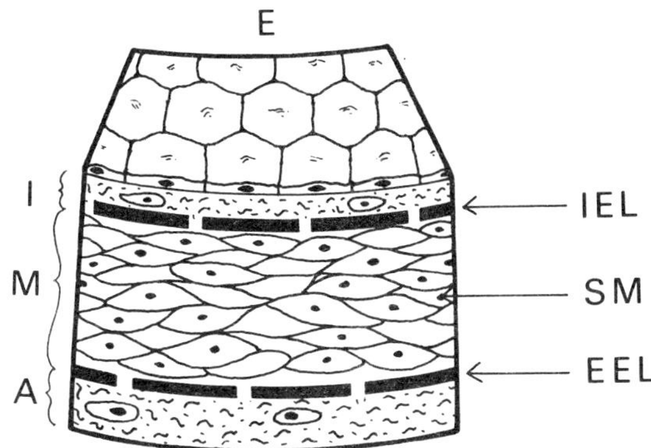

Apart from loss of elasticity in old age and some disorders of comparatively minor importance, the two outer layers of the artery wall, the media and the adventitia, are remarkably trouble free. The trouble-prone part of the artery, the structures responsible for nearly half of all deaths in advanced countries, are those constituting its innermost layer, the intima. This consists of a layer of flat epithelial cells which are in immediate contact with the blood carried by the artery. Underneath them there is a small space, loosely filled with connective tissue, the subendothelium. This space contains a few scattered cells of the same type which constitute the smooth muscle of the medium layer, except that these are individual, motile cells, capable of secreting various types of fibre. Nominally the internal elastic lamina is a part of the intima. In fact, both structurally and functionally the elastic lamina belongs to the muscular layer. The trouble-prone part of the artery consists of nothing more than a single layer of endothelial cells and an adjoining small space with a few intimal smooth muscle cells in it.

Before considering the disorders of the intima, a few words are needed on the supply of the artery wall with nutrients and other essentials of life. Like all living cells, those constituting the artery wall must be supplied with oxygen and nutrients, and their waste products have to be carried away from them. For this purpose small blood vessels, the *vasa vasorum*, penetrate the outer layer of the artery wall and form a capillary bed there. These supply the outer half of the artery wall, the adventitia and a part of the media. The inner half of the wall takes its nutrients from the blood carried by the artery.

Disorders of the Artery Wall

The most important disorder of the artery, atherosclerosis, is the accumulation of lipids in the intima. Lipid deposists accumulate in the subendothelium, the space immediately beneath the layer of epithelial cells. The space is originally small, but can be greatly distended by fatty deposits. The accumulating lipids are mainly cholesterol esters, namely cholesterol with an attached fatty acid molecule. Cholesterol can act as as weak base, and combined with a weak fatty acid constitutes the equivalent of an inorganic salt. This is a cholesteryl ester, and as there are many types of fatty acids capable of combining with cholesterol, there is a correspondingly large number of esters. Two are of particular importance. Cholesterol combined with linoleic acid forms a linoleate, and with oleic acid, an oleate.

Cholesterol is a highly stable, waxy substance, an essential constituent of the animal body. Thus for insects, which cannot synthesise it, it is a vitamin. The flexibility of the animal body, in comparison with the more rigid structure of plants, is largely due to the fact that the outer shell of plant cells is cellulose, while that of animal cells is a complex three-layered construction consisting of lipids and proteins. These cell membranes combine toughness and flexibility, make the cells watertight but also permit controlled exchange of water, oxygen and nutrients between the cell's interior and its environment. Beside the cell itself, its organelles have similar membranes of their own. Cholesterol is a part of these membranes, hence a vitally important part of every single cell in the body. In addition, the cholesterol nucleus is also the nucleus of steroid hormones, some of the most important chemical messengers in the body.

The usefulness of cholesterol does not alter the fact that its accumulations in the walls of arteries ultimately become obstructions to blood flow, much the same way as the usefulness of bricks, as a building material, would not diminish their obstructive properties when dumped in a canal.

The lesions of the artery wall, in all of which cholesterol plays a part, are classified as fatty streaks, fibrous plaques and complicated

Figure 4.2: Schematic Diagrams of the Inner Part of the Artery Wall. Upper left: Normal artery. Upper right: Artery wall with fatty streak. Lower: Artery wall with fibrous plaque.

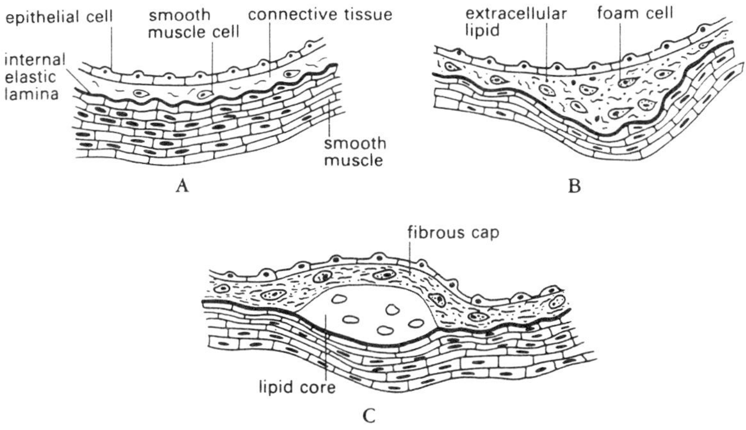

Source: Reproduced from D.L.J. Freed (ed.), *Health Hazards of Milk* (Baillière-Tindall, London, 1984), p. 216, by permission of the publisher.

lesions. These could be progressive stages of the atherosclerotic process, thus the complicated lesions undoubtedly arise from the fibrous plaques, but there is some doubt whether the fibrous plaques develop from fatty streaks.

The fatty streaks are visible, without magnification, as yellowish lines or small patches on the luminal surface of the artery. The lines are flat or slightly raised, they cause no obstruction to blood flow and no clinical symptoms. When magnified, the earliest lesions are seen to consist of lipid-laden intimal smooth muscle cells which are present in greatly increased numbers in some areas of the subendothelium. The cells appear to have imbibed so much lipid, that it fills their entire cytoplasm and gives them a foamy appearance. At a later stage lipid droplets also appear between cells in subendothelial space; these are probably the remains of dead cells. The intracellular lipid is cholesteryl ester, mainly oleate. Fatty streaks appear in large arteries, particularly the aorta, at a very early age, probably in infancy, and continue to occupy increasing areas, mainly in the aorta, in childhood and early adult life. They are universal in children of all races in all parts of the world; the aorta of young females is more heavily affected than that of young males.[2] Fatty streaks in childhood occupy about 10 per cent of the aorta, in early adult life the affected area may increase to 30–50 per cent. The most heavily involved area of the aorta is its ascending and thoracic segments. The schematic diagram of the intima of normal arteries and those affected by lesions is shown in Figure 4.2.

In fibrous plaques, also shown in Figure 4.2, the intercellular lipid droplets of the fatty streak seem to have coalesced into small, encapsulated pools, 1–3 mm in diameter, which constitute the core of the plaque. Beside cholesteryl esters, the pools contain some free cholesterol, phospholipids and triglycerides, as well as dead and dying cells and other cell debris. The esterified cholesterol in these pools is mainly linoleate, in contrast with the oleate of fatty streaks. Cholesteryl linoleate is white in colour. While the oleate appears fatty, the linoleate is more waxlike. The core is surmounted by the fibrous cap, which, beside a greatly increased amount of connective tissue, contains two kinds of lipid-laden foam cells. One, as before, are smooth muscle cells, but beside them are lipid-laden macrophages. The part of the intima affected by the fibrous plaques is considerably thickened, so that the fibrous cap protrudes into the lumen of the artery. In heavily affected areas of arteries the fibrous plaques can be so numerous that they give the inside surface of the artery a porridge-like appearance, from which the disease takes its name.

Fibrous plaques are subject to various necrotic and degenetative changes, giving rise to the complicated lesions. Areas of the artery heavily affected by fibrous plaques tend to ulcerate and bleed, with consequent thrombus formation. Calcification of the lesion follows, presumably as a defensive measure to prevent rupture of the weakened artery wall. The resulting distorted, bone-like structures bear little resemblance to the normal artery, but they may still serve as conduits for years. The usual cause of death is the occlusion of the artery partly by the narrowing of the lumen due to intimal thickening and partly by thrombus formation. Particularly in the thin-walled cerebral arteries the endothelium is sometimes detached from the artery wall, resulting in fatal aneurysm, or the artery wall may rupture, resulting in cerebral haemorrhage.

One of the most curious features of atherosclerosis is its patchy distribution within the arterial system. Only a few arteries tend to be heavily infested with fibrous plaques, notably the aorta and the coronary and cerebral arteries, though arteries of the limbs, particularly the legs, the kidneys and the lungs may also be involved. Even within a given artery, distribution tends to be patchy. In coronary arteries atherosclerosis occurs mainly in the epicardial region, namely extramurally, outside the heart itself. In cerebral arteries atherosclerosis begins in the extracranial portion of the vessels, appearing normally only decades later in intracranial arteries. In the limbs the most common site is the femoral artery, and the popliteal artery just above the knee. It is this patchy distribution that makes atherosclerosis the deadly disease it is. Lesions concentrated in short sections of arteries endanger the blood supply of vital organs. If the plaques were evenly distributed in the arterial system, they would be harmless. The reasons for the peculiarities of distribution are not known. Generally, it can be observed that musculo-elastic arteries are more prone to atherosclerosis than muscular arteries and within individual arteries points of bifurcation are most vulnerable.

Equally puzzling is the epidemiology of the disease. Fatty streaks, as already pointed out, are universal, but fibrous plaques and complicated lesions are not. Coronary disease is essentially prosperity-related, it is virtually unknown in the poorer countries of the world and takes its highest toll in the most advanced countries. Cerebrovascular disease is similarly rare in the poorest countries and increases with prosperity, but the countries where mortality from cerebrovascular disease reaches its peak are not the same where the prevalence of coronary disease reaches its highest level. In Europe, for example, coronary mortality has a North–South gradient, being high in the North, low in the South, while in cerebrovascular mortality the gradient slopes in the opposite direction.

Male/female mortality rates vary in an equally capricious manner. Fatty streaks affect both sexes more or less equally, they may even be more pronounced in young females than young males. In coronary mortality there is an enormous difference in favour of women: in the 45–74 age group the male/female mortality ratio is of the order of 3/1. Cerebrovascular disease falls between the two extremes, the male/female mortality ratio in the 45–74 age group is about 3/2.

As will be explained later, the problem whether fatty streaks are the forerunners of advanced lesions, or represent a different disorder, is of some importance from the point of view whether we are searching for one or two sets of causative agents. When atherosclerosis is induced in animals by the feeding of unnaturally large quantites of cholesterol-rich substances, they first develop a disorder resembling fatty streaks and subsequently one resembling advanced lesions, but the relevance of these experiments to human conditions is uncertain. In humans there are large and still unexplained differences between the two disorders.

Fatty streaks appear to be a disorder involving primarily (possibly exclusively) intimal smooth muscle cells, in fibrous plaques the foam cells are predominantly macrophages. The universality of fatty streaks points to a ubiquitous causative agent, possibly some genetic weakness of our species, while the prosperity-related prevalence of fibrous plaques to some environmental factor, or, indeed, two sets of environmental factors, one linked with coronary, the other with cerebrovascular disease. No satisfactory explanation exists for the large differences in the vulnerability of the two sexes for the various forms of lesions. Lastly, one of the most puzzling differences is that of the lipid accumulations in the two cases. As already pointed out, the accumulating lipid in both fatty streaks and fibrous plaques is cholesterol, but in the first case it is esterified with oleic acid, in the second case with linoleic acid, causing a change of colour from light yellow to white or light grey.

Theories of Atherosclerosis

Speculation about the causes of atherosclerosis began in the last century, long before adequate data regarding the physiology and nutritional requirements of normal arteries and the origin and progression of the pathogenetic process were available. The question debated by the early theorists was how lipids reached the subendothelium. The inhibition theory of Virchow assumed that the artery wall, for some reason, absorbed lipids from the circulation. The more imaginative, but entirely mistaken opposing view of Rokitanski was that lipids precipitated on the artery wall and became internalised by epithelial cells growing over them.

In 1913 two emigré Russian scientists, Anitchkov and Chalatov, produced atheroma-like lesions in egg-fed rabbits, the high cholesterol content of eggs being taken as the atherogenic agent. For the following 50 years coronary research was dominated by the cholesterol theory which proposed that it was the high quantity of cholesterol in Western diet that was responsible for the prevalence of coronary disease. Doubts began to be expressed in the 1950s, when it was pointed out that the cholesterol turnover in the human body was about 1 g per day, of which even a cholesterol-rich Western diet supplied only about a third, the rest being synthesised in the body. Omnivorous animals possessed a regulating mechanism which ensured that if the dietary intake of cholesterol was high, endogenous synthesis was reduced. The natural diet of herbivores contains virtually no cholesterol, so that they may lack such a regulator and may be ill-prepared for an artificial diet containing cholesterol in excess of needs. In such animals excess dietary cholesterol results in hypercholesterolaemia in the circulation and if the diet is maintained for some length of time, in rather more widespread fatty deposits in arteries than in the usual form of human atherosclerosis.

The cholesterol theory was defended by pointing out that the regulating mechanism did not reduce endogenous production exactly in accordance with intake. The serum cholesterol level of people living near starvation level was 80 mg/100 ml, that of well-fed Westerners between 120 and 200 mg/100 ml. The theory was extended by bracketing animal fats, particularly saturated fats, with cholesterol, on the basis that diets rich in fats also tended to raise serum cholesterol. Even then the cholesterol theory – virtually a doctrine of faith around the middle of the century – began to lose ground. The intense propaganda aimed at reducing the quantity of cholesterol and animal fats in Western diet did little to reduce coronary mortality. Some cholesterol-reducing diets, containing chemicals to reduce the absorption of cholesterol from the intestines or interfering with cholesterol metabolism in other ways, were tried with little success. Several large-scale intervention studies were conducted in various countries, notably the United States,[3] the UK[4] and Belgium,[5] in which thousands of middle-aged men were advised to keep to a 'prudent' low-fat, low-cholesterol diet, with the finding that coronary mortality in these groups did not differ from that in control groups, who were not given any dietary advice and presumably consumed the normal diet for the country. It is not doubted that cholesterol has some connection with atherosclerosis, but the disease is more likely to result from some error of cholesterol metabolism than from the quantity of its dietary intake.

A more recent theory is the *reaction to injury* hypothesis.[6] The endothelium of arteries is a slowly renewing structure, dead cells can occasionally be seen among living cells. Tissue renewal may be faster, hence necrotic cells more common, in areas where the shearing stress on endothelial cells is high, e.g. at the point of branching or bifurcation. Beside mechanical stress, chemical or immunological injuries may occur in arteries. Such injuries may result in the proliferation of intimal smooth muscle cells and in the production of connective tissue fibres. The main argument against the theory is that it does not explain the lipid-laden state of smooth muscle cells in atherosclerotic lesions which is thought to be the initial event of the atherogenic process. Intimal smooth muscle cells, when engaged in the repair of injuries, fulfil the same function and presumably use the same techniques as fibroblasts in the skin. Fibroblasts do not become lipid-laden in the repair of wounds.

The *monoclonal hypothesis*[7] points to the finding that the smooth muscle cells found in a fibrous plaque are probably the descendants of a single smooth muscle cell, and hence suggests that the increased number of such cells in an atherosclerotic lesion is the result of a neoplastic mutation, the cellular components of the plaque representing a benign tumour. Like the injury hypothesis, it fails to explain the lipid-laden state of the cells. Multiple benign tumours of smooth muscle cells occur in other tissues, without the mutated cells containing the lipid inclusions characteristic of atherosclerotic lesions.

The *lysosomal theory*[8] suggests that atherogenesis may be initiated by the malfunction of lysosomes, the digestive organs of cells. This hypothesis will be mentioned again when the role of the lysosome in cholesterol metabolism is discussed.

The Role of Cholesterol in Artery Disease

The lipid accumulation in fatty streaks as well as the lipid core of fibrous plaques consist of various esters of cholesterol. This is why the understanding of the pathogenesis of artery disease seems to centre on discovering how excessive quantities of cholesterol find their way into the artery wall. But while the connection between cholesterol and artery disease is not in doubt, the nature of this connection, its causes and its mechanism have eluded a century of research.[9,10]

In spite of voluminous literature on the subject, few writers make it clear what exactly the problem is. Cholesterol is needed by every single cell in the body, so that if its synthesis or transport were unavoidably hazardous, error-prone, accident-prone processes, any organ in the body could be the site of lesions similar to those in artery walls. In some diseases this is exactly the case, granules containing cholesterol crystals can appear anywhere in the body. In normal persons, however, such lesions appear only in arteries, in fact, only in some arteries and only in certain locations within those arteries. The analogy that offers itself is that of a large network of roads subject to accidents, but the accidents restricted to a 50 mile stretch of the roads. The observation that serum cholesterol density is a risk factor means, in terms of the analogy, that road accidents are more probable if traffic density is high.

This may well be true, but in normal persons, even in cases of moderate hypercholesterolaemia, cholesterol deposits are still restricted to artery walls. Arteries are only a small part of the body, what singles them out as sites for cholesterol-related disorders? An added mystery is that while most organs in normal persons are free of any kind of disorder involving cholesterol, the artery wall is subject to more than one kind, ranging from the harmless fatty streaks to lethal fibrous plaques.

Let us consider how cholesterol is normally delivered to tissue cells and how it is utilised by them.[11,12] As already mentioned, cholesterol is a hydrophobic substance, its transport in a water-based system is by means of carrier proteins. Those involved in cholesterol transport are mainly the low-density lipoproteins (LDL). Tissue cells capture plasma lipoproteins by means of surface receptors which bind them on contact. The LDL receptors are located in a special area of the cell's surface, in the so called coated pits. When receptors have captured a certain quantity of lipoproteins, the coated pit sinks into the cell and cuts itself off from the surface to form an endocytotic vesicle. This moves to a lysosome, the digestive organ of the cell, and unites with it. In the lysosome the carrier protein breaks down and its lipid load is subjected to the action of various digestive enzymes. Most of the cholesterol content of the lipoprotein is in the form of esters, mainly linoleates. In the process of digestion these are de-esterified, and the resulting free cholesterol is discharged to form an intracellular pool on which the cell can draw for its requirements. A schematic diagram of the events of this process is shown in Figure 4.3.

When cells utilise cholesterol for the construction of cell membranes, or the membranes of their organelles or of endocytotic or exocytotic vesicles, they need free cholesterol. However, they are apparently unable to store free cholesterol for any length of time, so that the quantity not immediately used is re-esterified with the aid of the enzyme ACAT (Acyl CoA:cholesterol acyltransferase). In this process cholesterol is esterified with oleic acid, so that the resulting ester is cholesteryl oleate, the characteristic ester of fatty streaks.

The cell regulates its intake of cholesterol by varying the number of LDL receptors appearing on its surface.[13] These receptors are not normally destroyed in lysosomes, but are recycled and used repeatedly. However, when necessary, the cell can synthesise additional receptors or destroy (or store) superfluous ones. The recycling or synthesis of receptors is controlled by some regulating mechanism within the cell which apparently monitors the size of the free cholesterol pool in the

Figure 4.3: The Internalisation and Digestion of Plasma Lipoproteins. Abbreviations: CS = cell surface, CP = coated pit, L = lipoproteins, EV = endocytotic vesicle, Lys = lysosome, H = hydrolases.

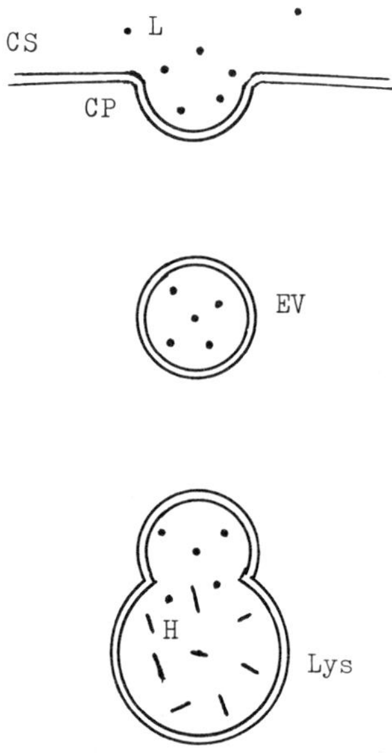

cell and determines further activity accordingly.[14] The same mechanism also controls other activities connected with cholesterol synthesis or utilisation. Thus it suppresses endogenous production of cholesterol in the cell, if adequate supplies reach it from the blood. It also controls ACAT synthesis, taking care of the storage of surplus cholesterol. However, the synthesis of LDL receptors is also influenced by various hormones, the production of which is not under the cell's control, such as thyroxine, insulin and platelet-derived growth factor.

In the genetic disorder familial hypercholesterolaemia cells fail to produce surface receptors capable of binding lipoproteins.[15] The lipoproteins are still produced in the body in the usual manner, but with the lack of acceptors they accumulate in the blood stream. In hypercholesterolaemic monozygotes the plasma concentration of cholesterol can rise to 4–5 times its normal level (about twice normal in heterozygotes). At such a high concentration cells are capable of taking up plasma lipoproteins by means of a secondary, non-specific mechanism. Persons suffering from this disorder tend to develop extensive atherosclerosis of the arteries at an early age. Another characteristic site of cholesterol deposits in hypercholesterolaemiacs are tendon sheaths, notably on the back of the hands and at the heels. Subcutaneous deposits (xanthomas) are also common.

In some rare disorders (Schüller-Christian syndrome; xanthoma disseminata) widespread cholesterol-containing granulomas can appear in many parts of the body, e.g. in bones or internal organs. The disorder does not appear to be of genetic origin, its causes are unknown.

Turning to the specific case of arteries, there is one notable difference between their inner layers and most other tissues from the point of view of cholesterol supply. Most tissues receive nutrients from the blood via capillaries, and if they do, they are rarely troubled by cholesterol-related disorders. Similarly, the outer part of the artery wall is supplied with nutrients from a capillary bed, as small blood vessels (the vasa vasorum) penetrate into large arteries and supply their *outer layers* with blood. These outer layers are also remarkably trouble free. The inside part of the artery wall has no capillaries, it is supplied with lipoproteins from the blood carried by the artery by transmission through endothelial cells. Similarly, there are few, if any, capillaries in tendon sheaths. Cholesterol-related disorders seem more likely to arise in tissues supplied with lipoproteins by some other means than in the usual manner through capillaries. Hence the examination of the process, whereby endothelial cells submit plasma lipoproteins to the tissues below them, may be of interest.[16,17]

Endothelial cells, which are in direct contact with arterial blood, have surface receptors, like other cells, which can capture plasma lipoproteins on contact. Some of these form endocytotic vesicles, as shown in Figure 4.3, to supply the cell's own needs. Others, however, form *transcytotic* vesicles, the contents of which are discharged by exocytosis to the subendothelial space. This process is shown diagrammatically in Figure 4.4. The few cells normally populating the subendothelium, the intimal smooth muscle celis, have direct access to these lipoproteins, but in order to reach the smooth muscle cells in the inner part of the media, the nutrients have to pass through the internal elastic lamina. This is a perforated sheet and nutrients presumably pass through the perforations.

The trouble spot is the subendothelium. This suggests that its cells are oversupplied with nutrients that are actually intended for the smooth muscle cells of the media. Instead, these pile up before the bottlenecks presented by the perforations of the internal elastic lamina, so that the few cells in the subendothelium exist in a permanent state

Figure 4.4: The Transmission of Plasma Lipoproteins by Transcytosis. Abbreviations: CW = cell wall of endothelial cell, L = lipoproteins, TV = transcytotic vesicle.

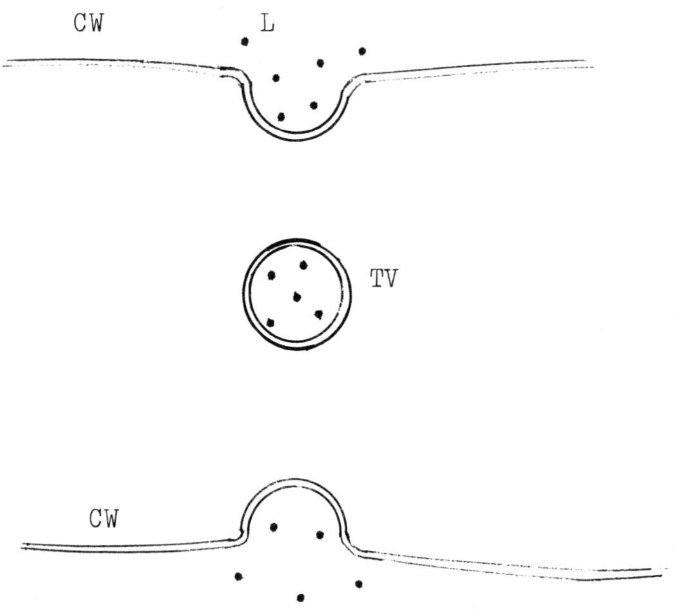

of mild hypercholesterolosis. The degree of this depends mainly on the size of the artery, as in large arteries a thicker bundle of smooth muscle cells relies on supplies transmitted through the endothelium. Furthermore, in large elastic arteries, like the aorta, several elastic laminae are interposed between muscle cells located at around the midline of the artery wall and their source of supply. Generally, the bigger the artery, the greater is the concentration of gradient of lipoproteins between the subendothelium and the midline of the artery wall.

As already pointed out, cells can regulate their cholesterol intake by varying the number of their LDL receptors, but uptake by secondary, non-specific acceptors may cause difficulties in an environment containing a higher than normal concentration of lipoproteins. The most onerous case is that of the aorta, followed, in order of decreasing severity, by other elastic arteries. This is also the order in which fatty streaks affect the arterial tree.

Cholesterol needs are higher in a growing animal than in an adult.

Cholesterol in the body is a building material, not a nutrient, hence its consumption is higher when the body is still in the process of building itself, than when cholesterol is needed only for replacement and repair. Hence the problem of the cholesterol supply not being readily accessible to tissues eases with age. This may be the explanation of the fact that fatty streaks arise mainly in infancy and childhood.

Veins are constructed essentially on the same plan as arteries, with a three-layered structure, but unlike arteries, they are free of atherosclerosis. The possible explanation is that they are much thinner walled and are mechanically weaker. The structure separating the subendothelium and the media – that corresponding to the internal elastic lamina in arteries – is more like an open network of fibres than a continuous perforated sheet. Hence the difficulty of supplying cells in the middle of the wall of veins with lipoproteins is not so pronounced as in the case of arteries.

Summarising, fatty streaks may arise in marginal cases owing to a concentration gradient of lipoproteins in the inner half of the artery wall. If cells in a comparatively inaccessible position near the midline of the artery wall are supplied with an adequate quantity of lipoproteins, those nearer the endothelium may be oversupplied. There is ample room for individual variations, as cells can synthesise cholesterol from water-soluble precursors, so that it is not essential to provide an adequate supply for cells in the most inaccessible position. The cells most exposed to hypercholesterolosis are intimal smooth muscle cells, some of which may become gradually overloaded with lipids and ultimately die. Until they do, they are presumably capable of processing their lipoprotein intake by lysosomal digestion and esterification, so that when the cells dies, they liberate cholesteryl oleate into subendothelial space.

Another point to note about intimal smooth muscle cells it that their function is the repair of injuries. They guard the most vital supply routes in the body where major injuries are irreparable. If the aorta or one of its main branches suffers substantial damage, the animal is dead before repair can even begin. The only useful function intimal smooth muscle cells can perform is to sense incipient injuries and react to them instantly. This means that they must be very sensitive to injury signals reaching them from other cells. In order to be able to react to such signals without delay, they must carry a large store of nutrients. The difference between a store that enables instantaneous action and one that represents an intolerable overload, may be a very fine one.

The injuries which intimal smooth muscle cells may be able to repair are those of the endothelium. The sheet of endothelium is in a constant process of slow renewal, occasionally a dead cell can be seen among living cells. Sometimes a part of the endothelium is torn away from the connective tissue supporting it, so that blood flows into the space between the torn part of the sheet and the internal elastic lamina, tending to tear away further parts of the endothelium. The lesion (aneurysm), unless it remains small, is usually fatal and it is presumably the intervention of smooth muscle cells that can keep it small. When intimal smooth muscle cells receive injury signals, they proliferate and make a temporary repair of the injured area with their fibres. It is, however, conceivable that when intimal smooth muscle cells become overloaded with lipids and die in consequence, they also emit injury signals which cause their neighbours to proliferate, with the possibility of a snowball effect. When a few cells die and cause others around them to proliferate, they all have a preferential claim for supplies intended for median smooth muscle, and so the mass of cells, all overloaded with lipids and constituting a fatty streak, may arise.

Differences Between Fatty Streaks and Fibrous Plaques

Fatty streaks are universal in all races in all parts of the world. They affect mainly infants and children and affect both sexes approximately equally. Their primary target is the aorta. The predominant lipid of the fatty streak is cholesteryl oleate. The cells affected by lipid overloading are intimal smooth muscle cells. In contrast, fibrous plaques develop at a later age, are prevalent only in prosperous countries, are probably diet-related and cause a large excess of male mortality. They also begin in the aorta, but even there the mainly affected areas are not quite the same as those most vulnerable to fatty streaks. The latter appear mainly in the ascending and thoracic segments of the aorta, the fibrous plaques tend to be most extensive in its abdominal region. The predominant lipid of the fibrous plaque is cholesteryl linoleate, and the lipid-laden cells are partly intimal smooth muscle cells and partly macrophages. In view of such a large number of differences it is still a debated point whether fibrous plaques develop from fatty streaks or represent an independent lesion, resulting from a different set of causes. Cholesterol-fed animals develop fatty streaks which never develop into fibrous plaques. When they do, it is after a prolonged and excessive feeding of an unnatural diet, pointing towards the conclusion that the causes differ only quantitatively, not in kind. But even if the causes are the same, it is clear that fatty streaks do not inevitably progress to fibrous plaques. They appear to do so only in prosperous countries. In poorer countries they stop developing, and possibly retrogress in later childhood. It can be assumed that beside a natural predisposition of arteries to cholesterol-related disorders there must be some additional factors, probably nutritional and probably linked with overnutrition rather than undernutrition, that cause fatty streaks to progress to fibrous plaques.

Considering the many differences between the fatty streak and the fibrous plaque individually, the first is the intriguing difference in lipid composition. How does the cholesteryl oleate content of fatty streaks change into the cholesteryl linoleate of plaques? As already explained, cholesterol in the blood is mainly in the form of linoleates, oleates are produced in peripheral cells. Two explanations seem possible. One is that intimal smooth muscle cells are overwhelmed by the influx of lipoproteins and their lysosomes become incapable of producing the hydrolases necessary to de-esterify the linoleates obtained from the LDL particles.[7] Instead of free cholesterol, the lysosome must be assumed to discharge linoleates, and when the cell dies, these are liberated into the subendothelium. Note that the lysosome is apparently still capable of digesting the protein carrier of the plasma lipoproteins as well as lipids, other than cholesterol, which they may have contained. The second possibility is that endothelial cells discharge more lipoproteins into the subendothelium than the quantity needed by smooth muscle cells, so that there are no takers for a part of the discharge. The problem in this case is, what happened to the protein carriers of the lipoproteins transmitted by the endothelial cells? Such questions are not intended to indicate that the suggested solutions are impossible, but that details of the process are still inadequately explored. Cholesteryl esters are highly stable subtances, when cells die, they remain like bones in a cemetary, but little is known about the method of disposing of less stable substances in extracellular space.

Another major difference between fatty streaks and fibrous plaques is the presence of macrophages in the latter. The intervention of macrophages is normally corrective or restorative, even if not necessarily successful. Macrophages can ingest foreign matter, dead cells and cell debris. If they invade fatty streaks, their presumable task is the removal of excess lipids. However, while they can digest most substances found in dead cells, they cannot break down cholesterol, and for a long time it was a matter of speculation what exactly they did with it. At one time it was thought that they ingest as much lipid as they can hold and bodily carry it away from the lesion. The problem was clarified by

Brown, Ho and Goldstein in 1980,[18] who found that macrophages subject cholesterol esters and cell debris containing cholesterol to lysosomal digestion and, like other cells, produce a pool of free cholesterol. If the environment contains an acceptor for free cholesterol, notably HDL carrier proteins, this, or a part of it, is excreted, if not, it is stored. Apparently macrophages are just as unable to store free cholesterol for any length of time as tissue cells, so that if the available free cholesterol cannot be quickly unloaded to acceptors, it is re-esterified. Thus begins a slow cycle, in the course of which cholesteryl esters are repeatedly de-esterified and re-esterified. Whether the phagocyte is ultimately able to dispose of its store of cholesterol, depends on the availability of HDL, the limiting factor in the clearance of fatty deposits. The macrophage itself does not act as a carrier. HDL lipoproteins move through endothelial cells in the reverse direction, but otherwise in the same manner as LDL. While the HDL molecule is still in the bloodstream, a plasma enzyme LCAT (lecithin: cholesterol acetyltransferase) converts its load of free cholesterol into cholesteryl linoleate, the predominant plasma lipoprotein. The destination of HDL is the liver, but before arriving there it may unload its cargo to an IDL (intermediate density lipoprotein) carrier. That, in turn, is ultimately transformed into LDL, completing the cycle.

Another area of uncertainty is the assumed structural organisation that takes place if and when fatty streaks are converted into fibrous plaques. The function of the fibres is presumably defensive. An unorganised mass of cholesteryl esters and other lipids between the endothelium and the internal elastic lamina would be under continuous pulsating pressure, tending to flatten it and increase the area occupied by it. Ultimately subendothelial space might be converted into a continuous lipid sheet, weakening the anchorage of the endothelium, probably predisposing to aneurysms, and at the same time cutting off smooth muscle cells from their source of nutrients. This is the presumable reason for breaking up a contiguous mass of lipids into distinct, encapsulated granules, even if at the expense of creating potential obstacles to blood flow.

Lastly, from the practical point of view the most important problem is the probable connection of fibrous plaques with the diet. Fatty streaks are universal in infants and children in all parts of the world, fibrous plaques occur only in the population of prosperous countries. In poorer countries fatty streaks cease to grow, probably retrogress, in later childhood, while in more prosperous communities they persist and may be superseded by fibrous plaques. Clearly, some factors must be active in one case which are inactive or non-existent in the other. Most probably the difference is in the diet. The goal we are ultimately aiming for is the complete understanding of the atherogenic process, but that is a long-term project. In the meantime literally millions of lives could be prolonged, if it were possible to identify the critical items of diet which are responsible for advanced artery disease in prosperous countries.

Speculating on the nature of the possible connection between diet and artery disease, there seem three possibilities to be explored. (1) Plasma lipoprotein density is of the order of 80 mg/100 ml at starvation level, while in Western countries 200 mg/100 ml is regarded normal, and can be as high as 1000 mg/100 ml in familial hypercholesterolaemia patients. Such a high density of lipoproteins could be the most important factor to cause an over-abundant supply of cholesterol to reach the arterial subendothelium. This seems such an obvious possibility that it was virtually the only one to receive attention in the past. (2) Another possibility is that the key role in atherogenesis is played by HDL carrier proteins. The mechanism for removing surplus cholesterol from arteries as well as from any other organ exists. Its failure to function satisfactorily in arteries is due to the scarcity of the appropriate carrier proteins in the appropriate place. There could be something in Western diet that interferes with the synthesis of HDL carrier proteins. (3) The diet may contain some unsuspected toxin which interferes with an unknown aspect of cholesterol transport or utilisation. Plant metabolites seem to have an uncanny ability of finding the weak spots of biological processes in animals and the target of many of them is the circulatory system.

Let us consider the second of these possibilities. It seems inherently improbable that people living on poor, barely adequate diets have a better ability to synthesise a sufficient quantity of HDL carrier proteins than those living on abundant diets, but the possibility should not be dismissed too lightly. Living under natural conditions involves storage of body fat when conditions are good and their mobilisation and re-use in the lean seasons. The searching out of re-usable matter plays a more important part in the life of the ill-nourished than of the well-nourished. Cholesterol deposits in artery walls represent a waste. If other parts of the body are starving, it is more important to mobilise them and use them elsewhere than if the waste as such is immaterial, much the same way as trade in second-hand goods is a more important part of the economy of poor than of rich communities. If this argument is correct, there may be nothing in Western diets to retard the synthesis of HDL carrier proteins, more of them may be produced under conditions of semi-starvation because then they represent a more important item of the body economy and a larger proportion of resources are used to produce them.

The same considerations may apply to women who, even on Western diets, have a much higher resistance to artery disease than men. Women in their reproductive period live in a state of readiness to mobilise stored nutrients in pregnancy and lactation, eventualities non-existent in the lives of men. The concentration of HDL is in fact higher in the plasma of women than in men. The concentration is equal in the two sexes – about 53 mg/100 ml – up to the age of 14. After that it drops to about 45 in men, while in women it slowly rises to about 60, dropping slightly only after the age of 65. In women who use oestrogens as oral contraceptives in their reproductive period and as hormone replacement after the menopause, plasma HDL level rises to about 65 mg/100 ml, and reaches it peak a few years later than in non-users. In men heavy exercise raises HDL level, possibly because in heavy exertion fat depots are used as sources of energy.

The next question to be investigated is whether epidemiological studies can help in the identification of food items connected with artery disease.

Epidemiology

Whenever there is reason to believe that a disease could be connected with some pathogenic agent in the diet, epidemiological studies can provide valuable evidence whether the assumed connection is likely to be true, and at least some clues pointing to the causative agent. The general reasons for believing that atherosclerosis is a diet-related disease, have already been explained in Chapter 2. The main evidence is that immigrants moving from low risk to high risk areas tend to be assimilated in respect of vulnerability to atherosclerosis by their host country. It was also pointed out that ethnically similar groups show great differences in the prevalence of artery diseases depending on the conditions under which they live. Diet is presumably an important contributor to such differences.

There are two basic ideas as to how to obtain leads which may result in the identification of dietary pathogens. One is to investigate whether the diet of people who suffer from a given disease and ultimately die of it, differs from the diet of those who do not suffer from it and ultimately die of some other disease. The great difficulty is to obtain reliable data of the food intake of a large number of people for many years, possibly decades, so that such studies are immensely expensive and take decades to produce results.

If a short list of suspected dietary pathogens is already available, a group of people, usually in the early phase of atherosclerotic artery disease, can be persuaded to abstain from the consumption of the suspected food items, and their fate can be compared with a matched group of controls who were not given dietary instructions and presumably consume the normal diet of the country. The method is expensive, takes a long time to produce results and the assumption that the intervention group really consumes less of the suspected foodstuffs than the control group, is not necessarily correct.

The second basic idea is to compare the geographical distribution of a disease with that of various foodstuffs on the basis of published mortality and food consumption statistics, looking for the dietary item the geography of which best matches that of the disease. The advantage of the method is that it is comparatively inexpensive and can be carried out in a reasonably short time, but it also has its limitations and is subject to errors which have already been pointed out earlier in the book. The obvious function of the statistical method is to carry out preliminary surveys, attempting to reduce a large group of potentially suspect food items to a short list which subequently should be checked by prospective or intervention studies. In fact, not nearly enough use was made of the method in the past, suspected foodstuffs were tended to be selected on the basis of superficial evidence rather than of a systematic statistical survey.

As both mortality and food consumption statistics contain errors and as mortality is caused by food consumption in the past, not in the period immediately preceding death, a perfect match between the geographical distribution of a disease and that of the consumption of a certain foodstuff is unobtainable, one has to look for the best match. For this purpose a yardstick is needed to compare imperfect matches and judge which of them are better than others. One such measure is the calculation of the so called product-moment correlation coefficient, which denotes lack of correlation between an independent variable, in the given case the consumption of a given foodstuff, and a dependent variable, in the given case mortality from a disease, by zero, and perfect correlation by 1. Actual values range between these two limits for positive correlation, and between 0 and –1 for negative correlation. In practical cases a correlation coefficient of 0.9 denotes a degree of positive correlation when causal connection is probable.

It has already been pointed out, but it must be repeatedly stressed, that a prosperity-related disorder, like coronary disease, is likely to show a degree of positive correlation with virtually any index of material advance, because the populations of prosperous countries consume more of all luxury foods (even modest luxuries), than those of poor countries. In a country where, let us say, chocolate consumption is high, that of coffeee or spices or sugar or fruit is also likely to be high. If coronary mortality were caused by one such luxury food, a degree of positive correlation would exist between it and all other luxury foods due to indirect connection. A modicum of positive correlation between mortality from a disease and the consumption of a foodstuff is insufficient evidence, the epidemiologist is obliged to find the foodstuff the geographical distribution of which has the *strongest* correlation with that of artery disease.

On this principle, I went through, some years ago, the most detailed international food consumption statistics available at the time: that issued by the Organisation of Economic Cooperation and Development (OECD)[19] for its member countries, comparing the geographical distribution of *all* items, one by one, with mortality in the same countries from coronary heart disease, obtained from World Health Organisation Statistics Annuals.[20] Some of the results[21–23] were as follows. The correlation coefficients (r) between male coronary mortality rates in the 45–75 age groups and the consumption of various foodstuffs were:

meat	$r = 0.58$
eggs	$r = 0.60$
animal fats	$r = 0.76$
animal proteins	$r = 0.81$
sugar	$r = 0.84$

tending to incriminate sugar. However, a puzzling feature of the list is that the correlation coefficient between coronary mortality and the total consumption of animal proteins is a comparatively high 0.81, whereas with meat and eggs, the major sources of animal proteins in the diet, it is only 0.58 and 0.60 respectively. This calls attention to the last remaining major source of animal proteins in the diet, milk.

Milk and dairy products $r = 0.91$.

OECD statistics include data on the protein and fat content of dairy products, on the basis of which correlation coefficients can be calculated for milk proteins and milk fats separately.

Milk fats (including butter, cream, etc.)	$r = 0.88$
Milk proteins	$r = 0.86$

As both are lower than the correlation coefficient for whole milk and all dairy products, both milk proteins and milk fats may contain some atherogenic agent.

A surprising result obtained when it was intended to check whether fermentation had an effect on the apparent atherogenic effect of milk and dairy products. OECD statistics separate cheese from other milk products, hence it is possible to exclude it from milk consumption. Results were:

Milk fats, excluding cheese	$r = 0.88$
Milk proteins, excluding cheese	$r = 0.93$

putting milk proteins in the lead. It may be noted that OECD statistics do not include data on the consumption of yoghurt and similar products as separate items, so that it is not certain that it is fermentation that destroys apparent atherogenic properties. An atherogenic agent may remain in the whey when milk solids are coagulated. This could be decided if data were available for the consumption of yoghurt and similar products, which are fermented but uncoagulated, and cottage cheese which is coagulated but not fermented. This, however, is not the case and demonstrates one of the limitations of statistical analysis. Nor do the results make it entirely clear whether milk fats can be exonerated. An atherogenic agent could be associated both with milk proteins and milk fats, but to a greater extent with the former.

When food consumption data are correlated with mortality from a disease, a time interval should be allowed between them, the food consumption figures predating mortality statistics by several years, since a disease, if it is caused by a dietary pathogen, must be caused by food eaten a long time before the appearance of clinical symptoms. It is not possible to know in advance what this interval should be; the time lag which gives the best correlation has to be found by trial and error. In the case of milk and coronary disease I have tried several possibilities, in one case correlating mortality statistics with food consumption statistics which pre-dated them by three years, in another case with the average consumption of 21 years (the entire period for which

Table 4.1: Coronary Heart Disease Mortality Rates (1977-80) and the Consumption of Unfermented Milk Proteins (average consumption of 6 years, preceding mortality statistics by 7.5 years)

Country	Male mortality rates in age groups 45-54	55-64	65-74	Female mortality age group 65-74	Milk proteins (g/day)
Finland	380.1	976.0	1926.1	760.8	29.0
New Zealand	265.0	754.6	1724.9	790.4	22.9
Ireland	263.1	784.3	1703.9	765.8	25.1
UK	218.5	733.8	1623.0	686.5	17.1
Sweden	159.1	575.9	1622.0	599.5	24.6
USA	260.4	704.4	1577.2	712.1	19.0
Denmark	181.7	597.3	1517.6	598.5	16.1
Australia	215.6	592.6	1506.3	637.1	18.8
Canada	224.5	642.8	1442.9	623.3	18.0
Norway	191.4	590.3	1328.7	505.3	19.8
Germany	150.4	448.0	1169.7	435.1	14.3
Netherlands	165.4	479.5	1119.9	427.9	17.8
Austria	160.5	413.3	1017.9	413.0	15.4
Belgium	158.1	435.7	968.9	419.2	11.5
Italy	135.5	340.3	765.9	348.4	6.8
Portugal	94.7	225.8	601.4	283.7	5.2
Spain	80.8	218.3	503.4	202.8	9.5
France	78.7	197.8	501.2	200.3	10.5
Yugoslavia	112.6	254.8	500.8	298.4	7.6
Japan	29.6	92.8	270.5	143.7	3.8

statistics were avaiable). The result of this study was that the time interval was not critical. The correlation coefficient varied, but not to a great extent. A reasonable interval is 5-10 years, and it seems advantageous to eliminate the effect of year to year random variations in milk consumption by averaging the consumption of two or more years in that period.

Data based on the latest available statistics are shown in Table 4.1. Mortality rates for men are shown for three decennial age groups, 45-54, 55-64 and 65-74 separately. The rates represent the number of deaths in a country per 100,000 of the living population of the same age group. The correlations with the consumption of milk proteins (excluding cheese) is stronger in the older age groups, in the given case the correlation coefficients for men in the three decennial age groups are 0.87, 0.92 and 0.93 respectively. The presumable reason is that the group dying of coronary disease at an early age includes a larger proportion of people suffering from diabetes or from a genetic

Figure 4.5: Male Coronary Mortality Rates 1977-80, age group 65-74, and the Consumption of Unfermented Milk Proteins. Food consumption statistics predate mortality statistics by 7.5 years.

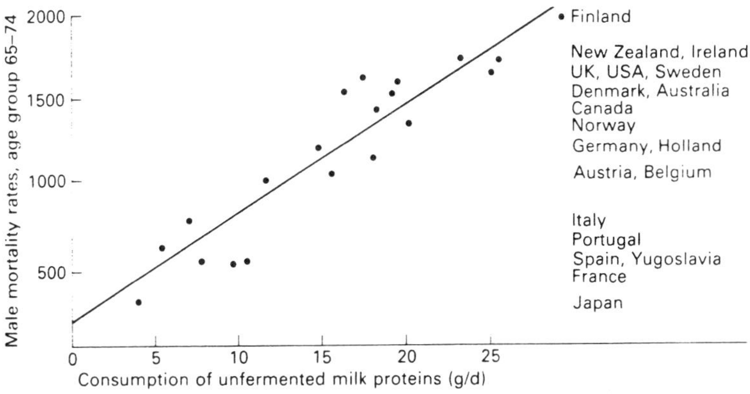

Source: Reproduced from D.L.J. Freed (ed.), ***Health Hazards of Milk*** (Bailliere Tindall, London, 1984), p. 222, by permission of the publisher.

defect like familial hypercholesterolaemia, than the older groups, so that their illness and death is only partly diet-related.

Female mortality rates from coronary disease between ages 45 and 74 are about a third of the corresponding male rates in most Western countries. Table 4.1 shows female mortality rates for the 65-74 age group. The correlation coefficient also tends to be somewhat lower than for men, thus in the given case for the 65-74 age group it is 0.88.

The connection between milk protein consumption and coronary mortality is shown graphically in Figure 4.5[21] for the male age group of 65-74. The same can be more accurately expressed by equations of the form $y = ax + b$, where y is the dependent variable, namely mortality, x the independent variable, namely food consumption, and a and b are constants. These equations for the four groups in Table 4.1 are

male mortality,	65-74 age group	$y = 66.4x + 131$
	55-64 age group	$y = 30.5x + 25.7$
	45-54 age group	$y = 10\ \ x + 19.2$
female mortality,	65-74 age group	$y = 25.7x + 90.4$

The constant b in these equations, which can also be seen in Figure 4.1, is the intercept on the Y axis, namely the mortality that would remain if milk consumption were reduced to zero. It shows the fact which, in any case is obvious in case of a multicausal disorder, that milk consumption does not account for the entire mortality from coronary disease, but it appears to account for a very high proportion of it, about 90 per cent in men, 80 per cent in women.

It has already been mentioned that the epidemiological distribution of the three main forms of atherogenic artery disorders, the fatty streak, coronary disease and cerebrovascular disease are different. Fatty streaks have the simplest geography: they are universal in infants and children of all races in all parts of the world. They are presumably also correlated with milk consumption. A disorder universal in infants is likely to be connected with milk, the universal diet of infants, and it can be assumed that in countries where milk remains a part of the diet throughout life, they persist, whereas in countries where it is exclusively an infant food, they slowly regress.

Other data which may provide a pointer to the causation of artery disease are those indicating an association between coronary disease (and, to a lesser extent, cerebrovascular disease) and female sex hormones. As already pointed out, female mortality in the 45-74 age group from coronary disease is only a third of the corresponding male mortality. This suggested the possibility that oestrogenic hormones had a protective effect against artery disease. On this basis the administration of natural oestrogens to male coronary patients was tried in the 1950s. Conjugated equine oestrogens (Premarin) were used for this purpose in the US with doses ranging from 1 to 10 mg per day.[24] Originally good results were reported, but when these claims were checked later in the Coronary Drug Project[25,26], adverse effects were noted and the group of male patients treated with oestrogens (2.5-5 mg/day) were withdrawn from the study before its completion because of excess mortality from cardivascular causes. Later, in the 1960s the synthetic oestrogen diethylstilboestrol was tried in the palliative treatment of prostatic cancer, which is a hormone-dependent disease whose progress can be temporarily checked by castration. Earlier in this century castration was, in fact, used in the treatment of the disease, until it was suggested that treatment with female sex hormones may provide a form of chemical castration in place of the physical one. Stilboestrol did have a palliative effect on prostatic cancer, but after some years it was noted that an unduly large proportion of the stilboestrol-treated patients died of coronary and cerebrovascular disease.

A large case and control study was initiated in the United States by the Veterans Administration.[27] This and many later studies showed that more patients died in the treated group from artery disease than in the control group from cancer. The quantity of diethylstilboestrol administered to male patients in the original trials was 5 mg per day. Such results indicate that whatever the effect of oestrogens may be on women, they have an adverse effect on men.

More recent studies,[28–31] including one on the Framingham cohort,[31] found raised oestrogen levels in the circulation of men suffering from coronary diseases in comparison with men free of the disease. Thus the serum level of 17β-oestradiol, the most important female sex hormone, found by Phillips *et al.*[31] in male coronary patients of all age groups up to 75 was 37.8 ± 10 pg/ml, in comparison with 32 ± 7 pg/ml in controls. Luria *et al.*[30] found that plasma oestradiol levels of 46, 51 and 52 pg/ml in three groups of coronary patients compared with an average of 30 and 38 pg/ml in two groups of controls.

Oral contraceptives appear to have an adverse effect on the circulatory system. Oral contraceptives have two major ingredients, oestrogens and progestogens. The latter are synthetic hormones with progesterone-like properties which prepare the female body for pregnancy. Oral contraceptives were introduced into clinical use in the early 1960s and their ill effects on the circulatory system, particularly from venous thrombosis, soon became apparent. These effects were generally ascribed to the oestrogen component, hence the oestrogen content of 'the pill' was quickly reduced to a low level, generally to 30–50 μg of oestradiol – a small quantity in comparison with that produced endogenously by the female body. After about a decade of use, however, it became apparent that progestogens also had an adverse effect on the circulatory system. The most important of these is high blood pressure, depending not only on the quantity and composition of the progestogen, but also on the length of its use. The high blood pressure persists after the use of oral contraceptives is discontinued and constitutes a risk factor for both coronary and cerebrovascular disease.

In 1949, about the time when oestrogens were first tried on male coronary patients in the US, Ratschow[32] in Germany began to investigate the treatment of such patients with androgens (testosterone). He and his followers working mainly in Germany, Denmark, Belgium, Austria and Japan, pointed out that the effect of male hormones is not exclusively androgenic, they also influence protein metabolism, muscle development, increase haemoglobin synthesis and tend to counteract diabetes. They also have an effect on serum lipoprotein level, but this is to decrease the quantity of high density lipoproteins (HDL) in the bloodstream, which carry surplus cholesterol away from peripheral cells. At least in this respect the effect of oestrogens, which increase HDL level, is beneficial and that of androgens is adverse. Another potential risk of the application of testosterone, already appreciated in the 1950s, is its possible carcinogenic effect on the prostate. For this reason much work was done on modifications of the testosterone molecule to produce a steroid with reduced androgenic effect; but with the retention or possible enhancement of its anabolic properties.

Many successes have been claimed for the application of anabolic steroids to male and female patients at high risk of coronary disease. Goto and Tsushima,[33] for example, have reported on a trial involving 320 male and female hypercholesterolaemic subjects of whom 160 were treated with the steroid ethylnandrol and 160 with placebo. After 7 years the number of deaths from all causes were 13 in the steroid group, 17 in the placebo group. Of these only one death in the steroid group was caused by coronary disease and none by cerebrovascular disease, while in the placebo group three deaths were from coronary disease and two from cerebrovascular disease. Work with the application of testosterone and related steroids to patients suffering from circulatory disorders is still continuing in many countries.[34]

What Could Make Milk Atherogenic? The Oestrogen Hypothesis

Milk is the unique (or near-unique) source of several substances in the human diet. If there is reason to believe that a connection exists between milk and artery disease, its first constituents to look at are obviously those that make it different from other foods.

The previous section also drew attention to the apparent connection between artery disease and female sex hormones. The two lines of inquiry become convergent by noting that milk contains several kinds of female hormones (oestradiol, oestrone, progesterone), cow's milk probably more than others, because the cow is artificially kept in a state of lactation well into its next pregnancy. During pregnancy the placenta is a site of strong hormonal activity, the main source of progesterone in milk. As commercial milk is mixed from the yield of many cows, it contains all important female sex hormones. This is one of its unique properties, cow's milk is the only important source of natural oestrogens in Western diet.

Figure 4.6a: Some Natural Female Sex Hormones and Their Mimics

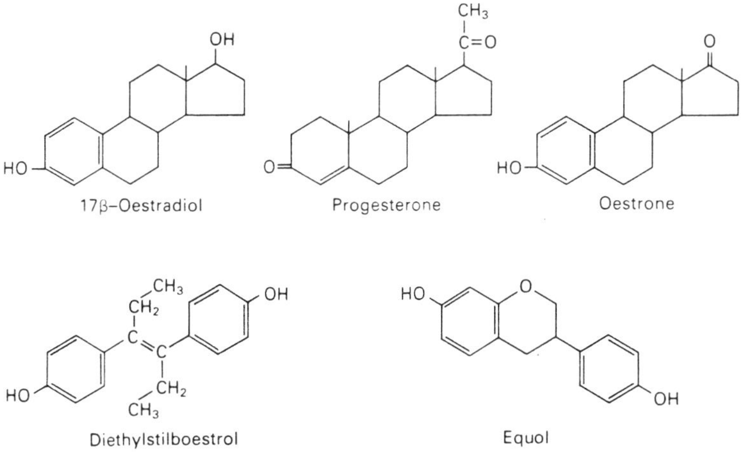

17β–Oestradiol

Progesterone

Oestrone

Diethylstilboestrol

Equol

Source: Reproduced from D.L.J. Freed (ed.), *Health Hazards of Milk* (Baillière-Tindall, London, 1984), p. 225, by permission of the publisher.

Figure 4.6b: Cholesterol

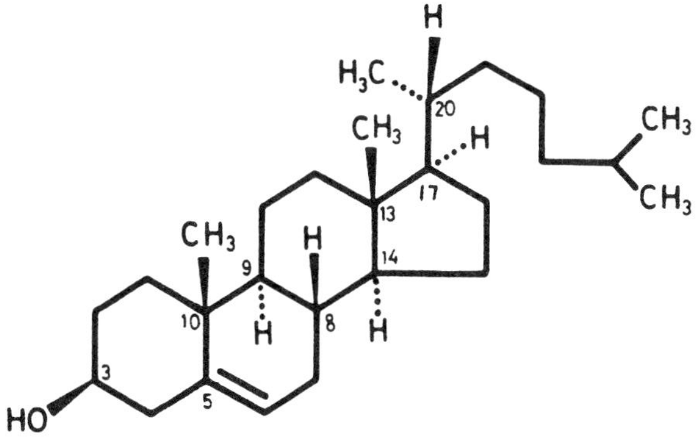

There is no readily appreciable evidence to show whether any particular oestrogen has a stronger connection with artery disease than others. The chemical structure of some of the more important natural oestrogens, as well as that of diethylstilboestrol and cholesterol is shown in Figure 4.6. When oestrogens were administered to men, diethylstilboestrol had a stronger atherogenic effect than natural hormones, but the probable reason was that it was applied in a larger effective dosage. The usual dose in both cases was 5 mg/day, but the oestrogenic effect of stilboestrol is several times as high as of oestradiol. The reason is that natural sex hormones are quickly oxidised or otherwise modified in the liver, whereas stilboestrol is so stable that the liver is apparently unable to break it down and its normal mode of disposal is by excretion. Consequently it makes more circuits in the blood stream than natural hormones, hence its greater oestrogenic and probably also its greater atherogenic effect.

The oestrogen content of milk has been the subject of many studies. A report by Lunaas[35] puts its average 17β-oestradiol content at 0.27 μg/l. The total oestrogen content of milk, including progesterone, is about 1.3 μg/l. The oestradiol content of milk is approximately the same as that of the plasma in women. The plasma level varies with the menstrual period, and highest (about 6 μg/l) just before ovulation. Its average value over the whole period is about 0.25 μg/l. Men also produce a small quantity of oestrogens (just as women produce a small quantity of androgens). The mean level of oestradiol in the plasma of men is of the order of 0.02–0.04 μg/l, tending to increase with age. The oestradiol content of milk is high in comparison, the quantity contained in one litre of milk is about 3 times as much as that in the circulatory system – namely about 3.5 litres of plasma – of a man. However, sex hormones are short-lived in the body, the quantity produced daily, both in men and women, could be 300 times as much as that contained in the circulatory system at any given time. The daily production of oestradiol in a man is of the order of 30–50 μg, to which the intake from 1 litre of milk would add less than 1 per cent. The effect seems negligible.

A possible reason why it may not be negligible is the poor utilisation of endogenous hormones. These are discharged into the bloodstream, a small fraction finding their way to their target organs, while the rest is destroyed by the liver usually after a single circuit. A much smaller quantity would be equally effective if better directed to target organs. The question, therefore, is, whether dietary oestrogens could be in a better position to reach coronary arteries than endogenous hormones.

The fate of dietary oestrogens when absorbed from the digestive tract is probably similar to the chemically related cholesterol, which, in the presence of fatty acids, bile and pancreatic juice, is absorbed in the small intestine by cells of the intestinal mucosa. These pass short-chain fatty acids unchanged into the hepatic circulation, but other lipids are passed into the lymphatic system in carrier packages. Lymphatic vessels take them to the point where the thoracic duct – the main trunk of lymphatic channels – unites with the venous system. From there the combined contents are delivered to the right atrium of the heart and from there their route takes them to the lungs, to the left atrium and finally out into the arterial system. The heart apparently contains oestrogen receptors, because concentrations of tritium-labelled oestrogens have been found in both atria. No similar concentrations have been detected in the lungs, but tritiated oestrogens have been found again in coronary arteries.[36–38] Apparently, therefore, dietary oestrogens can find their way to the heart and its blood vessels. They seem to have no ill effect on the heart itself, but they may have an ill effect on the arteries. Only a very small ill effect is needed to produce a disorder which, in the average case, needs 50 or more years to develop into clinical disease.

The possible effect of oestrogens on the arterial system was the subject of much research and speculation. One of their known effects is that they promote LDL receptor synthesis in cells. As discovered by Davis and Roheim[39] in 1978 and confirmed by other observers since, the administration of a large dose of 17β-oestradiol to rats caused the virtual disappearance of all lipoproteins from the plasma. The cause of the phenomena was found to be a tenfold increase in the number of lipoprotein receptors in the liver. This is the opposite of the effect obtaining in familial hypercholesterolaemia. If cells fail to produce surface receptors, there are no takers for lipoproteins circulating in the blood, hence there is a large increase in cholesterol level. If cells produce an abnormally large number of surface receptors, the competition for circulating lipoproteins increases and their level in the plasma is reduced. Both extremes are likely to have an adverse effect on artery disease. In the familial hypercholesterolaemia type of disorder plasma cholesterol level increases to such an extent that cells can secure their needs by a secondary, non-specific mechanism. This probably lacks the fine regulator which ensures that individual cells can take up plasma lipoproteins in accordance with their needs. If there is no such regulator, some cells are likely to be inadequately supplied, while others are oversupplied. Similarly, in the other type of disorder the synthesis of surface receptors, hence the uptake of plasma lipoproteins is controlled not by the cell's needs, but by an extraneous factor, the presence of oestrogens in the plasma. The likely consequence is, once more, an inadequate supply of lipoproteins for some cells, an oversupply for others.

In my previous writings[21] I have attempted to formulate a speculative explanation, how oestrogens might interfere with the synthesis of surface receptors. The increase of receptors is the presumable result of interference with the control mechanism which normally regulates the synthesis of recycling the LDL surface receptors in individual cells. As already described in this chapter, the regulator monitors the quantity of free cholesterol discharged from the lysosome and forming a pool inside the cell. Probably two mechanisms are involved in this process, a receptor mechanism which admits only free cholesterol to the pool, and a monitoring mechanism which surveys its continually varying size. It is conceivable that the receptor mechanism can be misled to admit some cholesterol-like substance to the pool which the monitoring mechanism refuses to accept as such. Some foreign substances mixed in the pool, as far as the regulator is concerned, may break up its continuity and lead to a misjudgement of its size, resulting in receptor synthesis in excess of needs. As is shown in Figure 4.6, the steroid skeleton of cholesterol is the same as that of oestrogens. It is conceivable that an oestrogen (probably one particular oestrogen) could be the cholesterol-like substance admitted to the pool and leading to regulatory errors.

Another possible effect of oestrogens, at least on women, is that they appear to promote the synthesis of HDL carrier proteins. As pointed out already, plasma HDL concentration is approximately equal in the two sexes (53 mg/100 ml) before puberty, but then it drops to 45 mg/100 ml in men and rises to about 60 mg/100 ml in women. As HDL is the vehicle for the transport of cholesterol *from* peripheral tissues to the liver, a high HDL level decreases the risk of cholesterol accumulation in arteries and provides the only known mechanism which might heal cholesterol-containing lesions. It is, however, possible that the HDL-increasing effect of oestrogen applies only to women, indeed, the opposite effect may obtain in men. Female hormones prepare women ultimately for pregnancy, which involves a large-scale mobilisation of the resources of the body for the nutrition of the fetus, hence creates a need for HDL carrier proteins. In men the only apparent effect of oestrogens is to counteract the effect of male hormones, resulting in placidity and obesity, conditions which do not throw an extra burden on HDL proteins, so that there is no reason for them to promote HDL synthesis.

Among other possible explanations Luria *et al.*[30] called attention to the thrombogenic effect of oestrogens. A finding of the Coronary Drug Project[26] was that among men treated with natural oestrogens there was a higher incidence of thrombophlebitis and pulmonary embolism as well as of myocardial infarction. The terminal event in coronary disease is often thrombosis. In the advanced state of atherosclerosis arteries tend to ulcerate and bleed, with the possibility of clot formation. At the same time the lumen of the artery is reduced by plaques. When it is reduced to about half of its original size, a blood clot may completely occlude it, sometimes with fatal consequences. It is conceivable that the diet contains an agent or agents which promote atherosclerosis and another agent which promotes blood clotting, but the statistical correlation between coronary mortality and a thrombogenic agent is likely to be weak, because the dietary item containing it can be consumed throughout life with impunity, only in the most advanced stage of atherosclerosis does it have a harmful effect. If the atherogenic effect of milk were due to its oestrogens, the strong statistical correlation between it and coronary mortality would support the view that oestrogens were primarily atherogenic and only to a lesser extent thrombogenic.

Hitherto attention was focused on *male* coronary mortality. Death rate among women, even if much lower than in men, is still considerable, particularly in old age. Oestrogens are unlikely to have the same adverse effect on women as on men and the quantity of dietary oestrogens is an even smaller proportion of endogenous production than in men. The question is, what causes coronary disease in women?

Two possible answers can be offered. One is that dietary oestrogens account only for that part of male mortality that is in excess of female mortality, approximately two-thirds. This would leave one third of male mortality and the whole of female mortality to be accounted for by some other causative agent. That agent would be still something that is active only in prosperous countries and probably contained in some item of the diet. An epidemiological check on this point is possible by attempting to correlate female mortality statistics with food consumption. The ranking list of female mortality among OECD countries in the age group 55-64 is shown in Table 4.2.

The reason for taking the 55-64 age group for this table is that the few cases of female coronary mortality which occur below the age of 55, are likely to be associated with disorders like familial hypercholesterolaemia or diabetes, while in old age female mortality gradually assumes the pattern of male mortality, showing a high degree of correlation with milk consumption. The most conspicuous difference between Table 4.2 and the ranking order of male mortality is that Finland is displaced from its leading position in the latter to sixth place,

Table 4.2: Ranking List of Female Mortality in OECD Countries in the 55-64 Age Group

1. Ireland	12. Belgium
2. USA	13. Austria
3. New Zealand	14. Germany
4. Australia	15. Yugoslavia
5. UK	16. Italy
6. Finland	17. Portugal
7. Canada	18. Switzerland
8. Denmark	19. France
9. Sweden	20. Spain
10. Norway	21. Japan
11. Netherlands	

the other changes seem of minor importance. I have not yet carried out the work of finding out whether this list can be correlated with the consumption of some specific food item, there are certainly no obvious candidates. In the consumption of animal fats, for example, the leading countries are New Zealand, Ireland, Denmark, Germany, Canada, England, Belgium, Austria, which are poorly correlated with the ranking list of female mortality.

The other possibility for the cause of coronary disease in women is that exogenous oestrogens (and possibly progestogens) have the same tendency to be deposited in coronary arteries in women as in men, the lower mortality in women being due to a better clearance rate which, in turn, is the consequence of the higher concentration of HDL in their plasma. This, as already pointed out, is about 30 per cent higher in women in their reproductive period than in men of similar age. In old age the level of HDL in the plasma of women drops, with a corresponding increase in coronary mortality.

There are two pieces of evidence in favour of this alternative. One is that oral contraceptives, particularly in the 1960s when their oestrogen content was higher than in the more recent preparations, though still low in comparison with the endogenous production of oestrogens in women, were found to have adverse cardiovascular effects,[40-42] the other is that in old age the correlation between milk consumption and female coronary mortality is nearly as strong as with male mortality. As already mentioned, the correlation coefficient in women in the 65-74 age group is 0.88 as compared with 0.92 in men of the same age.

It may be pointed out that another cholesterol-related disorder, gallstones, is more frequent in women than in men. Cholesterol stones tend to form in the gall bladder if the proportion of cholesterol, bile salts and lecithin in the bile is outside certain limits. The better transport of cholesterol from peripheral tissues to the liver in women may result, on occasions, in a surplus of cholesterol in the gall bladder, hence in a tendency of gallstone formation. While it is by no means certain that the high resistance of women to one cholesterol-related disease, atherosclerosis, is complementary to vulnerability to another cholesterol-related disorder, gallstones, the assumption is, at least, plausible and might be taken as an indication that the higher serum level of HDL in women could be an important factor in both cases.

Other Theories Linking Cow's Milk with Atherosclerosis

Several workers have noticed the close country-by-country correlation between coronary mortality and cow's milk consumption, and developed theories to explain the presumed causal connection. The various theories are not mutually exclusive; all, some or none might be correct.

The Lipid Hypothesis

This is based on the classic theory that cholesterol deposits in the arteries arise from a surfeit of dietary cholesterol. Milk and milk products are, of course, rich sources of cholesterol and saturated fats. Milk fat, together with beef fat and mutton fat, contains 60 per cent saturated fat and is among the most saturated of all food fats. It is rich in stearic and myristic fatty acids which promote thrombosis in test tubes and raise blood cholesterol levels in experimental animals. They retard the metabolism of the essential (unsaturated) fatty acids by competition for the same enzymes.

Against the lipid hypothesis stands the fact that, in spite of enormous and costly trials in many countries, it has not been convincingly demonstrated that the 'prudent diet' of low animal fats and cholesterol actually reduces the severity or prevalence of coronary disease, except in cases of severe hypercholesterolaemia.

The Xanthine Oxidase Hypothesis

Drs K.A. Oster and D.J. Ross have drawn attention to the fact that milk is a rich source of the enzyme xanthine oxidase. This is attached to the membranes that surround the fat droplets, and when milk is homogenised, some of these membranes are turned inside out, so that, on swallowing, the enzyme escapes proper digestion in the intestine. Still bound to its inverted fat droplet, the enzyme passes into the lymphatic drainage of the intestine, bypassing the normal filter of the liver. Once in the circulation, it deposits small spots of enzyme in the blood vessels, dissolving away the normal phospholipids (plasmalogens) of the vessel walls and perhaps generating harmful free radicals, thus initiating the damage to the vessel endothelium that ultimately leads to atherosclerosis.[43,44] Homogenised milk, according to this theory, is more harmful than untreated milk. Pasteurisation damages the enzyme to some extent but does not destroy it. UHT and sterilised milk, on the other hand, contain no xanthine oxidase and should be safe in this regard; this is also true of fermented milk products such as cheese and yoghurt. No attempt is made to explain why the damage is more extensive in some arteries than in others or why women are more resistant to the disease than men.

The Immunological Hypothesis

Dr D.F. Davies and Mr G. Rees, of Carmarthen, Wales, have made the observation that men who had severe heart attacks, have significantly higher levels of antibodies against cow's milk in the bloodstream than healthy controls or men who had mild heart attacks.[45] This antibody also seems to bind to, and activate human platelets, thus acting as a thrombogenic agent.

These antibodies would also combine with milk-derived antigens every time the man ingests milk, forming circulating immune complexes. It is known from animal experiments that such complexes tend to settle in the walls of arteries, causing inflammation there. This might be another initiator of eventual atherosclerosis. The milk antigen in question appears to reside on the membrane that surrounds the fat globule, just like xanthine oxidase, but it is not thought to be the same as xanthine oxidase.

Dr P.J. Gallagher, of Southampton, has shown in experimental animals that if he maintained two groups of similar animals at the same blood cholesterol level, but fed one group a food to which they had circulating antibodies and the other group a food against which they did not have such antibodies, the first group developed more atherosclerosis than the latter.

Other Theories

Dr J.C. Annand, a general practitioner in Edinburgh, points out that the real upswing in coronary mortality appears to have happened at the same time as pasteurisation of milk became widespread in the UK, and wonders whether the heating process might be the dangerous factor.[46]

Dr J.J. Segall,[47] another general practitioner in London, noting the apparent harmlessness of fermented milk products, suggests that the milk sugar (lactose), which is destroyed by fermentation, might be the real risk factor. Dr T.H. Crouch, a general practitioner in France, points the finger of accusation at the practice of bottle-feeding newborn babies on milk products that are derived from cow's milk and share many of its immunological characteristics. Bottle feeding became the norm only in the 1950s in the UK though it was steadily increasing in popularity from about the 1930s. Apart from this theory, Dr Crouch was one of the investigators[48] who carried out a pilot study on coronary patients on a milk-free, egg-free diet, with promising results.

Cerebrovascular Disease

Cerebrovascular disease (stroke), apart from the fact that it affects arteries of the brain instead of those of the heart, is essentially the same atherosclerotic disorder as coronary disease, consisting of a slow accumulation of fibrous plaques which tend to obstruct blood flow. After coronary disease and cancer it is the third largest killing disease in many advanced countries. In England and Wales, for example, there were 150,000 deaths from coronary disease, 130,000 from all types of cancer and 70,000 from cerebrovascular disease in 1980. Apart from the mortality it causes, the narrowing of cerebral arteries due to the slow accumulation of plaques is largely responsible for mental deterioration in the elderly, and a non-lethal attack can leave its victim with the most grievous loss of faculties.

The walls of cerebral arteries are notably thin in comparison with their size, so that they are mechanically weaker than other arteries. Whereas in coronary disease the terminal event is usually the occlusion of an important artery, in cerebrovascular disease the rupture of the artery wall, followed by massive haemorrhage, is a not infrequent alternative to occlusion as the cause of death. Consequently hypertension is considerably more important in the aetiology of cerebrovascular disease than of coronary disease. In Chapter 3 attention was called to the so-called pressor amines, present in a large variety of common foods, ranging from cheese and fish products to fruit (pineapples, oranges, lemons, plums, grapes), vegetables (potatoes, broad beans) and beverages (red wine, beer and tea). Pressor amines constrict blood vessels, hence lead to a rise in blood pressure. Their effect is capricious, because the enzyme monoamine oxidase (MAO) normally renders them harmless. Some plants, however, contain a MAO inhibitor, so the two types of plant together can have a pathogenic effect. Beside nutrients, microorganisms in spoilt food, or fungi, like ergot, may contain potent vasoconstrictors.

The geographical distribution of cerebrovascular disease is substantially different from that of coronary disease. The latter is non-existent in the poorest countries of the world, its prevalence rising in direct proportion to prosperity. Cerebrovascular disease reaches its peak in moderately prosperous countries and declines again with further rise of affluence, so that its connection with prosperity is parabolic. In Europe, for instance, there is a North/South gradient in coronary disease, mortality being high in the North and low in the South, in cerebrovascular disease the gradient is the reverse. The world leaders in cerebrovascular mortality are Bulgaria and Portugal. The male/female mortality ratio is also different in the two cases, in cerebrovascular disease in the 45–74 age group it is about 3/2, in coronary disease 3/1.

Cerebrovascular disease is *not* correlated with the consumption of milk or with that of any other foodstuff of animal origin, meat, fat or eggs. In a previous statistical study[49] I reported a fair degree of positive correlation between cerebrovascular mortality and the consumption of plant proteins, excluding the protein content of cereals. The results of this study are reproduced in Figure 4.7. The 21 countries shown in the figure are member states of the Organisation of Economic Cooperation and Development and the mortality rates apply to the latest year, ranging from 1977 to 1980, for which data were available from World Health Organisation Statistics Annuals. Food consumption data were obtained from OECD Food Consumption Statistics. The average consumption of 8 years, between 1970 and 1978 were used, immediately preceding the year of the mortality statistics. The best correlation, with a correlation coefficient of 0.8, was obtained for men in the 65–74 age group, this is shown in Figure 4.6. For women in the same age group the correlation coefficient was 0.72.

Whenever the causative agent of some pathological condition in the central nervous system is different from agents inducing similar conditions in other parts of the body, a possible reason can be that one pathogenic agent cannot pass the blood/brain barrier, the other can. This would imply that atherosclerosis in coronary and cerebral arteries is caused by two different agents, both of which may bear some resemblance to cholesterol, one associated with milk, one with plant proteins. Women appear to have a higher resistance to both agents than men,

Figure 4.7: Male Cerebrovascular Mortality Rates 1976-9, Age Group 65-75, and the Consumption of Plant Proteins, Except Cereal Proteins. Note: Food consumption is the average of eight years preceding the date of mortality statistics.

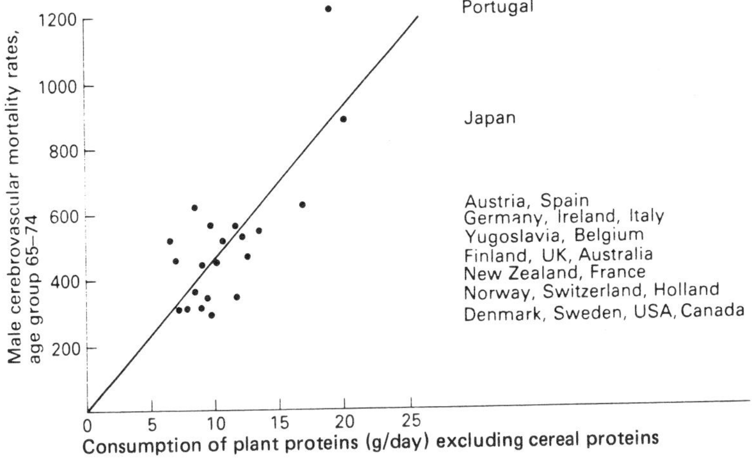

Source: Reproduced from D.L.J. Freed (ed.), *Health Hazards of Milk* (Baillière-Tindall, London, 1984), p. 223, by permission of the publisher.

particularly to the one associated with milk. The blood/brain barrier arises from a different construction of capillaries in the brain than in other organs. As the innermost part of the artery wall is not supplied by capillaries, the blood/brain barrier as such does not apply in that case, but it can be assumed that the arterial endothelium which does supply it, also differs in transmittivity in various parts of the circulatory system, giving rise to the highly uneven distribution of atherosclerotic lesions in its various branches.

A possible clue to the identity of the substance which may be the causative agent of cerebrovascular disease is the observation that when the synthetic oestrogen diethylstilboestrol was administered to men in the treatment of prostatic cancer,[26,27] it caused an increase in mortality from both coronary and cerebrovascular disease. Another possibly relevant observation is that mortality from both disorders tends to be higher in areas where the water supply is soft than where it is hard, so that the two pathogens must be different in some respects but similar in others.

The group of substances to which these clues seem to point are oestrogen-mimicking substances (phyto-oestrogens) produced by a number of plants, particularly by leguminous plants.[50,51] In chemical structure they are isoflavones, bearing a resemblance to stilboestrol. In the digestive tract they are converted into equol, in which form they are absorbed from the gut. Equol is a weak oestrogen but still capable of competing for receptor sites with natural oestrogens.[51] The highest known concentration of phyto-oestrogens appears in some varieties of clover. Among plants used for human consumption the richest source are soya beans. Another leguminous plant, peanut, is probably in second place. It seems possible that the statistical correlation between cerebrovascular disease and the consumption of plant proteins is due to indirect effects: protein-rich plants also tend to be sources of phyto-oestrogens. No statistical data are available which would enable the epidemiological to correlate cerebrovascular mortality directly with the consumption of phyto-oestrogens. It is conceivable that in the same way as the heart and its arteries are 'target organs' for natural oestrogens, cerebral arteries have an affinity for equol.

Summary

Atherosclerotic artery disease is the first-ranking killer disease in advanced countries, its worldwide toll is of the order of 2 million deaths per year. In spite of intensive research, its causes and pathogenesis are still obscure. Atherogenesis is apparently a process of great complexity. The simple presumptions on which early research was based, for instance that cholesterol precipitated onto artery walls, or that the amount of cholesterol appearing in fibrous plaques depended on the quantity of dietary cholesterol, were incorrect.

Cholesterol-containing deposits are possible, but uncommon, in other organs beside arteries. Artery disease can be induced in some animals but rarely (if ever) occurs under natural conditions. It is also rare in humans in third-world countries. It is a major killing disease only in the prosperous parts of the world.

The comparative rarity of cholesterol-related disorders contrasts with the fact that in the population of advanced countries major arteries are subject to two or possibly three different kinds of such disorders. The two basic forms are the fatty streaks and the fibrous plaques, which differ from each other in a number of respects, e.g. in the composition of their cholesterol esters. Fibrous plaques in cerebral arteries differ, at least epidemiologically, from those in other arteries.

One of the most puzzling features of atherosclerosis is its patchy distribution within the arterial system. Only a few arteries, and only short lengths in those, are affected. In the affected areas cholesterol containing fibrous plaques, usually of 1-3 mm diameter, can be so densely packed that they give the inside of the artery the porridge-like appearance from which the disease takes its name. It is exactly this uneven distribution that makes atherosclerosis the deadly disease it is. A given quantity of plaques evenly distributed throughout the arterial system would be harmless, but concentrated in short lengths of a few vital arteries they gradually present an obstacle to blood flow and ultimately reduce the lumen of the artery to about half its original diameter. In such cases an aggregation of platelets and blood corpuscles, a thrombus, can completely occlude the artery.

The core of the plaques contain lipids, mainly cholesterol esters. Cholesterol, a substance insoluble in water, is transported in the blood in association with protein molecules, the carrier protein with its lipid load constituting a lipoprotein. Cells draw their cholesterol requirements from the blood by means of surface receptors which can bind specific lipoproteins on contact. In addition they have a secondary, non-specific mechanism of uptake, but this can satisfy their needs only if the lipoprotein density of the blood is several times its normal value.

The immediate cause of atherosclerosis is probably the malfunction of the uptake mechanism. Certain cells, notably smooth muscle cells in the innermost layer, the intima, of the artery wall capture far more lipoproteins than they need. The affected cells become grossly overloaded with lipids and die. The accumulations of lipids in atherosclerotic plaques are the remains of such dead cells. Both the primary and the secondary mechanisms of lipoprotein uptake can malfunction in this manner.

There is no theory that can explain all the peculiarities of atherosclerotic artery disease: their patchy distribution, the differences between fatty streaks and fibrous plaques, the difference between coronary and cerebrovascular disease and the like, but there are some important clues. One such clue is that artery disease is likely to have some connection with male and female sex hormones, androgens and oestrogens. Mortality from coronary disease is much higher in men than in women, hence it seemed reasonable to assume that oestrogens had a protective effect on the arteries. On this basis the administration of natural oestrogens to male coronary patients was tried in the US at around 1950. The attempt was a failure. After many years a large-scale check, the Coronary Drug Project found that oestrogens, in fact, had an adverse effect on men. At the same time the synthetic oestrogen diethylstilboestrol came into use in the palliative treatment of prostatic cancer, until another large trial conducted under the aegis of Veterans Administration found that more stilboestrol-treated patients died of coronary and cerebrovascular disease than placebo-treated controls of cancer.

While in the US male coronary patients were treated with oestrogens, Ratschow in Germany tried to treat them with androgens (testosterone). He and his followers pointed out that the effect of male sex hormones was not exclusively androgenic, they also influenced muscle development, haemoglobin synthesis and other biological processes. The group made no attempt to explain the paradox that if oestrogens were atherogenic and androgens had a protective effect, why was mortality from artery diseases so much higher in men than in women. But whatever the theoretical aspects, the many trials in which testosterone or related steroids were applied to male and female patients at a high risk from coronary disease, demonstrated a better chance of survival in the steroid groups than in the placebo groups.

Many experiments have been performed on animals with the administration of natural or synthetic, labelled or unlabelled oestrogens, invariably showing adverse effects on the arteries. Some of the more notable experiments found that the heart was apparently a target organ of oestrogens, accumulations of tritium-labelled oestrogens being demonstrated in both atria as well as in coronary arteries. A large dose of oestradiol applied to rats resulted in a large increase in lipoprotein receptors in some liver cells.

Beside the apparent connection with sex hormones, atherosclerotic artery diseases are strongly linked with the diet. Hence the question arises, how the two contributory factors, the hormonal and the dietary, are interrelated.

The two factors could be coincident if some items of the diet contained female sex hormones (or their mimics, like phyto-oestrogens), so that their consumption would be equivalent to the continuous slow administration of oestrogens to the consumer. None of the popular suspects linked with coronary disease, like cholesterol, saturated fats, sugar, coffee, etc. contain oestrogens, but in the last two decades evidence began to accumulate to the effect that coronary mortality was more strongly linked with the consumption of milk and dairy products than with any other item of the diet. Milk *does* contain a significant quantity of natural oestrogens and it is the only known significant source of such oestrogens in the diet. The oestradiol content of commercial cow's milk is approximately the same as its serum level in women and about eight times as high as its serum level in men. The oestradiol content of 0.5 litres of milk, which is approximately the average British daily consumption, is roughly equal to that contained in the entire circulatory system of a man at a given point of time.

However, the life of sex hormones in the blood is short, a daily oestradiol intake in milk of the order of 0.1 μg is a small part of the endogenous production of oestradiol even in a man. Furthermore, coronary mortality in women is also strongly correlated with milk consumption, in spite of the fact that the intake in their case is an even smaller fraction of the endogenous production.

This difficulty, and more importantly, the apparently paradoxical resistivity of women and vulnerability of men, can be resolved by the assumption that only *exogenous* oestrogens have an atherogenic effect, possibly because they have a different pathway in the circulation from natural hormones. Dietary oestrogens enter the circulation through the lymphatic system where they may become associated with different carriers than endogenous hormones. Similarly, synthetic hormones, like diethylstilboestrol, and oestrogen mimics present in some plant foods, are not comparable in some respects to endogenous oestrogens. Natural hormones are normally destroyed in the liver after a single circuit in the blood stream, whereas the liver is unable to destroy or neutralise stilboestrol, which keeps circulating in the blood until excreted by the kidneys. It can be assumed that exogenous hormones have an influence on the arteries in both men and women, which depends only on the quantity of their intake, not on the relative quantity of the intake to endogenous production.

The effect of exogenous oestrogens could be counteracted by exogenous androgens by competition for receptor sites. When captured by specific receptor sites in arteries, testosterone or related steroids may prevent the entry of exogenous oestrogens, without having an adverse effect on the arteries themselves.

Oestrogens appear to possess the specificity of reacting only with a few receptor sites which must be a distinctive feature of the pathogen of atherosclerosis. As already mentioned, the heart and coronary arteries appear to be target organs of oestrogens. The apparent effect of oestrogens on some recipient cells is an increase of lipoprotein receptor synthesis which would cause the cells to take up plasma lipoproteins in excess of their needs. The cells which react to oestrogens in this manner are not necessarily intimal smooth muscle cells, they could be the endothelial cells which supply smooth muscle cells with nutrients by a process of transcytosis. The effect of exogenous oestrogens could be an increase in the quantity of plasma lipoproteins transmitted to the subendothelium, where smooth muscle cells could be oversupplied with nutrients and take up an excess quantity of lipoproteins by overloading their secondary uptake mechanism.

The higher resistivity of women could be due to their better ability to dispose of surplus cholesterol in peripheral tissues. Oestrogens prepare a woman's body ultimately for pregnancy which involves much re-location of stored nutrients. Hence sex hormones promote high density lipoprotein (HDL) synthesis in women which can move unneeded cholesterol from peripheral tissues back to the liver. They do not have a similar effect on men. Plasma HDL concentration is approximately equal in men and women before puberty, but after puberty its level rises in women and drops in men. Exogenous testosterone induces a further drop, partly counteracting its beneficial effect due to the assumed competition with oestrogens for receptor sites. Prevention of artery disease would probably be better served by abstention from oestrogen-containing foods than their counteraction with androgens.

The specificity of exogenous natural oestrogens appear to be such that they may have an effect on coronary, but not on cerebral arteries. It is, however, possible that oestrogen mimics produced by some plants (phyto-oestrogens) may have the same effect on cerebral arteries as exogenous natural oestrogens on coronaries. The synthetic oestrogen diethylstilboestrol affects both.

References

1. DeVries, W.C., Anderson, J.L., Joyce, L.D., Anderson, F.L. *et al.* 'Clinical Use of the Total Artificial Heart', *New England Journal of Medicine* (1984), *310*, 273–8.
2. Bierman, E.L. 'Disorders of the Vascular System' in R.G. Petersdorf, R.D. Adams, S. Braunwald *et al.* (eds.) *Harrison's Principles of Internal Medicine* (McGraw Hill, New York, 1983).
3. Multiple Risk Factor Intervention Research Group. 'Multiple Risk Factor Intervention Trial: Risk Factor Changes and Mortality Results', *Journal of American Medical Association* (1982), *248*, 1465–77.
4. Rose, G., Turnstall-Pedoe, H.D. and Heller, R.F. 'UK Heart Disease Prevention Project: Incidence and Mortality Results', *Lancet* (1983), *1*, 1062–6.
5. Kornitzer, M., Dramaix, M., Thilly, C. *et al.* 'Belgian Heart Disease Prevention Project: Incidence and Mortality Results', *Lancet* (1983), *1*, 1066–70.
6. Ross, R. and Glomset, J.A. 'The Pathogenesis of Atherosclerosis', *New England Journal of Medicine* (1976), *295*, 369–77; 420–7.

7. Benditt, E.P. and Benditt, J.M. 'Evidence for the Monoclonal Origin of Human Atherosclerotic Plaques', *Proceedings of the National Academy of Sciences of USA* (1973), *70*, 1753–6.
8. Wolinsky, H. and Fowler, S. 'Participation of Lysosomes in Atherosclerosis', *New England Journal of Medicine* (1978), *299*, 1173–8.
9. Bondy, P.K. and Rosenberg, L.E. (eds.) *Metabolic Control and Disease* (Saunders, Philadelphia, 1980).
10. Myant, N.B. *The Biology of Cholesterol and Related Steroids* (Heinemann, London, 1981).
11. Brown, M.S., Kovanen, P.T. and Goldstein, J.L. 'Regulation of Plasma Cholesterol by Lipoproteins Receptors', *Science* (1981), *212*, 628–35.
12. Anderson, R.G.W., Brown, M.S., Beisiegel, U. and Goldstein, J.L. 'Surface Distribution and Recycling of the Low Density Lipoprotein Receptors as Visualised with Antireceptor Antibodies', *Journal of Cell Biology* (1982), *93*, 523–31.
13. Anderson, R.G.W., Brown, M.S. and Goldstein, J.L. 'Role of the Coated Endocytotic Vesicle in the Uptake of Receptor-bound Low Density Lipoprotein in Human Fibroblasts', *Cell* (1977), *10*, 351–64.
14. Goldstein, J.L. and Brown, M.S. 'The Low-density Lipoprotein Pathway and its Relation to Atherosclerosis', *Annual Review of Biochemistry* (1977), *46*, 897–930.
15. Goldstein, J.L., Kite, T. and Brown, M.S. 'Defective Lipoprotein Receptors and Atherosclerosis: Lessons from the Animal Counterpart of Familial Hypercholesterolaemia', *New England Journal of Medicine* (1983), *309*, 288–96.
16. Simonescu, N., Simonescu, M. and Palade, G.E. 'Recent Studies on Vascular Subendothelium', *Annals of the New York Academy of Sciences* (1976), *275*, 64–75.
17. Schwartz, C.J., Gerrity, R.J., Lewis, L.J., Chisholm, G.M. and Bretherton, K.N. 'Arterial Endothelial Permeability to Macromolecules' in G. Schettler and A. Weizel (eds.) *Proceedings of the Fourth International Symposium* (Springer Verlag, Berlin, 1977), pp. 1–11.
18. Brown, M.S., Ho, Y.K. and Goldstein, J.L. 'The Cholesteryl Ester Cycle in Macrophage Foam Cells. Continual Hydrolysis and Reesterification of Cytoplasmic Cholesteryl Esters', *Journal of Biological Chemistry* (1980), *255*, 9344–52.
19. Organisation of Economic Cooperation and Development. Food Consumption Statistics. Paris, 1954–1975.
20. World Health Organisation. *World Health Statistics Annuals*, Geneva, 1976–1981.
21. Seely, S. 'Milk and Atheroma II. Epidemiology and Theoretical Aspects' in D.L.J. Freed (ed.) *The Health Hazards of Milk* (Baillière-Tindall, London, 1984), pp. 214–30.
22. Seely, S. 'Diet and Coronary Heart Disease: a Survey of Mortality Rates and Food Consumption Statistics in 24 Countries', *Medical Hypotheses* (1981), 7, 907–18.
23. Seely, S. 'Diet and Coronary Heart Disease: a Survey of Female Mortality Rates and Food Consumption Statistics in 21 Countries', *Medical Hypotheses* (1981), 7, 1133–8.
24. Marmorston, J., Moore, F.J., Hopkins, C.E. *et al.* 'Clinical Studies of Long-term Estrogen Therapy in Men with Myocardial Infarction', *Proceedings of the Society of Experimental Biology and Medicine* (1962), *110*, 400–8.
25. The Coronary Drug Project Research Group. 'The Coronary Drug Project: Initial Findings Leading to Modifications of its Research Protocol', *Journal of the American Medical Association* (1970), *214*, 1303–13.

26. Carlson, L.A. and Roessner, S. 'Results of the Coronary Drug Project – an Interpretation', *Atherosclerosis* (1975), *22*, 317–22.
27. Veterans Administration Cooperative Urological Research Group. 'Treatment and Survival of Patients with Cancer of the Prostate', *Surgery, Gynecology and Obstetrics* (1967), *124*, 1011–18.
28. Phillips, G.B. 'Evidence for Hyperoestrogenaemia as a Risk Factor for Myocardial Infarction in Men', *Lancet* (1976), *2*, 487–90.
29. Klaiber, E.L., Broverman, D.M., Haffajee, C.L. *et al.* 'Serum Estrogen Levels in Men with Acute Myocardial Infarction', *American Journal of Medicine* (1982), *73*, 972–81.
30. Luria, M.H., Johnson, M.W., Pego, R. *et al.* 'Relationship Between Sex Hormones, Myocardial Infarction and Occlusive Coronary Disease', *Archives of Internal Medicine* (1982), *142*, 42–4.
31. Phillips, G.B., Castelli, W.P., Abbott, A.D. and McNamara, P.M. 'Association of Hyperestrogenemia and Coronary Heart Disease in Men in the Framingham Cohort', *American Journal of Medicine* (1983), *74*, 863–9.
32. Ratschow, M. 'Leistungen und Leistungsgrenzen der Sexualhormone als Kreislaufmittel', *Endokrinologie* (1949), *26*, 157–71.
33. Goto, Y. and Tsushima, M. 'Primary Prevention of Atherosclerotic Vascular Disease with Ethylnandrol', *Bulletin of the European Organisation for the Control of Circulatory Diseases* (1977), *2*, 94–100.
34. Einfeldt, H. and Møller, J. *The Treatment of Cardiovascular Disease with Testosterone* (Springer Verlag, Heidelberg, 1984).
35. Lunaas, T. 'Transfer of Oestradiol-17β to Milk in Cattle', *Nature* (1963), *198*, 288–9.
36. Stumpf, W.E., Sar, M. and Aumuller, G. 'The Heart: A Target Organ for Estradiol', *Science* (1977), *197*, 319–21.
37. Harder, D.R. and Coulson, P.B. 'Estrogen Receptors and Effects of Estrogen on Membrane Electrical Properties of Coronary Vascular Smooth Muscle', *Journal of Cell Physiology* (1979), *100*, 375–82.
38. McGill, H.C. and Sheridan, P.J. 'Nuclear Uptake of Sex Steroid Hormones in the Cardiovascular System of the Baboon', *Circulation Research* (1981), *48*, 238–44.
39. Davis, R.A. and Roheim, P.S. 'Pharmacologically Induced Hypolipidemia. The Ethinyl Estradiol-treated Rat', *Atherosclerosis* (1978), *30*, 293–9.
40. Plunkett, E.R. 'Contraceptive Steroids, Age and the Cardiovascular System', *American Journal of Obstetrics and Gynecology* (1982), *142*, 747–51.
41. Mann, J.I. 'Progestogens in Cardiovascular Disease: An Introduction to the Epidemiologic Data', *American Journal of Obstetrics and Gynecology* (1982), *142*, 752–7.
42. Meade, T.W. 'Oral Contraceptives, Clotting Factor and Thrombosis', *American Journal of Obstetrics and Gynecology* (1982), *142*, 758–61.
43. Ross, D.J., Ptaszinski, M.P. and Oster, K.A. 'The Presence of Extopic Xanthine Oxidase in Atherosclerotic Plaques and Myocardial Tissue', *Proceedings of the Society for Experimental Biology and Medicine* (1973), *144*, 523–6.
44. Oster, K.A. 'Plasmalogen Disease: a New Concept of the Etiology of the Atherosclerotic Process', *American Journal of Clinical Research* (1971), *2*, 30–5.
45. Davies, D.F., Rees, B.W.G. and Davies, P.T.G. 'Cow's Milk Antibodies and Coronary Heart Disease', *Lancet* (1980), *1*, 1190–1.
46. Annand, J.C. 'Further Evidence in the Case Against Heated Milk Protein', *Atherosclerosis* (1972), *15*, 129–33.
47. Segall, J.J. 'Hypothesis: Is Lactose a Dietary Risk Factor of Ischaemic Heart Disease', *International Journal of Epidemiology* (1980), *9*, 271–6.

48. Crouch, T.H. and Freed, D.L.J. 'Milk-free, Egg-free Diet in Symptomatic Coronary Disease', *The Practitioner* (1984), *228*, 623–4.
49. Seely, S. 'Diet and Cerebrovascular Disease: Search for Linkages', *Medical Hypotheses* (1982), *9*, 509–16.
50. Seely, S. 'Diet and Cerebrovascular Disease', *Nutrition and Health* (1983), *2*, 173–9.
51. Seely, S. 'The Changing Face of Cerebrovascular Disease', *Ecology of Disease* (1983), *2*, 125–8.
52. Axelson, M., Clark, J.B., Eriksson, H.A. *et al.* 'Estrogen Binding in Target Tissues: a GC/MS Method for Assessing Uptake, Retention and Processing of Estrogens in Target Cell Nuclei *in vivo*', *Journal of Steroid Biochemistry* (1981), *14*, 1253–60.

5 CANCERS OF THE DIGESTIVE TRACT

S. Seely

If food contains carcinogenic substances, the part of the body which immediately comes into contact with them is the alimentary canal. Some parts of the digestive tract are, in fact, highly vulnerable to cancer, presumably caused by dietary pathogens.

Epidemiological studies also support the view that human diet probably contains carcinogenic agents. The great differences in diet in various parts of the world are presumably responsible for the distinct, sometimes capricious geographical distribution patterns of cancers of the various organs of digestion, sometimes with large differences in the incidence of cancers of such organs in neighbouring countries, or in various socio-economic groups within a country. The differences sometimes cut across ethnic boundaries. Cancer of the liver, for example, is common in some parts of the world, rare in others. Similarly changes in dietary habits are presumably responsible for the sometimes considerable changes in mortality from a given type of cancer within a few decades. In Western countries, for example, mortality from cancer of the stomach was rising up to the 1930s when it was one of the leading causes of cancer mortality. A decline then started in the United States, gradually spreading to other Western countries. Mortality from this cause in the United States is about a third of what it was in the early thirties. In some other Western countries mortality halved in about 40 years. The causes of the decline are still obscure, but changes in dietary habits provide the most likely explanation.

Immigrant studies have demonstrated that settlers tend to be assimilated by the host country in respect of vulnerability to cancers of the digestive tract. Thus in the United States mortality from cancer of the stomach is low, from that of the colon high, whereas in Japan the relation between the two sites is the opposite. In population groups of Japanese descent living in the United States mortality from cancer of the stomach is lower, from cancer of the colon higher than in Japan, complete assimilation usually taking about two generations. Another example, already mentioned in Chapter 2, is that when Okinawa Island was returned to Japanese sovereignty in 1972 after 27 years of

American occupation, mortality rate from gastric cancer was about a quarter of that prevailing in Japan.

Lastly it may be pointed out that in the animal world only the human species is highly vulnerable to cancers of the digestive tract. Spontaneous cancers of digestive organs are rare in animals.

From the point of view of carcinogenic influences, the digestive tract can be divided into three sections. The oral cavity, the oesophagus and the stomach can be grouped together in the first section, the small intestine constitutes the second and the large intestine the third.

Organs in the first section come into contact with food esentially as it is in the diet, food is still only slightly processed when it reaches the stomach. Of these, the oral cavity is in contact with solid foods only during the short period of mastication, and with liquids for an even shorter time. The contact the oesophagus makes with food, solid or liquid, is of the most cursory nature. The gullet, like other parts of the alimentary canal, is, in fact, capable of propelling food by a wave of peristaltic contraction, but owing to our upright posture food falls to the bottom of the oesophagus in advance of the peristaltic wave. While, therefore, the small and large intestine are permanently in contact with food or food remains, the mouth and oesophagus are normally empty. The stomach is in an intermediate position. Its upper part, the fundus, normally contains only gases, its body and its lower parts, the antrum and the pylorus, contain food and digestive juices secreted by the stomach. The importance of this can be judged from the fact that gastric cancer normally originates in the lower parts of the stomach, particularly its terminal part, the pylorus.

The question, how the epithelial cells lining the stomach are protected not so much from possible carcinogens in food, but from the acid secreted by the stomach itself, was the subject of many studies. Some protection is provided by mucus covering not only the gastric epithelium but that of the entire alimentary canal. The mucus secreting cells, together with other glandular cells which secrete a variety of digestive juices, are in the mucosa, the layer of the intestinal wall immediately underneath the sheet of epithelial cells lining the wall. These discharge mucus to cover the epithelial cells, through minute canals. Older literature on the subject tends to overestimate the protective power of the mucus, the main protection of the epithelial cells is apparently provided by their own membranes, but the mucus undoubtedly contributes to their defence. The fact that it is also likely to provide some shielding from dietary carcinogens, is an added bonus.

The small intestine is a tube of about 3 metres in length, though after death, when its muscles relax, its length doubles. Its inside surface is covered with finger-like projections 0.5 to 1 mm in length, the so called villi, which give it a velvety appearance. The villi, in turn, are covered with microvilli, presenting an immense surface in contact with food. The total inside surface of the human small intestine is about 300 square metres. By the time food reaches the small intestine, combined with bile and digestive juices from the salivary glands, the stomach, and the pancreas, it is in a liquid state. As nutrients are extracted from it, every food particle must come into intimate contact with some part of the intestine wall. By that time digestive juices may have destroyed some, but not all carcinogenic substances in food. Some liver cancers, for example, are known to be caused by dietary carcinogens (like the dye butter yellow mentioned in Chapter 1) and those could have reached the liver only via the small intestine, with their carcinogenic potency at least partly intact.

By the time food remains reach the colon, most nutrients as well as most of the digestive juices have been extracted or reabsorbed from them. Some carcinogens, no doubt, have been absorbed by the body, but the residue reaching the large intestine may still contain others. In the process of further dehydration which food undergoes in the large intestine, some more carcinogens may be absorbed by the body, while others may become concentrated into the faeces. In the large intestine food remains are invaded by bacteria, some of which are useful to the host animal, but others are not. These may add their own, possibly toxic waste products to the contents of the large intestine.

This brief account of the passage of food through the alimentary canal is sufficient to indicate that the contents with which various digestive organs come into contact, vary considerably, so that if food does contain carcinogenic substances, exposure to them can be entirely different in, let us say, the oesophagus and the colon. It is, therefore, not surprising that some parts of the digestive tract are highly vulnerable to cancer, while others enjoy near immunity. The surprise comes when it is found that the sections that are cancer-prone and cancer-free, are not those one would expect to find vulnerable to, or well protected from cancer. It would be reasonable to expect that the oesophagus, the part of the alimentary tract which makes the briefest contact with food, would be free of cancer. In fact, oesophageal cancer is one of the leading causes of mortality in some parts of the world, causing more deaths in such areas than any other form of cancer. Similarly one would expect to find the small intestine, with its large surface and close contact with food, highly cancer prone. In fact, it is the most trouble free section of the digestive tract. Cancers of the small intestine are rare. These examples are sufficient to demonstrate that carcinogenesis is a complex process and that the identification of dietary carcinogens is an immensely difficult undertaking.

In the following sections some of the more important parts of the digestive tract and their cancers will be discussed separately.

The Oral Cavity

Cancers can arise in all parts of the oral cavity; the lips, tongue, salivary glands, the floor of the mouth and the pharynx. In Western countries the prevalence of the disease is low, thus in England and Wales it accounts for about 2 per cent of all cancers, though it may be as high as 5 per cent in some other Western countries. Prevalence is particularly high in India, in some regions of which it may account for half of all cancers. Other areas with high prevalence are Sri Lanka, Singapore, Brazil and Puerto Rico. This is a cancer where there is little doubt about the causative agent: betel and tobacco chewing in the worst affected areas. In India the chewing quid is called 'pan'. Its main constituents are betel leaf, betel nut and lime, to which some aromatic substances and tobacco leaf may be added. In Soviet Central Asia and parts of Afghanistan the chewing mixture, called 'nass' consists of betel, tobacco leaf and lime treated with some oils, notably cotton and sesame oil. Betel leaf and betel nut come from different plants. Betel leaf comes from the plant *Piper betle*, which belongs to the family of peppers. It is the dried leaf of this plant which stains saliva bright red. Betel nut is the fruit of the areca palm. In other areas where mouth cancer is prevalent, tobacco chewing and snuff taking are implicated. In Western countries oral cancers are associated with heavy alcohol consumption combined with heavy smoking. It is a disease which its victims inflict on themselves.

The Oesophagus

Cancer of the oesophagus is usually a rapidly fatal disease even for those receiving good medical care. Among its victims there is a large excess of males, though in the parts of the world where prevalence is high, female mortality is also heavy.

The regions where oesophageal cancer is a leading cause of mortality, are mainly in Asia. Ethnic groups of Mongolian and Turkic origin appear to be particularly prone to the disease. Mortality rates are very high in Soviet Central Asia, notably in the large area between the Caspian and the Aral Sea, including parts of Kazakhstan, Uzbekistan and Turkmenistan. Other regions of high mortality are parts of Northern and Eastern Siberia, Northern Iran and Northern Afghanistan. Mortality is also high in some provinces of China. Within these regions there can be great variations, e.g. population groups of Russian origin in Siberia and the Persians in Iran are less affected than those of Mongolian origin in the same areas, for instance the Turkoman in Northern Iran.

Outside Asia mortality is high among urban blacks in South Africa. Lower, but still fairly high rates obtain in the Caribbean, Latin America and the blacks in the United States. In the medium range are some parts of Japan, India and Singapore. In Europe and in the white population of the United States mortality is low, but no country is entirely free of the disease.

There is only weak correlation between cancer of the oesophagus and that of the oral cavity, stomach or lungs, though cancer of the oral cavity is somewhat more frequent in areas where oesophageal cancer is common. Day and Munoz[1] express the opinion that the oesophagus is an organ of particularly high susceptibility to cancer. Given an equal exposure to dietary or inhaled carcinogens, the oesophagus is more likely to develop cancer than the mouth, stomach or lungs.

An interesting observation regarding the possible connection between oesophageal cancer and the chewing of betel and tobacco is presented by Jussawalla.[2] Pan (betel) chewing in India is a risk factor of cancer of the oesophagus, while nass (tobacco) chewing in Central Asia and Iran apparently does not increase the risk. The explanation suggested by Jussawalla is that tobacco chewers spit out the liquid produced by chewing, whereas betel chewers usually swallow it.

The causative agents of oesophageal cancer must possess properties which can inflict damage on tissues – even if only on more than usually sensitive tissues – during a brief contact, hence their identification ought to be comparatively easy. Possible suspects are hot foods, particularly hot liquids. If the liquid also contains some highly reactive chemicals, like tannin, suspicion seems even more justified. Alcohol is more likely to have a damaging effect if consumed in a concentrated form, rather than in a diluted form as wine or beer. Highly seasoned foods could be possible suspects. Less obvious suspects are carcinogenic substances in food plants, for instance the precursors of quercetin, a mutagen, present in tea, red wine, bracken fern (consumed as food only in Japan) and onions.[3] With the exception of spices, these are, in fact, the main suspects considered in connection with oesophageal cancer. The high mortality in Soviet Central Asia is generally attributed to the consumption of strong, hot tea. Similarly, tea consumption is also high in northern and eastern Siberia[4] and northern Iran.[5] In Japan rice gruel cooked in hot tea is associated with a high incidence of oesophageal cancer.[6] The heavy consumption of alcohol is a risk factor, particularly when combined with heavy smoking. The probability that spirits represent a greater risk than drinks with a less concentrated alcohol content, is supported by a French study[7] comparing the correlation of oesophageal cancer with alcoholism on one hand and cirrhosis of the liver on the other. In France alcoholics are mainly consumers of spirits, while cirrhosis is associated mainly with wine drinking. The correlation was found to be much stronger with alcoholism than with cirrhosis of the liver.

Bracken fern has been suspected for some time as a carcinogenic agent implicated in oesophageal and possibly gastric cancer in Japan. Notably Hirayama[8] has found that individuals who eat bracken fern daily are three times as likely to develop cancer of the oesophagus as those who avoid it.

The Stomach

Cancer of the stomach is one of the major disorders that plagues humanity. At the beginning of the century it was the leading cause of cancer deaths in men in Western as well as some Far Eastern countries. Female mortality is about half of that obtaining in males, gastric cancer in women was the third large killing disease among cancers, preceded by cancers of the uterus and breast.

In the United States mortality from gastric cancer reached its peak at around 1935 when its former upward trend reversed and a steady decline began. Current mortality in the US is about a third of the peak figure in the mid-thirties. A recession in Canada began about 5 years later and in some countries of Western Europe another 5 or so years later. The decline in these countries was not as pronounced as in the US, in a few countries mortality approximately halved, in others the drop was about 30 per cent. The decline, however, was not universal, there was little change in Japan, the country with the highest mortality from gastric cancer, and in some European countries, like Hungary or

Table 5.1: Gastric Cancer Mortality Rates in OECD Countries

Country	Year of mortality statistics	Male mortality rates in age groups 45-54	55-64	65-74
Japan	1980	53.5	139.5	345.8
Portugal	1979	37.4	99.4	211.7
Austria	1980	22.9	68.1	179.4
Finland	1978	20.3	53.5	169.2
Italy	1978	23.7	69.8	168.6
Yugoslavia	1979	23.1	67.3	154.5
Germany	1980	17.7	58.3	152.0
Spain	1978	21.1	65.4	148.5
Belgium	1977	12.4	39.6	135.2
England & Wales	1980	13.4	49.0	131.4
Ireland	1978	17.5	49.9	121.0
Holland	1980	17.0	43.5	114.8
New Zealand	1979	12.0	33.3	103.7
Norway	1980	9.7	35.8	99.0
France	1978	11.9	33.7	92.5
Sweden	1980	11.6	25.7	88.9
Switzerland	1980	12.1	31.0	86.8
Australia	1980	10.5	29.9	72.5
Canada	1978	10.2	30.1	71.2
Denmark	1979	14.7	30.3	70.5
USA	1978	7.3	18.7	42.1

Portugal, where mortality is still very high. Male mortality in the 55-74 age groups is shown in Table 5.1. Female mortality is consistently around the halfway mark of male mortality in all countries.

In spite of the decline, 14,000 people die of gastric cancer in a year in the United States, 12,000 in the UK, 18,000 in Germany, and 50,000 in Japan. The worldwide toll is of the order of a quarter of a million. There is little need to enlarge on the desirability of discovering the causes of the decline and help the process on its way.

Many suggestions have been made regarding possible causative agents. Smoked and highly salted fish and meat products have been blamed. Smoking, alcohol and radiation could be risk factors. The theory currently in favour suggests nitrosamines as causative agents. Some foods, like cured meat, green vegetables and some cheese contain nitrates and so does the water supply in some areas. Bacteria convert nitrates into nitrites which then may combine with amines in cooked fish and meat products, tea, cereals, or, more distantly, from drugs or pesticides, to form nitrosamines, which are potent carcinogens. Nitrosamines as such can be found in minute amounts in mushrooms, smoked fish, bacon, sausages.[9]

The bacteria which convert nitrates into nitrites may be present in the mouth or in achlorhydric (non-acidic) stomach.[10] Hence achlorhydria is thought to predispose to gastric cancer.

Evidence in favour of the theory is the observation that mortality from gastric cancer tends to be higher in areas where the nitrate content of the water, and possibly of the soil, hence vegetables, is high.[11,12] A higher than normal concentration of nitrite was found in the gastric juice of achlorhydric patients.[13]

Vitamin C can prevent the formation of nitrosamines, hence is thought to have a preventative effect on gastric cancer. It has been suggested that the decline began with the discovery of vitamins in the 1920s and the increasing awareness of their importance, resulting in increased consumption in prosperous countries.

It may be pointed out in this connection that H_2-(acid secretion) inhibiting drugs, like cimetidine and ranitidine, obviously result in achlorhydria. These drugs came into use for the relief of gastric and duodenal ulcer about a decade ago, and the next decade is likely to show whether there will be an increase of gastric cancer among patients receiving them.

An alternative theory, put forward at least a hundred years ago, is that gastric cancer, or pre-cancerous lesions, are produced by hot food. Though the theory has fallen from favour in the recent past, it has a high biological plausibility and it may be worthwhile to recapitulate the arguments in its favour.

The main reason for subjecting the upper part of the digestive tract to injuriously high temperatures, is its insensitivity to heat. While the maximum tolerable temperature for a bath is 43°C, and the lethal temperature for cell cultures, tissue transplants and the like is 47°C, fluids in the mouth feel lukewarm at 50°C. Several tests have been carried out on various groups regarding the preferred temperature of hot drinks, results ranging from 51 to 68°C.[14]

The best example to illustrate the carcinogenic effect of repeatedly applied high, but still tolerable temperature is that of the so-called kang body heaters used at one time in the Himalyan regions of China and India. These were containers filled with charcoal embers and ash, carried strapped to the body, and were notable causes of skin cancer where they were in contact with the skin.

The reason why the core temperature of the mammalian body has to be kept within the narrow limits of about 32–42°C is that the enzymes used in homeotherm metabolism work faultlessly only in this range. Poikilothermal (cold-blooded) animals have developed different enzymes which have a larger temperature range. Mammalian tissues not engaged in metabolic activities, like the skin, can tolerate a wider temperature range. However, the digestive tract is obviously engaged in metabolic activities, hence the damaging effect of higher than normal temperature is, at least, plausible. Apart from the effect of hyperthermia as such, any potentially harmful chemical is likely to be more effective when dissolved in hot water than at body temperatures.

A hypothesis attempting to make carcinogenesis in the stomach understandable, has to explain not only how a hypothetical carcinogen affects the stomach, but also, why it ceases to be carcinogenic by the time it reaches the small intestine. What happens to nitrosamines there, for example? Hot foods obviously cool to body temperature in the stomach, so that their sphere of influence does not extend beyond it.

The reason for the decline of gastric cancer, in this light, is the partial supplanting of the traditional hot drinks, tea and coffee, with soft drinks.[15] In warm climates the only natural drink available to large sections of the population is lukewarm and often polluted water. Efforts to find something more wholesome and palatable go back thousands of years. Thus beer-brewing was practised in Babylon 6,000 years ago, the Bible attributes the discovery of wine making to Noah. The boiling of water and flavouring it with tea was practised by the Chinese 2,000 years ago. Tea and other flavouring substances, like coffee and cocoa, were introduced into Europe in the fifteenth century. In cold countries clean and palatable water is more easily obtainable than in hot countries. In their case the attraction of hot beverages is simply their warmth.

The bactericidal properties of dilute carbonic acid was discovered towards the end of the last century. Dilute carbonic acid has the great advantage that it makes water free of bacteria and is neither intoxicating, nor carcinogenic. Its disadvantage is that it is unstable at normal atmospheric pressure, so that its storage and transport requires pressurised containers, hence makes it comparatively costly. Soda water appeared in Europe early in this century, but did not enjoy great popularity until it began to be flavoured. This was the great American invention, starting the soft drink industry. The largest manufacturer of soft drinks, the Coca-Cola Company, was incorporated shortly after the turn of the century. The downward trend of gastric cancer mortality in the United States seems well matched, allowing for a time lag of a decade or so, by the upward tend of soft drink consumption. Thus in the early 1930s the annual per capita consumption of soft drinks was estimated at 40 bottles, in 1960 at 190 bottles, in 1970 at 300 bottles. From the United States the use of soft drinks spread to countries with close cultural ties with the United States, where the per capita consumption of soft drinks is second only to US, then gradually to Western Europe. The introduction of such drinks to Okinawa during its US occupation, partly replacing the traditional tea, may have been a contributory factor in the reduction of gastric cancer mortality.

The main difficulty of the hot food hypothesis is that its testing by epidemiological means is almost impossible. How would it be possible to demonstrate that those suffering from gastric cancer consumed their hot drinks hotter than their neighbours a decade or two before they were stricken by the disease? Those protagonists of the theory who attempted the impossible by questioning cancer patients retrospectively about their dietary habits, did more harm than good. Questioning patients about past dietary habits tends to produce peculiar results even regarding items of diet. When the questions concern the temperature of food in the distant past, never measured by the patient, the case is that one cannot answer questions to which one does not know the answer. Consequently all surveys produced different results, good, bad and indifferent. The hypothesis has to stand or fall with its biological plausibility and the circumstantial evidence that the increase in the popularity of cold drinks at the expense of hot drinks correlates well with the recession of gastric cancer mortality.

The Small Intestine

In comparison with other parts of the digestive tract the small intestine is highly resistant to cancer. In the United States in 1979 for instance, cancer of the stomach caused 14,000 deaths, colorectal cancer over 50,000, cancer of the small intestine about 2,000. These may have little connection with the diet. Other diseases, notably Crohn's disease (an inflammatory bowel disease of unknown causation) and coeliac disease (see Chapter 1) appears to predispose to cancer of the small intestine.

The most intriguing problem in connection with cancer of the small intestine is to find the reason for its comparative rarity. The small intestine is just as exposed, if not more exposed, to pathogenic influences as any other part of the digestive system, as demonstrated by the frequency of ulcers in its proximal part, the duodenum. The small intestine represents 90 per cent of the total absorptive capacity of the digestive tract. Attention has already been called to its enormous surface, some 300 square metres for a tube 3 metres in length.

Among possible reasons for the high resistivity is the dilution of its contents. The volume of food entering the body daily is about 2 litres, that entering the small intestine about 9 litres. Of this about 1.5 l originate in the salivary glands, the gastric juice supplies 3 l, the pancreative juice 2 l and bile about 500 ml per day. Thus the volume entering and leaving the stomach daily is about 30 per cent lower than that in the small intestine. Most of these fluids are withdrawn in the ileum (the distal part of the small intestine), reducing the volume passing through it to 1–2 litres per day.

The turnover of mucosal cells in the small intestine is very high, the average life of the cells is about five days. It has been suggested that the high rate of turnover may have a protective effect, namely that cancer cells may be suppressed when they have to proliferate in competition with other fast-dividing cells. However, mucosal cells in the stomach also have a high turnover, which does not prevent cancer there. Conversely, non-proliferating tissues are not unduly cancer-prone. The brain, for example, is only moderately vulnerable to cancer and skeletal muscles are among those most resistant.

It has already been pointed out that the small intestine is not subjected to heat shocks, like the stomach. Temperature is also higher than the normal level of the body in the colon, where the bacterial degradation of food residues is a heat generator. It is probable that heat enhances the pathogenic effect of carcinogenic agents, hence their damaging effect may be less in the small intestine than in its proximal and distal neighbours.

Other possible factors in the favour of the small intestine could be its ability to detoxify some pathogenic agents and its ability to produce immunoglobulins, so that its immunological protection is probably good. However, when the enumeration of possible protective effects is finished, the cancer resistance of the small intestine still remains remarkably high. It remains to be said, therefore, that the small intestine is a particularly cancer-resistant tissue in the same way as the oesophagus is particularly susceptible. Translated into plain language, this means that we don't know why one of them is highly resistant, the other highly vulnerable.

The Liver

It is intended to mention liver cancer only briefly. Though it is the most important form of cancer and one of the leading causes of death in some countries, particularly Africa and parts of Asia (notably China), in Western countries primary liver cancer is rare. In Europe and North America tumours found in the liver are usually secondary cancers, originating from a primary in some other organ.

The main causes of primary liver cancer are known with a fair degree of certainty. These are aflatoxins, hepatitis B virus, cirrhosis of the liver (hence excessive alcohol consumption), and some hormonal effects. Aflatoxins are the natural products of some mildew-forming micro-organisms notably *Aspergillus flavus* and *Aspergillus parasiticus* which spoil various grains and other plant seeds (notably peanuts). Their carcinogenic effect on the liver seems universal in the animal kingdom, thus spoilt animal feeds resulted in the death of a large number of turkey poults in England in the early 1960s and there was a similar liver cancer epidemic of rainbow trout in a fish farm in the United States caused by contaminated fish meal. Aflatoxins are thought to be mainly responsible for the high mortality caused by liver cancer in Africa.

Hepatitis B virus is probably the most important worldwide factor in the occurrence of liver cancer. A recent development in this field is the production of a hepatitis B vaccine, holding the promise of eventual control of virus-induced liver cancer. This is a field of intense study at present.

The connection between cirrhosis of the liver and liver cancer has been firmly established on the basis of numerous studies. In the Western world alcoholism is probably the most important cause of primary liver cancer.

Oral contraceptives increase the risk of a benign tumour, hepatic adenoma, in young women. The risk is small; it has been estimated[16] that one in 80,000 oral contraceptive users develop such adenomas per year. The tumour may regress if the use of oral contraceptives is discontinued. Similarly, androgen-anabolic steroids used in the treatment of some rare diseases also increase the risk of primary liver tumours.

The Colon and Rectum

The main function of the colon is the absorption of water, sodium and other minerals from the intestinal contents. About 90 per cent of the fluid reaching the colon from the ileum is absorbed there, reducing the volume of chyme entering it from the small intestine from 1 to 2 litres per day to about 150 g of semi-solid faeces. Certain vitamins are also absorbed in the colon, some of them synthesised by intestinal bacteria.

The most notable feature of the large intestine is its teeming bacterial population. There are only a few bacteria in the small intestine, beginning to appear in its distal portion, the ileum. The only part of the digestive tract where large colonies of bacteria exist is the colon. The main types are *Escherichia coli* and *Enterobacter aerogenes*, but many other organisms are present in smaller numbers, including, for example, gas gangrene bacilli which can cause serious illness outside the intestines. A large part of the bulk of the faeces consist of dead or alive bacteria.

At one time it was thought that bacteria produce a number of vitamins which the host animal can utilise. In fact, they produce those vitamins mainly for their own use. Folic acid seems to be the only vitamin produced by them which experimental animals can absorb in appreciable amounts. If the immune system which prevents intestinal bacteria from entering other parts of the body falters, for example due to radiation damage, the massive bacterial invasion that follows can result in death from general sepsis.

Various mechanisms have been proposed whereby intestinal bacteria may convert dietary pro-carcinogens into more active carcinogens. One example, confirmed by experiment, is that of the potent carcinogenic substance, methylazoxymethanol (MAM), the naturally occurring glycoside of which, cycasin, is found in plants of the Cycadeceae. When cycasin was administered to germ-free rats, it was harmless, when fed to normal rats, it was carcinogenic. The reason was that only bacteria could split the glycoside, liberating MAM.[17]

In advanced countries the large intestine is the most cancer-prone part of the digestive tract. The cancers of the colon and rectum are often grouped together as colorectal cancers, but there are epidemiological differences between the two. Both are prosperity-related, but cancers of the colon more so than those of the rectum. In countries where mortality from colorectal cancers is high, about two-thirds of the deaths are caused by cancer of the colon, about one-third from that of the rectum. Where the prevalence is low, rectal cancer represents a large proportion. In the United States colon cancer mortality was essentially steady during the last decades, but there was a small, gradual decrease in rectal cancer.

Male and female mortality rates from cancer of the colon are equal in most countries. In rectal cancer male mortality generally tends to exceed female mortality.

In advanced countries colorectal cancer causes about 12 per cent of all cancer deaths. The yearly toll from this cause in the recent past was over 50,000 in the United States and of the order of 10,000 in England and Wales, France, Germany, Italy and Japan. If the US mortality rate is taken as 100, most Western European countries range from 60 to 100. Male mortality rates from cancer of the colon in these decennial age groups between 45 and 74 years are shown in Table 5.2.

Many epidemiological studies have been carried out on migrant populations as well as on various ethnic groups and social classes within a country, all consistent with the view that the main causative agent of cancers of the large intestine are of environmental, probably dietary origin. Apart from the great favourite of epidemiologists, the Japanese population of Hawaii, Puerto Ricans as well as immigrants of Polish origin have been studied in the United States, and the differences between the white and black populations are under constant observation. What seems to emerge from all these studies is that if colorectal cancer is caused by the diet, the causative agent is some modest luxury, little of which is consumed in poor countries and then by the wealthier social groups, while in prosperous countries it gradually becomes an item of the normal diet. Before 1950 in the United States, for example, mortality from cancer of the colon was twice as high in whites as in blacks. Since then mortality among blacks has been rising year by year, now approaching parity with whites, presumably due to their better socio-economic standard. In the US and in Europe white collar workers are at a somewhat higher risk than manual workers. In Japan cancer of the colon is associated with the Western style of living and in India with the higher social classes.

There cannot be many medical problems more studiously investigated than the aetiology of colorectal cancer. It is, however, probable that the further food travels in the digestive tract and the more it is subjected to the action of digestive juices, loss of nutrients and finally to bacterial action, the more difficult it becomes to trace its carcinogens to the items of the diet from which they originated. The identification of carcinogens is difficult enough in any part of the alimentary canal, but becomes increasingly difficult in its distal part.

Table 5.2: Colon Cancer Mortality Rates and the Consumption of Selected Food Items

Country	Year of mortality statistics	Male colon cancer mortality rates in age groups: 45–54	55–64	65–74	In year 1970 per caput consumption of: Animal fats	Vegetable fats	Meat proteins (g/day)	Fish proteins	Combined meat and fish
USA	1978	14.4	43.6	106.6	101.4	65.2	41.3	2.4	43.7
Canada	1978	14.9	41.8	100.0	123.5	24.6	35.3	2.0	37.3
Australia	1980	17.8	40.2	85.7	106.4	24.4	43.6	2.2	45.8
Ireland	1978	16.2	38.1	89.8	126.6	22.3	29.0	1.1	30.1
New Zealand	1979	19.0	37.2	93.6	134.4	12.6	40.1	1.7	41.8
Denmark	1979	12.9	36.8	90.9	130.8	26.3	21.5	8.9	30.4
France	1978	9.6	34.9	94.0	107.5	45.4	32.8	5.4	38.2
Austria	1980	14.1	33.4	90.4	111.8	43.0	24.1	1.4	25.5
Germany	1980	11.0	33.3	90.5	125.3	45.3	23.2	3.7	31.9
Italy	1978	11.9	32.1	77.6	54.3	69.7	20.7	3.6	24.3
UK	1980	11.1	30.2	75.6	113.9	29.2	26.3	2.5	28.8
Belgium	1977	11.6	30.1	91.2	115.3	50.2	28.8	4.6	33.4
Holland	1980	9.0	28.3	81.0	94.7	79.1	22.2	3.7	25.9
Portugal	1979	9.5	27.0	64.9	51.4	59.6	13.8	16.4	30.2
Switzerland	1980	6.9	26.9	89.4	98.7	53.4	25.2	2.2	27.4
Sweden	1980	7.4	24.8	69.5	90.4	38.1	18.6	7.1	25.7
Norway	1980	9.7	21.6	75.3	106.8	32.3	14.7	11.3	26.0
Spain	1978	5.5	19.0	48.8	49.3	53.2	17.0	7.6	24.6
Japan	1980	6.1	16.4	40.8	31.0	28.7	6.8	14.0	20.8
Finland	1978	8.1	13.8	44.2	102.2	23.8	18.1	4.0	22.1
Yugoslavia	1979	5.2	11.9	31.3	57.6	34.6	12.9	0.6	13.5

Table 5.2, beside male colon cancer mortality rates in three decennial age groups between 45 and 74, shows the daily per capita consumption of the two main classes of foodstuffs with which the disease is thought to be correlated,[18-20] namely animal fats and animal proteins. The 21 countries in the table are member countries of the Organisation of Economic Cooperation and Development, whose food consumption statistics[21] are the sources of the consumption data. Mortality figures, the source of which are World Health Statistics Annuals,[22] apply to the latest year for which statistics were available at the time of writing, 1979 or 1980 for most countries. Food consumption data apply uniformly to the year 1970, to give a 9-10 year time lag between mortality and food consumption statistics. These figures confirm only the correlation between animal proteins – not animal fats – and colon cancer. Best correlation obtains if the combined protein content of meat and fish is juxtaposed against colon cancer. The addition of egg or milk proteins makes the correlation weaker. The correlation with fat consumption, whether it is animal fat, vegetable oils or the two combined, is poor. This can be appreciated from the fact that the United States, which take the first place on the ranking list of colon cancer mortality, are in the thirteenth place among the 21 OECD countries on that of animal fat consumption. New Zealand, which leads the world in animal fat consumption, takes the fifth place on the ranking list of colon cancer mortality.

Among the three decennial age groups 45-54, 55-64 and 65-74, correlation is strongest with the middle group. If the correlation is assumed to be linear, expressed by the equation of the form y (colon cancer mortality) $= ax + b$, where x is the combined consumption of meat and fish proteins, the correlation coefficient (usually denoted by r) is 0.81 for the 55-64 age group, 0.76 for the 45-54 group and 0.78 for the 65-74 group. The correlation between the two variables, as shown in Figure 5.1 is, however, better approximated by a curving regression line, of the form $y = ax^2 + bx + c$. This line, for the age group 55-64, is represented by Figure 5.1. The correlation is more accurately expressed for the given age by the equation:

$$y = -0.024x^2 + 2.37x - 18.22$$

The correlation coefficient between the two variables in this case increases to 0.84. If the equation is taken at face value, it indicates that the tolerable intake of meat and fish proteins per day, at which colon cancer mortality would become zero, is about 8 grams. Note that the

Figure 5.1: Colon Cancer Mortality Rates and the Consumption of Meat and Fish Proteins

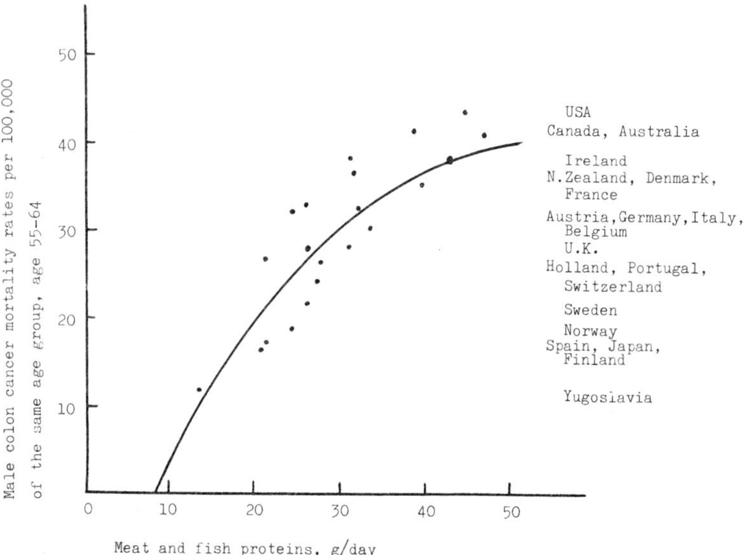

figure indicates protein content, not the weight of meat or fish.

It has also been suggested that the total calorie intake, rather than that of specific foodstuffs, could be the most important risk factor of colon cancer.[23] Comparison of total calorie intake and mortality in OECD countries does not support this theory.

One of the currently favoured theories[24-26] of interaction between food and colon cancer proposes that intestinal bacteria convert bile acids and cholesterol into some cancer-promoting substance. Primary bile acids, cholic and chenodeoxoycholic acids, are produced in the liver and discharged into the duodenum. More than 90 per cent is reabsorbed in the ileum, but a fraction reaches the colon. There bacteria convert cholic into deoxycholic acid and chenodeoxoycholic to lithocholic acid. The chemical formulae of these primary and secondary bile acids is shown in Figure 5.2. A certain quantity of free cholesterol also reaches the large intestine, where it is first converted by hydrogenation into coprostanol, then by oxidation to coprostanone. It has been claimed that there is a significant difference in the proportion of primary and secondary bile acids and of cholesterol and its

Figure 5.2: Human Bile Acids and Their Derivatives

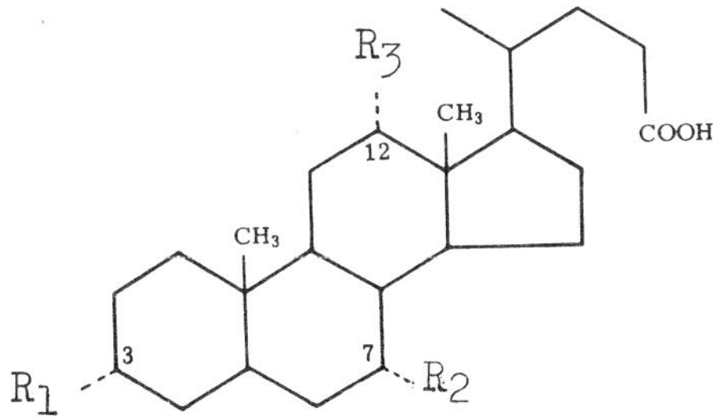

	R1	R2	R3
Cholic acid	OH	OH	OH
Chenodeoxycholic acid	OH	OH	H
Deoxycholic acid	OH	H	OH
Lithocholic acid	OH	H	H

degradation products in the stools of patients suffering from cancer of the colon and of controls, indicating higher bacterial activity in the former. There are similar differences in the stools of people in countries where mortality from cancer of the colon is high and where it is low.[27,28] In laboratory animals a high fat diet also increases the proportion of secondary bile acids in the faeces. These do not cause cancer themselves, but increase the effectiveness of other carcinogens administered to the animals.[29]

These investigations provide substantial evidence that there is a degree of correlation between colon cancer risk and faecal bile acid and cholesterol degradation patterns. It may be noted, however, that a high blood cholesterol level, which is another likely consequence of a high-fat diet, is not associated with the risk of developing cancer. On the contrary, low blood cholesterol levels seem associated with cancer risk at various sites.[29] It may also be pointed out that most theorists are concentrating on the effects of dietary fats, not of meat and fish consumption, with which the statistical correlation of cancer of the colon is much stronger. Meat and fish are, of course, sources of dietary cholesterol, but so are eggs and milk, with the consumption of which the disease is not correlated.

Lastly, no discussion of colon cancer would be complete without mentioning the vogue subject of dietary fibres. The apparent protective effect of fibre was first pointed out by Burkitt,[30] on the basis of the reasoning that rural Africans whose stools are soft, bulky and frequent, are free of cancer of the colon as well as of other ills of the digestive tract, like appendicitis, diverticulosis and intestinal polyps. As already pointed out, the differences between the diet of native Africans and of the population of Western countries are innumerable, and pointing to one difference as the root of all evils is simply a guess. However, the assumption is plausible. It is undoubtedly true that the faeces of carnivorous and herbivorous animals are different, and support a different bacterial flora. Even if carnivores under natural conditions are just as free of bowel cancer as herbivores, it is conceivable that the bacteria thriving on carnivorous diets produce more metabolites that could be carcinogenic to the human intestine, than those supported by the intestinal contents of herbivores.

The original theory of Burkitt was later modified by Trowell,[31] changing the term fibre so as to include not only crude fibres which pass through the human digestive tract entirely unchanged, like lignin, or largely unchanged, like cellulose, but also various plant polymers which are partly or largely degraded in the bowels, but still leave some undigested residue to give bulk to the faeces. Several epidemiological studies have been conducted since then to test the fibre hypotheses, notably one in Israel,[32] as well as other case-control studies,[33,34] comparing the dietary habits of colon cancer patients with that of controls. These claim significant differences between the fibre consumption of colon cancer patients and controls. The evidence may not be entirely convincing but, perhaps, deserves the benefit of doubt.

Animal experiments call attention to a number of substances, particularly anti-oxidants, which appear to have a protective effect when administered prior to, or simultaneously with carcinogens.[35] Apart from natural products, like ascorbic acid (vitamin C) and alpha-tocopherol (vitamin E), there are synthetic antioxidants, like carbon disulphide, butylated hydroxytoluene and butylated hydroxyanisole, which seem to have such a protective effect. Some of these substances are used as food additives. The trace element selenium, which is essential to normal metabolism, also appears to have an inhibitory effect on induced rodent tumours. Lastly vegetables of the cabbage family (Cruciferae) appear to have an anti-carcinogenic effect. The active substance is thought to be indole-3-acetonitrile[36] inactivating such carcinogens as those in bracken fern or in aflatoxin. A case-control study[37] reported negative correlation between the consumption of such vegetables and colon cancer risk.

Another suggestion that can be made in connection with the cabbage family is that their anti-thyroid action may be connected with carcinogenesis. Members of the cabbage family are well known to contain thiocyanate (see Chapter 3) which interferes with iodine metabolism and, under natural conditions, is a goitrogen. The thyroid gland is a regulator of oxygen uptake. Since virtually any metabolic activity requires oxygen, thyroid hormones tend to speed up the general rate of biological activity in the body. It is conceivable that cancer cells also need them for vigorous activity. Further, it is also conceivable that in affluent society the well-nourished body, supplied with iodine at three times the rate of the normal daily requirements, tends toward hyperthyroidism rather than hypothyroidism. Hence a goitrogenic agent, produced by plants as a defensive measure against animals, aimed at reducing the bioavailability of a scarce trace element, may act to our advantage in the given instance. Excessive iodine intake is not obviously harmful because the surplus can be excreted in the urine, but when a goitrogen appears to have a beneficial effect on us, the subject may deserve attention.

References

1. Day, N.E. and Munoz, N. 'Esophagus' in D. Schottenfeld and J.F. Fraumeni (eds.) *Cancer Epidemiology and Prevention* (Saunders, Philadelphia, 1982).
2. Jussawalla, D.J. 'Epidemiological Assessment of Aetiology of Oesophageal Cancer in Greater Bombay', *International Seminar on Epidemiology of Oesophageal Cancer*, Bangalore, India (1971).
3. Sugimura, T. and Nagao, N. 'Mutagenic Factors in Cooked Foods', *CRC Critical Reviews in Toxicology* (1979), *6*, 189-209.
4. Kolycheva, N.I. 'Epidemiology of Oesophagus Cancer in the USSR' in D. Levin (ed.) *Joint USA/USSR Monograph on Cancer Epidemiology in the USA and USSR* (1980).
5. Iran-JARC Study Group, 'Esophageal Cancer Studies in the Caspian Littoral of Iran: Results of Population Studies. A Prodrome', *Journal of the National Cancer Institute* (1963), *59*, 1711-12.
6. Segi, M. 'Tea-gruel as a Possible Factor for Cancer of the Esophagus', *Gan* (1975), *66*, 199-202.
7. Tuyns, A.J., Pequignot, G. and Abatucci, J.S. 'Oesophageal Cancer and Alcohol Consumption: Importance of the Type of Beverage', *International Journal of Cancer* (1979), *23*, 443-7.
8. Hirayama, T. 'Diet and Cancer', *Nutrition and Cancer* (1979), *1*, 67-81.
9. Editorial 'Environmental Nitrosamines', *Lancet* (1973), *2*, 1243-4.
10. Correa, P., Haenszel, W., Cuello, C., *et al.* 'A Model for Gastric Cancer Epidemiology', *Lancet* (1975), *2*, 58-9.
11. Cuello, C., Correa, P. and Haenszel, W. 'Gastric Cancer in Colombia I. Cancer Risk and Suspect Environmental Agents', *Journal of the National Cancer Institute* (1976), *57*, 1015-20.
12. Hill, M.J., Hawkworth, G. and Tattersall, G. 'Bacteria, Nitrosamines and Cancer of the Stomach', *British Journal of Cancer* (1973), *28*, 562-7.

13. Ruddell, W.S.J., Bone, E.S., Hill, M.J. *et al.* 'Gastric Juice Nitrite: a Risk Factor for Cancer in the Hypochlorhydric Stomach?', *Lancet* (1976), *2*, 1037–9.
14. Hunt, J.N. 'The Temperature of Choice for Hot Drinks, a Comparison of Men and Women', *Guy's Hospital Report* (1947), *96*, 60.
15. Seely, S. 'The Recession of Gastric Cancer and Its Possible Causes', *Medical Hypotheses* (1978), *4*, 50–7.
16. Jick, H. and Herman, R. 'Oral Contraceptive-induced Benign Liver Tumors – the Magnitude of the Problem', *Journal of the American Medical Association* (1978), *240*, 828–9.
17. Laqueur, G.L. 'The Induction of Intestinal Neoplasms in Rats with the Glycoside Cycasin and its Aglycone', *Virchow's Archives of Pathology and Anatomy* (1965), *340*, 151–63.
18. Armstrong, B.K. and Doll, R. 'Environmental Factors and Cancer Incidence and Mortality in Different Countries, with Special Reference to Dietary Practices', *International Journal of Cancer* (1975), *15*, 617–31.
19. Wynder, E.L. and Shigematsu, T. 'Environmental Factors of Cancer of the Rectum and Colon', *Cancer* (1967), *20*, 1520–61.
20. Kritchevsky, D. and Klurfeld, D.M. 'Fat and Cancer' in G.R. Newell and N.M. Ellison (eds.) *Nutrition and Cancer: Etiology and Treatment* (Raven Press, New York, 1981).
21. Organisation of Economic Cooperation and Development. *Food Consumption Statistics 1964-1978*, Paris (1981).
22. World Health Organisation. *World Health Statistics Annuals 1981 and 1982*, Geneva (1982–83).
23. Berg, J.W. 'Can Nutrition Explain the Pattern of International Epidemiology of Hormone-Dependent Cancers?' *Cancer Research* (1975), *35*, 3345–50.
24. Hill, M.J. 'Colon Cancer: A Disease of Fibre Depletion or Dietary Excess?' *Digestion* (1974), *11*, 289–306.
25. Reddy, B.S. 'Role of Bile Metabolites in Colon Carcinogenesis', *Cancer* (1975), *36*, 2401–6.
26. Reddy, B.S., Cohen, L.A., McCoy, D. *et al.* 'Nutrition and its Relationship to Cancer', *Advances in Cancer Research* (1980), *32*, 237–345.
27. Reddy, B.S. 'Nutrition and Colon Cancer' in H.H. Draper (ed.) *Advances in Nutritional Research* (Plenum Press, New York, 1979).
28. Mower, H.E., Ray, R.M., Schoff, R. *et al.* 'Fecal Bile Acids in Two Japanese Populations with Different Colon Cancer Risk', *Cancer Research* (1979), *39*, 328–31.
29. Doll, R. and Peto, R. *The Causes of Cancer* (Oxford University Press, Oxford, 1981), p. 1229.
30. Burkitt, D. 'Related Disease – Related Cause', *Lancet* (1969), *2*, 1229–31.
31. Trowell, H. 'Ischemic Heart Disease and Dietary Fiber', *American Journal of Clinical Nutrition* (1972), *25*, 926–32.
32. Modan, B., Barell, V., Lubin, F. *et al.* 'Low-fiber Intake as an Etiologic Factor in Cancer of the Colon', *Journal of the National Cancer Institute* (1975), *55*, 15–18.
33. Bjelke, E. 'Dietary Factors and the Epidemiology of the Cancer of the Stomach and Large Bowel' in: *Aktuelle Probleme der Klinischen Dietetik*, supplement to *Aktuelle Ernahrungsmedizin*. (George Thieme Verlag, Stuttgart, 1978).
34. Jensen, O.M., Mosbech, J., Salaspuro, M. *et al.* 'A Comparative Study of the Diagnostic Basis for Cancer of the Colon and Cancer of the Rectum in Denmark and Finland', *International Journal of Epidemiology* (1974), *3*, 183–6.
35. Wattenberg, L.W. 'Inhibitors of Chemical Carcinogens', in H.B. Demopoulos

and M.A. Mehlman (eds.) *Cancer and the Environment* (Pathotox, Park Forest South, Illinois, 1980).

36. Schottenfeld, D. and Winawer, S.J. 'Large Intestine' in D. Schottenfeld and J.F. Fraumeni (eds.) *Cancer Epidemiology and Prevention* (Saunders, Philadelphia, 1982).
37. Graham, S., Dayal, H., Swanson, M. *et al.* 'Diet in the Epidemiology of Cancer of the Colon and Rectum', *Journal of the National Cancer Institute* (1978), *61*, 709–14.

6 CANCERS OF THE BREAST AND PROSTATE

S. Seely

Cancers of the breast and prostate appear to be both hormone-dependent and diet-related diseases. Their hormone dependence is best illustrated by the fact that castration, by ovariectomy in one case and orchiectomy in the other, can, at least temporarily, check their growth. The reason for the only temporary relief secured by castration is that some cancer cells, sooner or later, mutate to make themselves independent of steroid hormones, and their descendants ultimately replace those which remain hormone dependent. At the same time the cancers are correlated with environmental factors, among which diet is likely to play a prominent part. The connection with exogenous factors can be surmised from epidemiological studies, observations on immigrant populations, case and control studies, on the same principles as employed in all diet-related or environment-related diseases.

The connection with diet in these two cancers could be direct or indirect. The simplest form of indirect connection would arise if it were found that abundant nutrition tended to result in an equally abundant production of male and female sex hormones, an increased level of which, in turn, promoted carcinogenesis in various organs of the reproductive system. This would be the simplest explanation of the finding that such cancers are more prevalent in prosperous than non-prosperous countries. However, indirect effects of a less obvious character are also possible. Diet could directly promote carcinogenesis if it contained substances with a specific effect on the organs concerned, like natural female sex hormones, oestradiol, oestrone, progesterone, etc. (see Chapter 4) in milk, or various oestrogen mimics (phyto-oestrogens) produced by a variety of plants.

The two highly cancer-prone organs, probably responsive to both hormonal and dietary influences, the breast and the prostate, will be considered separately.

The Breast

In Western countries breast cancer is one of the major causes of mortality in women. In England and Wales over 12,000 women die of this cause every year, in the United States over 40,000. Mortality rates are highest in some countries of Western Europe, notably the UK, the Netherlands and Ireland, decreasing towards the East and the South. Mortality is low in Asia and Africa. Mortality in American black women is still somewhat lower than in whites, but it has greatly increased in the last decades and is now approaching parity. Mortality rates are generally lower in rural than in urban areas and tend to increase with higher socio-economic status. Immigrants from a low risk to a high risk area are assimilated by the host country. Immigrants from Europan countries in the United States are usually assimilated in one generation; in Asiatic immigrants complete assimilation is slower, taking two generations.

A characteristic feature of breast cancer mortality is a peri-menopausal plateau in age-related increase. A few cases of breast cancer death begin to occur in girls shortly after the menarche, followed by a steady rise in mortality rates until the menopause. In that age group the curve seems to flatten out or may even decrease, constituting the peri-menopausal plateau. This is followed by a renewed increase of mortality into extreme old age. The probable explanation of the phenomenon is that there are two causative agents at work, one active mainly before the menopause, the other becoming active possibly 2–3 decades later and the peri-menopausal plateau arises when one of these factors has already started to decline while the other is not yet fully active. DeWaard *et al.*[1] suggested that pre-menopausal breast cancer was connected with ovarian hormones, post-menopausal cancer with hormones produced in the adrenals. It was found later that oestrogens in older women originate mainly in the ovary, and adrenals as androgens (androstenedione), which are converted into oestrogens (mainly oestrone) in peripheral tissues, notably adipose tissue.[2] My finding is that breast cancer in younger and older women is likely to be caused by two aetiological factors, the disease being hormone-related before the menopause and diet-related after the menopause. More of this will be said later when possible ideas on the causative process are discussed.

In view of the palliative effect of ovariectomy on the growth of breast cancer, it is reasonably certain that carcinogenesis is connected with hormonal factors, while the suspected effect of diet is only a surmise. Hence most work on the aetiology of breast cancer concentrated on hormonal effects, one line of thought being that it may be possible to identify some hormonal abnormality of breast cancer patients in comparison with controls. Thus it was found that in populations with a high prevalence of breast cancer, women excreted in the urine a larger total quantity of oestrogens, but a smaller quantity of oestriol, than women in low risk areas.[3] Oestriol is one of the many metabolites of the most important female sex hormone, oestradiol, which is normally metabolised to oestrone, then it may be further metabolised to oestriol. This finding stimulated further research on oestriol, but later investigators did not attribute much significance to this substance.[4] No demonstrable differences were found in the synthesis of various oestrogen fractions in women with or without breast cancer, or those living in high risk and low risk areas.[5,6] A later suggestion was[7] that breast cancer patients have a lower level of sex hormone binding globulin than controls. When oestrogens are produced, a certain proportion is bound to carrier proteins, namely hormone-binding globulins, the rest are released as free oestrogens into the circulation. The ratio of the two appears to be different in breast cancer patients and controls. The possible significance of this finding is now under investigation.

Other investigators[8] reported a *fall* in oestradiol levels in Japanese and Bantu women with breast cancer, a finding which seems difficult to reconcile with the palliative effect of ophorectomy. Are oestrogens implicated in the causation of, or in the defence against breast cancer? Yet another line of inquiry concerns the excretion of androgens in post-menopausal women. Higher rates of excretion were found in white than in Japanese women.[9]

Oral contraceptives have been suspected as possible promoting agents, but several investigators[10,11] have failed to detect increased risk in the case of pill users. Similarly, oestrogen replacement therapy received attention as a possible suspect. It was reported[12] that if the replacement therapy continued for a long time, 10–15 years, it resulted in an increase of breast cancer risk.

Women receiving diethylstilboestrol in the 1950s were followed[13] to establish whether breast cancer incidence in the group was higher than in controls. The risk appeared somewhat higher, but not significantly so.

I have considered the possibility that the dietary intake of natural oestrogens, like oestradiol, or other steroid sex hormones, like progesterone, may have an effect on the incidence of breast cancer. As already pointed out (Chapter 4), the most important source of natural oestrogens and progesterone in the diet is cow's milk, hence the subject of my inquiry was the possible correlation between breast cancer mortality and milk consumption. I found no correlation between them.

An alternative possibility is the connection between breast cancer and oestrogen mimics (phyto-oestrogens). The observation that first called attention to the phyto-oestrogen content of certain plants was that they induced lactation in unbred ewes. The example demonstrates that oestrogen mimics can induce changes in the breast. However, when the correlation of the dietary intake of phyto-oestrogens with breast cancer is examined, the result, once more, is disappointing. Phyto-oestrogens are produced mainly by leguminous plants, notably by soyabeans among those used for human consumption. The biggest consumer of soyabeans among OECD countries is Japan where mortality from breast cancer is notably low.

While, therefore, it is reasonable to believe that breast cancer must somehow be connected with female sex hormones, and is possibly caused by some abnormality in the synthesis, transport, uptake or metabolism of such hormones, little progress has so far been made in identifying the nature or cause of the assumed abnormality.

Turning to the possible connection between breast cancer and the diet, several suspect items have been put forward from time to time, like meat, eggs, milk and sugar, but the emphasis has always been on animal fats. The list seems to show little imagination, the suspected foodstuffs are the same as have been considered in connection with coronary heart disease, cancer of the colon and cancer of the prostate. In my opinion that is the consequence of the lack of systematic approach to the problem. The desirable method of searching for dietary pathogens is to scrutinise all foodstuffs and eliminate the obviously harmless items to arrive at a short list of potential suspects. Such a systematic approach is possible only if a quick and cheap method is available whereby the harmlessness of a foodstuff can be judged, otherwise suspected items have to be found largely by guesswork. If the confirmation or rejection of such guesses can be achieved only by immensely expensive case and control studies, there is a strong disincentive for imaginative guesses.

Within limits, there is a quick and inexpensive method whereby the harmlessness of a food item in respect of a given disease can be demonstrated, namely by showing that the geographical distribution of one does *not* coincide with that of the other. The main limitation of the method is that it can be applied only to countries for which both reliable mortality and food consumption statistics are available, and only to foodstuffs which are listed as separate items in those statistics. When searching for dietary items which may be connected with a disease, it is possible to go through the entire list of items in food consumption statistics and check the geography of each against that of the disease.

Returning to the case of animal fats, the suspicion falling on them was supported partly by tests on laboratory animals and partly by human studies. The former[14,15] indicate that a high-fat diet promotes spontaneous carcinogenesis in animals or enhances the effect of chemical carcinogens. There were numerous dietary studies on breast cancer sufferers and controls,[16–18] sometimes based on the dubious method of retrospectively questioning cases and controls about their past diets, and finding that cases consumed more animal fats, or a combination of animal fats and vegetable oils than controls. Other investigators report a high consumption of proteins,[19] amino acids,[20] dairy products[21] and sugar.[22] Several hypotheses have been advanced to explain the connection between fats and carcinogenesis. A high dietary intake of fats and proteins may result in increased hormone secretion which, in turn, may lead to fast growth and early sexual development. Rich diet predisposes to adiposity. It leads to increased bile secretion and the bacterial flora of the large intestine may convert bile salts into some carcinogenic agent.

In an attempt to check some of these suggestions, I and a collaborator[23] have conducted a statistical survey comparing the geographical distribution of breast cancer in OECD countries, item by item, with a list of food consumption statistics of the same countries. The source of mortality statistics were World Health Statistics Annuals[24] and that of food consumption statistics OECD publications.[25] The relevant figures are shown in Table 6.1. The consumption of animal fats and vegetable oils in the same countries can be found in Table 5.2. Food consumption statistics pre-date mortality statistics by 10 years.

The first finding of the survey was that there were considerable differences in the correlation between breast cancer mortality and food consumption in various age groups, good correlation obtaining only in older women. This confirms earlier reports[1] on the bimodal age distribution of patients with breast cancer and is in accordance with the view that in younger women hormonal effects, and in older women dietary effect may be the predominating influence.

The main finding of the survey was the outstandingly high correlation of breast cancer mortality in older women with *sugar* consumption. In the strongest case the correlation coefficient was 0.92. Animal fats were in second place, the highest correlation coefficient in this case being 0.83. This denotes a fairly good correlation, but it must be

Table 6.1: Breast Cancer and Sugar Consumption

Country	Year of mortality statistics	Mortality per 100,000 in age groups				Average consumption (g/day 1965–9)		
		35–44	45–54	55–64	65–74	Sugar	Glucose	Total
UK	1979	23.0	64.7	96.9	122.2	131.8	13.5	145.3
Holland	1979	20.7	56.5	94.2	117.6	125.1	13.8	138.9
Ireland	1977	19.3	69.0	72.2	112.5	126.8	11.3	138.1
Denmark	1979	17.7	49.0	96.9	109.0	135.0	–	135.0
Canada	1977	18.9	50.6	90.4	104.9	137.1	–	137.1
Switzerland	1979	19.4	48.2	88.1	103.9	121.1	–	121.1
US	1978	16.9	51.0	83.0	98.9	133.7	–	133.7
Belgium	1976	21.8	50.7	75.1	97.0	100.0	–	100.0
N. Zealand	1978	21.3	67.8	69.3	96.7	123.4	–	123.4
Norway	1979	11.3	40.6	68.9	95.1	120.4	–	120.4
Sweden	1979	13.4	33.9	66.2	94.0	117.4	–	117.4
Germany	1978	15.9	44.1	70.1	92.9	89.9	6.4	96.3
France	1977	13.4	39.5	64.1	85.6	92.2	4.1	96.3
Austria	1979	17.4	41.7	69.7	80.2	101.3	–	101.3
Finland	1977	11.3	35.6	52.8	77.7	114.4	–	114.4
Italy	1976	17.2	42.6	64.6	77.5	71.4	0.5	71.9
Spain	1977	14.4	33.5	45.2	51.0	66.4	–	66.4
Greece	1978	14.2	36.2	46.2	50.2	51.9	–	51.9
Portugal	1975	14.8	34.6	44.1	46.0	57.6	–	57.6
Yugoslavia	1977	13.4	30.4	39.7	44.0	67.0	–	67.0
Japan	1979	6.8	14.6	18.2	17.0	57.4	–	57.4
Mean	1978	16.3	44.5	67.4	84.5	101.9	2.4	104.3

remembered that in prosperous countries the consumption of several foodstuffs tends to increase in parallel. In countries, where sugar consumption is high, fat consumption is also likely to be high. Hence the importance of finding the foodstuff which gives the *best* correlation. It was interesting to note, however, that fats performed comparatively well in the younger age groups.

Detailed results were as follows. Denoting correlation coefficients in four decennial age groups as $r_{35\text{-}44}$, etc, the calculated coefficients were:

Sugar: $r_{35\text{-}44} = 0.57, r_{45\text{-}54} = 0.75, r_{55\text{-}64} = 0.86, r_{65\text{-}74} = 0.92$

Animal fats: $r_{35\text{-}44} = 0.58, r_{45\text{-}54} = 0.75, r_{55\text{-}64} = 0.75, r_{65\text{-}74} = 0.83$

The figures point to the possibility that if there is a causal connection between fats and breast cancer, that is more likely to exist in the younger age groups.

The regression line for sugar consumption and breast cancer mortality in the 65–74 age group is shown in Figure 6.1.

OECD statistics give sugar consumption in considerable detail: refined sugar, syrup, molasses, glucose, honey and maple sugar being listed as separate items. This made it possible to evaluate whether breast cancer was associated only with refined sugar (incriminated by Yudkin[26] as one of the root causes of ills in prosperous society) or all items with high sucrose content. The highest correlation with breast cancer mortality in older women obtained when all substances with a high sucrose content were included in sugar consumption in the proportion of their sucrose content. This is 80 per cent for syrup, 60 per cent for molasses, 64 per cent for maple sugar and 75 per cent for honey. This is how the sugar consumption figures in Table 6.1 were obtained. The only problematic item is glucose, the effect of which, according to our statistical analysis, is equivalent to twice its weight in sucrose. However, glucose consumption, as a separate item, is available for only a few OECD countries and, in any case, our statistical analysis should be confirmed by other observers before it can be set up as an observation of general validity. Hence glucose consumption in the case of the few countries, in the statistics of which it appeared as a separate item, was added to sugar consumption as equivalent to an equal weight of sucrose.

Even more important than the factual finding is the question whether it is possible to suggest a mechanism of interaction between sugar consumption and carcinogenesis specifically in the female breast.

Figure 6.1: Breast Cancer Mortality in the 65-75 Age Group and Sugar Consumption

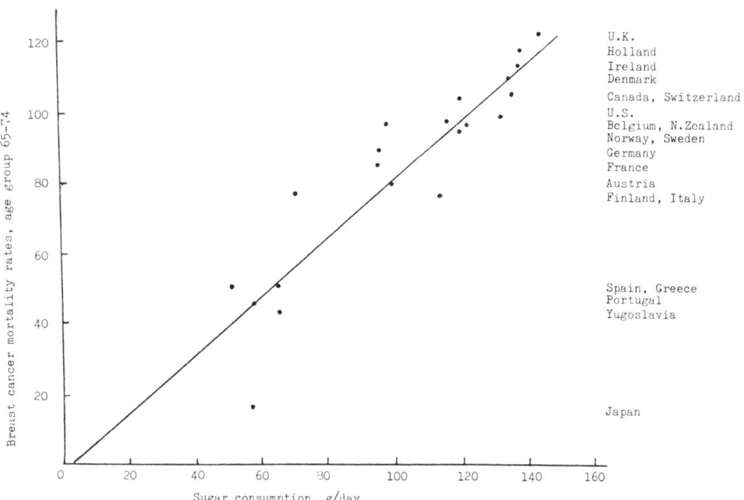

The probable connecting link between sugar and breast cancer is insulin. The growth and development of the various tissues of the female breast, and that of the breast as a whole, is dependent on several hormones, notably on insulin secreted by the pancreas and thyroxine secreted by the thyroid as well as on oestrogens and on pituitary lactogenic hormones. Mammary tumours, at least initially, are probably just as dependent on insulin as on female sex hormones. In experimental animals such tumours tend to regress if the insulin-secreting capacity of the pancreas is destroyed by streptozotocin.[27]

Insulin is produced by the pancreas in response to the rise in the level of blood sugar (glucose). The lay public is apt to think of insulin as an enzyme necessary for the digestion of sugar. In fact, it is more like a ration card. Remember, an age of plenty is a new development in biological history. The animal body has been designed for the more usual condition of seasonal variation in food supply, with periods of starvation interspersed with easier availability of food. The rationing of some key commodities, notably glucose, is presumably meant to ensure that in lean seasons vital and irreplaceable organs or tissues have first claim on the available supply, while less essential organs, if necessary, have to starve. The rationing system works by the pancreas monitoring blood glucose level and secreting insulin into the circulation accordingly. The highest priority tissues, like the brain, blood corpuscles, some cells in the intestinal mucosa, can draw glucose from the blood in the absence of insulin, some only in its presence, and low priority tissues may require a higher insulin level than those fulfilling more important functions.

The female breast is a low priority tissue. Its development can take place when food is plentiful. In periods of starvation its growth can come to a complete standstill or even regress without harm to the animal. Hence the insulin dependence of its tissues. It may be noted that rationing by insulin is so rigorous in the body that if the pancreas fails, as in diabetes, blood glucose runs to waste by being excreted by the kidneys rather than taken up by starving tissues in the absence of insulin.

While an overabundant dietary supply of sugar is an unnatural condition, within limits the body can deal with the situation. Notably the liver and other tissues, particularly muscles, can convert glucose into glycogen and store it for later use. Glycogen is a polysaccharide, composed of a large number of glucose molecules. Adipose tissue can convert glucose into fat which is another stable commodity. Difficulties seem to arise mainly in connection with the immediate response to the appearance of a large quantity of glucose in the bloodstream. Converting the surplus into a storable form takes time, while the body cannot tolerate more than a certain level of glucose in the blood. The magnitude of the problem depends primarily on the composition of dietary sugar.

Plants produce sugars in a variety of forms, consisting of one, two or more sugar molecules. One of the most important forms from our point of view is sucrose, a disaccharide, consisting of a glucose and a fructose molecule. The digestive system separates the two, and their absorption from the intestine follows two different pathways. The absorption of glucose is facilitated by the availability of sodium, a glucose molecule and a sodium molecule together being taken through the intestinal epithelium by a transport protein. In the presence of sodium the transport of glucose is rapid. Once absorbed, no further metabolic work is needed on glucose, the body can utilise it as such. The passage of fructose through the intestinal epithelium is slower and it does not need sodium for its transport. Its utilisation in the body can follow different pathways, notably it can be converted into glucose, or can be metabolised through a pathway which does not include glucose and permits utilisation by tissue cells without insulin.

The digestion of polysaccharides is a more complicated process, involving several steps which first break them into oligosaccharides and ultimately into monosaccharides. The body can synthesise fats from glucose, but the first and foremost uses of glucose is for energy production. What petrol is to the car engine, glucose is to the animal body. It is obviously not toxic, but it poses the problem that its concentration in the blood has to be kept within narrow limits.

The importance of this point is best illustrated by an example. In the mammary glands of all mammals (with the sole exception of the sea-lion) molecules of glucose, with the aid of various enzymes and co-enzymes, are converted into another, slightly different monosaccharide, galactose. This, with the aid of further enzymes, is combined with another molecule of glucose to form the disaccharide lactose. The digestive system of the infant goes through the same process in reverse, to obtain ultimately two molecules of glucose. The purpose in these manoeuvres would be difficult to understand if it were not for the necessity of interposing some barrier between the dietary intake of glucose and its appearance in the blood stream. If the intake is in a form which has to undergo transformation before it can be utilised, the organ performing the transformation, namely the liver, can act as a regulator, delaying the conversion until new supplies are needed. If milk contained glucose, no regulator would stand between its appearance in the intestine and its absorption straight into the bloodstream.

In this light the risk of excess sucrose consumption lies in the fact that its glucose fraction, constituting 50 per cent of the intake, is absorbed too quickly and may lead to an undesirably high level of blood glucose. This throws an unnatural function on the pancreas: instead of rationing a scarce commodity, it has to force excess glucose on low priority tissues. Even then the system has so many safeguards that serious ill effects rarely arise, unless sugar consumption is abnormally high or until in old age the system begins to falter and the various regulators involved in the process begin to fail in their duties. Under such conditions it is conceivable that excessive sugar consumption may lead to the hypertrophy of the breast, involving an increased cancer risk.

A particularly ill-judged development in the food industry in the comparatively recent past was the marketing of glucose syrup, used in place of sugar mainly in the manufacture of confectionery and similar products. As already pointed out, only half of the sucrose intake is glucose and only the glucose function is absorbed in an uncontrolled manner. If sugar is replaced by glucose, the risk is doubled.

The countries where glucose consumption is an appreciable part of the total sugar consumption, are the UK, Holland, Ireland, Germany and France. In the UK and in Holland glucose consumption is about 10 per cent of the total sugar consumption, in Ireland 8 per cent, in Germany 5 per cent, in France 4 per cent. The fact that the three countries with the highest glucose consumption occupy the first three places in the league tables of breast cancer, is in itself enough to tell a story.

As already mentioned earlier in this chapter, other hormones beside sex hormones and insulin participate in regulating the growth, development and functioning of the breast. One is growth hormone, secreted by the pituitary, another is thyroxine, secreted by the thyroid. As the thyroid is under pituitary control, both of these hormones are ultimately regulated by the pituitary. The effect of thyroxine is somewhat similar to insulin: it has a calorigenic action by the regulation of oxygen uptake by various tissues. It has a controlling action on the general level of energy use in the body. Hypothyroidism results in a slowing down of biological activity, mental retardation, dwarfism; hyperthyroidism results in excitability, overactivity, increased body temperature. It seems a possibility that abundant nutrition in prosperous countries has an effect on thyroxine output and in conjunction with insulin it may have a promoting effect on some forms of carcinogenesis. It does not seem possible to connect this effect with total calorie intake or specific items of diet. The only piece of shadowy evidence that I can suggest was mentioned in the previous chapter. Thyroid hormones control iodine and the diet is iodine-deficient in some parts of the world. In prosperous countries this was corrected by the addition of iodine to salt, in consequence of which normal iodine intake in these countries is about three times that necessary for thyroid function. Plants of the cabbage family produce thiocyanate, a substance which impedes the utilisation of iodine by the thyroid, hence, in bygone days, was a goitrogen. The apparent anti-carcinogenic action of vegetables of the cabbage family could be a pointer to the cancer-promoting effect of abundant thyroxine.

The Prostate

Cancer of the prostate is one of the most common neoplasms in men, accounting for about 10 per cent of male cancer deaths in Western countries. It is an old age disease, death rarely occurs from this cause

Table 6.2: Comparison of Mortality from Prostatic and Breast Cancer

Age Groups	25–34	35–44	45–54	55–64	65–74	Over 75
Breast cancer	3.9	23.4	67.3	97.8	122.3	182.9
Prostate cancer	—	0.1	2.2	18.4	89.1	298.3

before 40 and mortality is low before 60. From then onward, however, the rise of mortality with increasing age is the highest in all cancers. It is interesting to compare, for example, mortality in various age groups between prostatic cancer and breast cancer. The figures for England and Wales in 1980 are shown in Table 6.2 and graphically in Figure 6.2.

Figure 6.2: Breast and Prostatic Cancer Mortality Rates per 100,000 Living Population of the Same Age Group in England and Wales in 1980

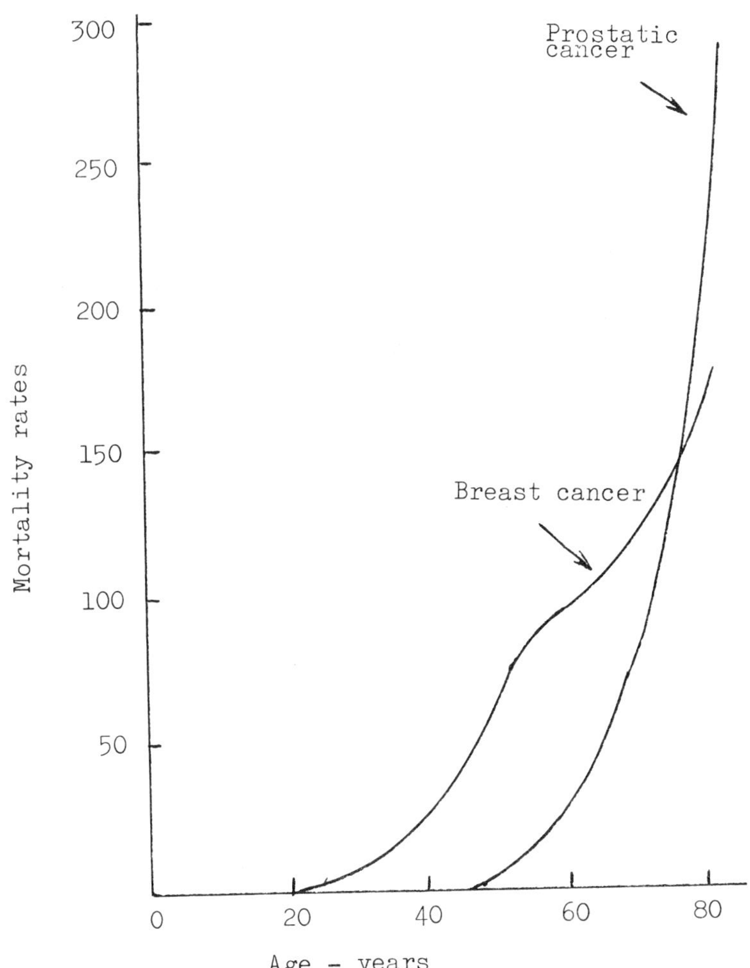

Another peculiarity of prostatic cancer is its long latency. Small latent (or silent) carcinomas are often found at autopsy in younger men. A survey on men over 44 years of age[28] found a latency rate of 20 per cent on autopsy. Possibly carcinogenesis in this case involves two sets of causative influences, one responsible for the original microscopic foci, and the other causing these, two decades later, to develop into invasive and metastasising carcinomas.

Prostatic tissue is just as much under hormonal control as the breast, and prostatic cancer can be checked by castration or by the administration of oestrogens. Hence prostatic cancer is obviously a hormone-related disease. Efforts of finding differences in the androgen level of prostatic cancer patients, however, have so far been unsuccessful. It was found, for example, that the plasma concentration of testosterone, dihydrotestosterone and androstene-3,17-dione were the same in men with benign hypertrophy of the prostate and with prostatic carcinoma.[29] The correlation with sexual activity seems more positive. For instance, interviews with prostatic cancer patients by Steele *et al.*[30] indicated a more frequent past history of venereal disease than reported by matched controls. A later study[31] found a more frequent history of venereal disease, higher coital frequency and more sexual partners in cases than in controls. It may appear paradoxical that a disease associated with sexual activity and male sex hormones takes it toll at an age of diminished hormone production and sexual function. The presumable explanation is the long latent period of the disease.

A negative correlation has been noted between prostatic cancer and cirrhosis of the liver.[32] Latent prostatic carcinomas found at autopsy in men who died from other causes were three times more frequent than in those dying from cirrhosis. The presumable connection between prostatic cancer and cirrhosis of the liver is due to hyper-oestrogenaemia induced by the latter condition.

The geographical distribution of prostatic cancer bears some similarity to that of breast cancer. Generally, where mortality in women from breast cancer is high, mortality from prostatic cancer in men is likely to be similarly high. There are a few exceptional cases, notably the very high mortality from prostatic cancer in American blacks, who are probably the world leaders. In comparison with breast cancer, prostatic cancer mortality is also exceptionally high in Scandinavian countries, notably Norway, Sweden and Denmark. Table 6.3 shows mortality rates of breast cancer and prostatic cancer in OECD countries in the 65-74 age group. The two are fairly close numerically in many countries.

Table 6.3: Mortality Rates from Breast Cancer and Prostatic Cancer in the 65–74 Age Group

Country	Mortality per 100,000 from		Country	Mortality per 100,000 from	
	Breast cancer	Prostate cancer		Breast cancer	Prostate cancer
Australia	90.9	105.4	Italy	75.2	77.0
Austria	88.3	109.7	Japan	18.2	19.0
Belgium	105.6	119.7	Norway	86.6	136.1
Denmark	128.8	129.1	N. Zealand	116.7	95.8
Canada	104.8	97.7	Portugal	60.4	101.1
Finland	66.0	98.8	Spain	49.3	87.6
France	82.1	101.3	Sweden	90.6	127.7
Germany	93.1	109.5	Switzerland	107.7	113.9
Holland	107.8	117.8	UK	122.3	89.1
Ireland	103.3	105.4	US	98.9	105.5
			Yugoslavia	53.0	68.5

The connection between prostatic cancer and the diet is indicated by the usual observations on immigrants or the great differences in mortality between ethnically related people living in different countries. Mortality from prostatic cancer in American blacks, for example, is six times as high as in those in Nigeria. Mortality in Japanese living in Hawaii is much higher than those living in Japan, though still only half the US rate.

In spite of the similarity between breast cancer and prostatic cancer mortality, the correlation of the latter with the two dietary items associated with breast cancer, sugar and animal fats, is poor. The correlation coefficient in the 65–74 age group with sugar consumption is 0.57, with animal fats 0.66. The possible reason for the difference is that in breast cancer hormonal and dietary effects separate in various age groups, whereas in prostatic cancer they are probably intermixed at all ages and mask each other's influence. Even allowing for these circumstances the correlation coefficient of 0.66 between fat consumption and prostatic cancer mortality is too low to assume causal connection between them, even if the possibility should not be excluded.

Several reports in the past have called attention to the possible connection between cadmium and prostatic cancer. Workers in industries involving cadmium exposure, like welding, electroplating, the production of alkaline batteries, are at an elevated risk of prostatic cancer.[33] The possible reason suggested by Greenwald[34] is that cadmium is a zinc antagonist. The normal prostate gland has a very high zinc content and zinc deficiency may have an adverse effect on it. The main source of cadmium in the diet is probably soft water passing through metal pipes.

References

1. DeWaard, F., Baanders van Halewijn, E.A. and Hurzinga, J. 'The Bimodal Age Distribution of Patients with Mammary Carcinoma. Evidence for the Existence of Two Types of Human Breast Cancer', *Cancer* (1964), *17*, 141-51.
2. Siiteri, P.K., Schwarz, B.E. and MacDonald, P.C. 'Estrogen Receptors and the Estrone Hypothesis in Relationship to Endometrial and Breast Cancer', *Gynecological Oncology* (1974), *2*, 228-38.
3. MacMahon, B., Cole, P., Brown, J.B. *et al.* 'Urine Oestrogen Profiles of Asian and North American Women', *International Journal of Cancer* (1974), *14*, 161-7.
4. Rudale, G., Apiou, F. and Muel, B. 'Mammary Cancer Produced in Mice by Estriol', *European Journal of Cancer* (1975), *11*, 39-45.
5. Bulbrook, R.D., Moore, J.W., Clark, G.M.G. *et al.* 'Plasma Oestradiol and Progesterone Levels in Women with Varying Degrees of Risk of Breast Cancer', *European Journal of Cancer* (1978), *14*, 1369-75.
6. Cole, P., Cramer, D., Yen, S. *et al.* 'Estrogen Profiles of Premenopausal Women with Breast Cancer', *Cancer Research* (1978), *38*, 745-8.
7. Siiteri, P.K. 'Extraglandular Estrogen Formation and Serum Binding of Estradiol: Relationship to Cancer', *Journal of Endocrinology* (1981), *89* Suppl., 119-29.
8. Hill, P., Wynder, E.L., Helman, P. *et al.* 'Plasma Hormone Levels in Different Ethnic Populations of Women', *Cancer Research* (1976), *36*, 2297-301.
9. Bulbrook, R.D. 'Urinary Androgen Excretion and the Etiology of Breast Cancer', *Journal of the National Cancer Institute* (1972), *46*, 1039-42.
10. Thomas, D.B. 'Role of Exogenous Female Hormones in Altering the Risk of Benign and Malignant Neoplasms in Humans', *Cancer Research* (1978), *38*, 3991-4000.
11. Vessey, M.P., Doll, R., Jones, K. *et al.* 'An Epidemiological Study of Oral Contraceptives and Breast Cancer', *British Medical Journal* (1979), *1*, 1755-8.
12. Hoover, R., Gray, L.A., Cole, P. *et al.* 'Menopausal Estrogens and Breast Cancer', *New England Journal of Medicine* (1976), *295*, 401-5.
13. Bibbo, M. 'Progress Report', *National Institute of Child Health and Human Development* (1977).
14. Carroll, K.K. and Khor, H.T. 'Dietary Fat in Relation to Tumorigenesis', *Progress in Biochemistry and Pharmacology* (1975), *10*, 308-53.
15. Hopkins, G.J. and Carroll, K.K. 'Relationship Between Amount and Type of Dietary Fat in Promotion of Mammary Carcinogenesis Induced by 7,12-dimethyl-benz(a)-anthracene', *Journal of the National Cancer Institute* (1979), *62*, 1009-12.
16. Armstrong, B. and Doll, R. 'Environmental Factors and Cancer Incidence and Mortality in Different Countries with Special Reference to Dietary Practice', *International Journal of Cancer* (1975), *15*, 617-31.
17. Wynder, E.L. 'Nutrition and Cancer', *Federal Proceedings* (1976), *35*, 1309-15.

18. Wynder, E.L. 'Dietary Factors Related to Breast Cancer', *Cancer* (1980), *46*, 899–904.
19. Ross, M.H. and Bras, G. 'Influence of Protein Over and Undernutrition on Spontaneous Tumor Prevalence in the Rat', *Journal of Nutrition* (1973), *103*, 944–7.
20. McSheehey, T.W. 'The Onset of Mammary Adenocarcinoma in Mice: A Possible Correlation with Nutrition', *Ecology of Food and Nutrition* (1974), *3*, 147.
21. Gaskill, S.E., McGuire, W.L., Osborne, C.K. and Stern, M.P. 'Breast Cancer Mortality and Diet in the United States', *Cancer Research* (1979), *39*, 3628–37.
22. Maruchi, N., Aoki, S., Tsuda, K. *et al.* 'Relation of Food Consumption to Cancer Mortality in Japan with Special Reference to International Figures', *Gann* (1977), *68*, 1.
23. Seely, S. and Horrobin, D.F. 'Diet and Breast Cancer: the Possible Connection with Sugar Consumption', *Medical Hypotheses* (1983), *11*, 319–27.
24. World Health Organisation. *World Health Statistics Annuals, 1981*, Geneva (1982).
25. Organisation of Economic Cooperation and Development. *Food Consumption Statistics 1964–1978*, Paris (1981).
26. Yudkin, J. 'Sugar and Ischaemic Heart Disease', *Practitioner* (1967), *198*, 680–3.
27. Shafie, S.M., Cho-Chung, Y.S. and Gullino, P.M. 'Cyclic Adenosine Monophosphate and Protein Kinase Activity in Insulin-dependent and Independent Mammary Tumors', *Cancer Research* (1979), *39*, 2501.
28. Breslow, N., Chan, C.W., Dhom, G. *et al.* 'Latent Carcinoma of the Prostate at Autopsy in Seven Areas', *International Journal of Cancer* (1977), *20*, 680–8.
29. Habib, F.K., Lee, I.R., Stitch, S.R. and Smith, P.H. 'Androgen Levels in the Plasma and Prostatic Tissues of Patients with Benign Hypertrophy and Carcinoma of the Prostate', *Journal of Endocrinology* (1976), *71*, 99–107.
30. Steele, R., Lees, R.E. and Kraus, A.S. 'Sexual Factors in the Epidemiology of Cancer of the Prostate', *Journal of Chronic Diseases* (1971), *24*, 29–37.
31. Krain, L.S. 'Some Epidemiologic Variables in Prostatic Carcinoma in California', *Preventive Medicine* (1974), *3*, 154–9.
32. Robson, M.C. 'Cirrhosis and Prostatic Neoplasms', *Geriatrics* (1966), *21*, 150–4.
33. Kolonel, L. and Winkelstein, W. Jr. 'Cadmium and Prostate Carcinoma', *Lancet* (1977), *2*, 566–7.
34. Greenwald, P. 'Prostate' in D. Schottenfeld and J.F. Fraumeni (eds.) *Epidemiology and Prevention* (Saunders, Philadelphia, 1982).

7 FOOD ALLERGY AND FOOD INTOLERANCE

D.L.J. Freed

Introduction

It would not be unreasonable to paraphrase the British Government health warnings on cigarette packs, and state that 'Food Can Seriously Damage Your Health!' I mean specific foods to which the unlucky individual happens to be sensitive. Bread, for example, is poison to the coeliac patient. Milk causes colic, flatulence and diarrhoea if drunk by a person who lacks the appropriate intestinal enzyme (lactase). A helping of broad beans (or even a dose of aspirin) can induce an attack of acute haemolytic anaemia in a person whose red blood cells lack the protective enzyme glucose-6-phosphate dehydrogenase. This illness is called 'favism'. Such reactions to foods are sometimes called 'food allergy', but this word may not be entirely appropriate. We shall discuss the precise meaning of the word allergy below. First we must consider the more general questions of food intolerance.

Does Specific Food Intolerance Exist?

Some children have an attack of asthma every time they eat eggs. The slightest trace of egg, even when hidden as a trace additive in puddings or cakes, may be sufficient to set off an attack, or even – in the most sensitive individuals of all – entering a room in which eggs have recently been beaten. Since exposure to eggs by these children is always followed by the illness, it is no coincidence. Conventionally, doctors require evidence that the illness has followed 'challenge' with the food on three separate occasions before accepting that coincidence has been ruled out (the Bellman's rule*). But can we rule out the patient's expectations? If, through past experience, a child has learned that

* Just the place for a snark! I have said it twice;
    That alone should encourage the crew
Just the place for a snark! I have said it thrice;
    What I tell you three times is true!

The Hunting of the Snark: Lewis Carroll

eating eggs always causes asthma, and then he is made to eat a cake and told that it contains egg (even if it does not), he may have an attack through Pavlovian reflex. This deceitful experiment has occasionally been done, and gleefully interpreted by sceptics to mean that asthma is 'all in the mind'. Of course that reasoning is fallacious, but in order to be sure that the outcome of challenge is not influenced by the patient's (or the doctor's) expectations, challenges should be done *double-blind*. The test food or drink is disguised, by mixing it into a flavoursome stew, or by giving it by stomach tube or in an opaque capsule, and consumed when both patient and medical attendants are ignorant of what the challenge contains. On other occasions an inert placebo is administered by the same route (though exactly what one can use as a truly inert placebo causes much difficulty – what about the flavouring of the stew, or the colouring pigment in the capsules?)

Many cases that satisfy the criterion of repeated provocation by double-blind challenge have been reported.[1–6] Coeliac disease is a classic example. Yes, specific food intolerance exists. The case histories given below are intended to give only a brief glimpse of an extraordinarily varied group of illnesses.

Case Histories

Case 1

A woman of 40 came to me with a long history of migraine. Since the age of 14 she had had several attacks of classic migraine, with severe one-sided throbbing headache, nausea and vomiting, and a strange visual disturbance in which she saw a shimmering pattern like castle walls dancing before her eyes ('teichopsia' or 'fortification spectra'). These attacks would last for between one and three days, and in between she was quite well. Fortunately the attacks only came once in every few months, so did not seriously interfere with her lifestyle. However, six weeks before coming to see me, she and her husband had entertained a foreign visitor at their home for a few days, during which time she had imbibed a good deal more alcohol than was her wont. She then had a very severe attack of migraine, with a lot of ill-defined malaise also, and since then she had been feeling constantly wretched with the illness. She could not go to work or attend to her family.

Over the years she had noted that attacks seemed to be triggered by sugar, alcohol, chocolate, and possibly by milk, onions and fatty fried foods. She had given up smoking at the age of 27. Since her acute flareup six weeks previously she had also found that she could not stomach coffee or the slightest trace of alcohol. Several close family members suffered from coeliac disease, so the concept of elimination dieting was familiar to her. She denied using the contraceptive pill.

On further questioning she considered it likely that she was addicted to bread, since whenever she went for a day without this food she felt a craving for it. She also had a craving for rich fatty foods, though she tried to avoid them for the sake of her figure (not very successfully; she was fighting a losing battle against encroaching obesity).

As well as the migraine, she had also suffered from hay fever since the age of 18.

Blood tests showed that she had a high concentration of IgE antibodies against grass pollen, a lower level of anti-wheat IgE antibodies, and a low but still significant level of IgE anti-mik antibodies (for discussion of IgE see p. 229).

I recommended a wheat-free, milk/meat-free diet, and after a week or so of this she began to feel better, though not entirely. On her own initiative she then began to avoid several other basic foodstuffs, without much benefit, though she felt that she became worse when she tried them again. When she returned some weeks later she was still rather ill, and now on a dangerously inadequate diet. Although she had lost some weight, she was deeply depressed and confessed that her constant illness (and her extreme diet) was placing her marriage under strain, and ruining her social life and that of her husband.

On this occasion she was seen not by me but by a female colleague at the clinic. To this lady doctor the patient now admitted that she was using the contraceptive pill. Since this is a well-known migraine trigger, my colleague had no hesitation in advising that she stop using the pill immediately and adopt a different mode of contraception. At the same time she advised that the patient's diet would have to be made less strict, for the sake of her health and her family, and arranged an appointment with the hospital dietitian.

Once the patient gave up using the pill, her constant feeling of illness departed completely and her depression lifted. She now cautiously experimented with items of diet, and discovered to her delight that she could tolerate many foods that she had previously been avoiding. She now takes a healthy balanced diet that includes all fish and shellfish, rice, potatoes and all pulses. She still has to avoid wheat and rye, corn, milk, chocolate, coconut and citrus fruits. She takes meats sparingly. On this regimen she is completely well.

This case can be reasonably described as a food allergy since the positive tests for IgE antibodies offer presumptive evidence of an immunological causation (see p. 226). The case also illustrates the additive roles of the contraceptive pill, and the alcoholic binge that precipitated her severe acute illness – not to mention the potential dangers of unsupervised dietary exclusions by partly-informed laymen.

Case 2

An unmarried girl of 24 had had catarrh every day, worse in winter months ever since an attack of glandular fever at the age of 19. The 'catarrh' consisted of thick mucus in the nose, which fell backward into the throat so that she had to swallow continually. She had some sneezing, but only in isolated attacks separated by several days. Every night her nose became completely blocked while she slept, sometimes waking her from sleep. She had episodes of deafness in one or the other ear, and she often had pains in the face suggestive of sinus inflammation. As a youngster she had had many and repeated attacks of tonsillitis, although (unusually) the tonsils had not been removed. She had never used the contraceptive pill.

On skin testing, she had the expected strong reaction to the house-dust mite but to nothing else. Her blood tests for IgE antibodies were uniformly negative. The apparent diagnosis was allergy to the house-dust mite, the routine treatment for which would normally either be sodium cromoglycate or a steroid, either or both to be given in the form of a nasal spray.

On questioning her about diet, I asked her what foods she really craved. She answered after careful thought, that there were none. I asked if there were any foods or drinks in her normal diet that she would feel really deprived of, if I said she had to avoid them. Again, she thought carefully and stated that she could easily give up anything I asked her to. I then asked specifically how much milk she would normally drink. Looking puzzled, she answered that she normally took about a pint-and-a-half of liquid milk daily, plus plenty of yoghurt and cheese; she considered this quite normal. In fact, an intake of that amount of milk is rare among adults in the UK (in spite of the advertising campaigns by the Milk Marketing Board) and I told her I considered milk to be a likely influence in her case. I was by no means sure of this, and told her so, but asked her nevertheless to stop taking milk and milk products for four weeks, just as an experiment.

She did as I asked, and was surprised to discover that she now had a very real craving for the substance. She was equally surprised to discover that within a week her catarrh dried up completely and she became completely well. She has remained well except for two occasions, when on holiday or attending a social function she took some milk or a food containing it; on both occasions her catarrh returned for a few days. Like the lady in Case 1, she is delighted by her new slim figure.

This case cannot strictly be described as an allergy, since both the skin test and the blood test for anti-milk antibodies were negative. If she has an allergy at all, it is to the house-dust mite. Nevertheless the crystal-clear association between milk ingestion and the illness makes this a probable case of cow's milk intolerance. The case also illustrates how careful a dietary history has to be, since there were no obvious clues in it – she denied any cravings, addictions, or indeed aversions, and thought that a daily milk intake of one-and-a-half pints was the norm. It is likely that a small dose of milk would indeed do her no harm, but her appetite for it is such that she would prefer not to have any than to tempt herself with small doses.

Case 3

A male doctor aged 39 complained of 'rheumatism', especially in the right knee, for about a year. On rising in the mornings his whole body felt aching and stiff, and all his major joints felt 'as if they were jigging with constant electric tingles'; however on sitting down to breakfast of a cup of tea and slice of toast these feelings slowly evaporated and he was able to function. Nevertheless, the right knee caused him pain throughout the day, so severe that he had to go up and down stairs on step at a time, like a toddler learning to walk. Blood tests for rheumatoid disease were negative, as were the joint X rays.

Being reluctant to embark on a lifetime of drugs, this patient began to read the popular paperback literature about arthritis and rheumatism, and found one book that explained the rudiments of food allergy. He could not think of any item or items of food to which he was addicted, or for which he had a craving, or indeed any aversions. But his wife pointed out that he had a 'thing' about peanuts and peanut butter. Although he did not eat these every day, he always made sure that there were some in the house. He never noticed if the Cornflakes packet was empty or the potatoes nearly gone, but well before the peanut butter jar was exhausted he would stroll out and buy some more. He was indeed quite an expert on different textures and types of peanut butter, and liked to be able to offer guests a choice. When she pointed this behaviour out to him, he denied the implication hotly, with vigour and scorn; he simply liked the stuff, he maintained, nothing more than that. Such was the vehemence of the denial that his wife retreated under the attack, and subsequently remained silent on the topic.

After more months of suffering, and much agonised introspection, the patient grudgingly conceded that he was indeed addicted, and voluntarily stopped consuming peanuts and peanut butter. At the same time he stopped taking bread, since his paperback had stated that wheat was a common trigger factor for arthritis. He found it extraordinarily difficult to keep up the diet, not only because of his craving but because of uncharacteristic lapses of memory. He would 'come to' to find himself standing at the kitchen cupboard with his teaspoon embedded in the peanut butter jar, having wandered absent-mindedly there while thinking of something else, totally forgetting about his diet. It took several weeks to discipline his mind so that these lapses stopped. Within a week after his last taste of peanuts or bread, he noticed to his astonishment that the pains in his knee were less, and the morning stiffness had quietly disappeared. After another two months, the rheumatism had virtually disappeared.

He methodically 'challenged' himself with peanuts. A 'small' (four ounce) helping caused no trouble, but a four ounce helping *daily for four days* brought on unmistakeable morning stiffness. Three slices of bread, on one day only, brought back the 'electric tingles' and stiffness, with reappearance of the knee pain. One slice of bread, on one day only, caused no symptoms. Because of the long timescale involved – two months to improve, several days to relapse – he has not attempted more rigorous, or blinded, challenges.

This case illustrates the fact that food addictions can disguise themselves just as thoroughly as alcohol addictions can, so that the sufferer himself is totally unaware of his abnormal need. The clue is provided by the excessive denials, when the possibility is suggested. In some cases the patient becomes deeply suspicious of those who mention his habit, even approaching paranoia. The case also illustrates the fact that sometimes there are no clues at all. This man gave up bread easily and without any cravings or problems, yet that was the more severe of his two dietary triggers.

Case 4

A married woman of 34 developed a distressing cough when about half way through her second pregnancy. After a few weeks of unsuccessful treatment by her general practitioner she was referred to a chest specialist in hospital, and very thoroughly investigated but without any cause being found. The cough persisted and now became associated with tightness of the chest and wheezing. A diagnosis of 'asthma, unknown cause' was made, and the appropriate medicated inhaler was prescribed, which controlled the symptoms adequately though not entirely. This state of affairs continued for the rest of the pregnancy, and gradually waned and disappeared a few months after the birth of the child. However, in the years that followed she found that whenever she caught a cold, the asthma returned and lingered for several weeks after the other symptoms had cleared up. It could also be triggered by inhaling paint fumes or other powerful smells.

A dietary enquiry disclosed an addiction to coffee. The amount consumed was not excessive – perhaps 4 or 5 cups daily – but she drank coffee daily and became distressed and scornful when the suggestion of addiction was made. Like the patient in Case 3, she strongly denied any possible connection between coffee and the asthma – after all, she pointed out, she had been drinking it for years, she did not get asthma every day, and anyway she knew what the triggers were (pregnancy, fumes and catching colds). However, I pressed her on this point on several separate visits, and eventually she reluctantly agreed to try coffee exclusion. After two days of this she had severe migraine for the first time in her life, and became very depressed. However, she persisted with coffee avoidance and by the end of the first week the withdrawal syndrome had abated. After a few weeks she cautiously tried drinking coffee again, and found to her relief that it caused no trouble. She returned to coffee drinking. Alas, she caught another cold, and the asthma returned in force. After a fortnight of this she stopped coffee again, and the asthma departed within 24 hours. Thereafter she noticed on three separate occasions that if she gave in to temptation and drank coffee *at a time when she was also in the early stages of catching a cold*, asthma inevitably followed. If she drank coffee at other times, or if she caught a cold but did not take coffee, there was no asthma. Curiously, she eventually developed a strong psychological aversion to coffee, even though she still finds the flavour and odour appetising. A subsequent pregnancy was uneventful.

This case illustrates the concept, borrowed from bacteriology, of 'opportunist pathogens'. Ordinarily harmless triggers, like pregnancy, paint fumes, or catching a cold, became capable of causing asthma only when she took coffee as well. None of these factors caused asthma unless she was also taking coffee. This phenomenon, in which two or more factors are required to act simultaneously before an effect is seen, is technically termed *synergism*. One needs to be quite lucky to identify these cases, though they are possibly very common.

This woman breast-fed her baby for several months. For the first few months, while she was still taking her daily coffee, the baby slept very little and cried incessantly while awake, refusing to be comforted. When she stopped taking coffee, the baby's behaviour and sleeping improved dramatically.

Case 5

Drs R. Finn and H.N. Cohen, in Liverpool, reported the case[4] of a man of 20 who complained of recurrent severe pains in the lower left abdomen, raising the suspicion of inflammatory bowel disease. However, thorough investigations failed to show a cause for the pains. On careful questioning they wondered whether the man's tea intake – about 10 cups a day – might be implicated. In hospital they put a thin tube into his stomach via the nose, ten times. On five occasions they injected water down the tube. On five occasions they administered cold tea. The order of the 'challenges' was randomised, and neither patient nor doctors knew on any one occasion whether tea or water was being given. Each time the challenge was tea, the patient experienced distressing palpitations and *the following day* had his typical abdominal pains. This never happened when the challenge was of water.

These two doctors were the first in the UK to use double-blind challenges for the diagnosis of food intolerances, thus proving the existence of the phenomenon beyond doubt and raising the possibility that *many* illnesses of unknown causation *might* be caused by it. In a brilliant series of studies they showed that symptoms as varied as palpitations, agoraphobia, nausea, constipation and chronic mouth ulcers were all caused by various common foods or drinks *in some patients* but not all. In the same year, 1978, Dr P.D. Buisseret, of London, reported[5] a series of no fewer than 79 children who had been ill as a result of cow's milk intolerance (as demonstrated by the Bellman's Criterion of three repeated relapses after three repeated challenges). The symptoms commonly caused were asthma, rhinitis (mainly blocked nose), eczema, abdominal pains, diarrhoea and vomiting. In several cases the pains came on shortly after a normal breakfast of cereal (with milk, of course) and had been commonly interpreted by parents and teachers as a variety of school phobia. Of these children 33 per cent had psychological or behavioural abnormalities which cleared up when milk was eliminated from their diets.

All of these cases show one central curiosity, that is, that food intolerance usually develops at some time after birth (sometimes even in the sixth decade of life and later), in people who had previously eaten or drunk that foodstuff for many years without any trouble.

Very occasionally babies are found who were apparently intolerant or allergic to a food at birth, having been sensitised in the womb, but this apparently is the exception. von Pirquet (see below) considered this element of *change* crucial for the definition of the word 'allergy'; ' "Allos" ', he wrote, 'implies deviation from the original state, from the behaviour of the normal individual'. In immunological terms, one or more sensitising doses are always required before allergy can occur. In toxicological terms, one may postulate a gradual accumulation of some mildly poisonous dietary component that does not reveal its toxicity by any obvious illnesses, or indeed in every person.

What Diseases are Caused by Food Intolerance?

No disease is *always* caused by food intolerance but a large number of diseases are *sometimes* caused by it. Take a look at the book rack in any health food store. Numerous books will be found extolling the virtues of this or that diet for hay fever, urticaria (hives), eczema, migraine, asthma, arthritis, rheumatism, depression, insomnia, excessive sleepiness, irritable bowels, constipation, colitis, lethargy, irritability, mental exhaustion, bad breath and hyperactivity. Some of the conditions you will probably never have heard of. Precisely the same list, curiously, features prominently in other books in the same shop: books that promote acupuncture, hypnosis, meditation, megavitamins, biofeedback, cell therapy and a host of 'fringe' practices. Are all of these claims wrong? No, each method works sometimes, and each method sometimes fails. The body has only a limited repertoire of disease states, and most of these can have more than one cause. Food intolerance is *sometimes* the cause of each of the conditions in this list, and is sometimes not the cause. The syndromes are sometimes bizarre.

New Causes for Old Diseases: Migraine, Irritable Bowel Syndrome

Pain is usually nature's protest against the physical damage of tissues or some harmful interference with biological processes. Like punishment fitting the crime, normally there is a fair degree of correspondence between the intensity of pain and the magnitude of the damage or the harmfulness of the underlying agent. Migraine is the exception. The severity of pains associated with it is out of all proportion to the presumable causes. There is no obvious abnormality connected with migraine. Apart from their periodic headaches, migraine sufferers seem normal and healthy. In fact, a recent survey by Professor W.E. Waters of London University has found that a group of women suffering from migraine lived longer than a corresponding group of non-sufferers.

The word migraine was taken by the French from the latin word hemicranium, to denote one-sided headaches. The term is not entirely appropriate, the headache is usually, but not necessarily one-sided. The French have a special name for the sufferer as well: migraineur.

The worst form of migraine usually begins with visual symptoms: focusing difficulties, flashes of light, an aura, or shimmering effects. The headache is dull to begin with, but becomes severe, of a throbbing quality, later. Most sufferers feel nausea, some vomit, some have diarrhoea – hence the term sick-headache. In the more frequent and somewhat less severe form the visual effects are absent. It is a common disorder – about one in five of the population have or have had it – and some sufferers have it once a week or more. An attack can last a whole day or even longer. In women it is sometimes associated with premenstrual tension or ovulation. The sufferers need rest and are best off if they can go to sleep, although some attacks, paradoxically, begin during sleep.

There are many theories regarding possible causes. Extracranial vasodilation, hence increased blood supply to some parts of the brain was suggested, but so was vasoconstriction, hence inadequate blood supply. Another idea was based on the observation that cheese and chocolates tended to precipitate migraine. Cheese and chocolates, as well as red wine, contain a potentially mildly toxic substance, tyramine, which is also produced by some intestinal bacteria. The most recent suggestion is that migraine could be a diet-related disorder, a form of food intolerance. If this is true we can forget about the blood vessels, and the consequences are important from the practical point of view. It may not be unduly difficult to identify the food items which precipitate attacks, so that even if the explanation is lacking, the sufferer can be given a chance to avoid food items with damaging properties.

Dr J. Egger and colleagues[16] conducted a trial in 1983 at the Institute of Child Health in London, in which 88 young migraineurs (and migrainettes) were put on a spartan diet of only six items: one meat (chicken or lamb), one carbohydrate food (rice or potatoes), one vegetable (cabbage), one fruit (banana or apple), water and vitamin supplements. If at the end of a period of 3 or 4 weeks they were free of migraine, other foods were introduced into their diets one by one, noting the item that caused the reappearance of headaches. If the original basic diet was unsuccessful, another basic diet was tried. By this means it was possible not only to construct a list of food items associated with migraine, but also to evaluate their order of importance, depending on the number of patients responding to a given item. The final list contained 55 items and brought some surprises. The most important items in their correct ranking order were: (1) cow's milk; (2) eggs, (3) chocolates, (4) orange, (5) wheat, (6) benzoic acid, (7) cheese, (8) tomato, (9) tartrazine, (10) rye. Further items were various kinds of meat and fish, tea, coffee, maize, soya beans, peanuts, potatoes, goat's milk. Many fruits and vegetables appear towards the end of the list. The most surprising feature of the list is that the popular suspects, chocolate and cheese, are in the third and seventh place respectively, while some items topping the list, like milk, eggs, orange, wheat, tomato, were unsuspected foods. It may be noted that alcohol was not among the tested items (these patients were considered too young).

The suspicion falling on two food additives, benzoic acid and tartrazine, should be sufficient to bring pressure on the food industry for their withdrawal. Tartrazine is a yellow colouring agent, serving no useful purpose beside its cosmetic effect. Benzoic acid is a preservative which is useful in keeping down bacterial and fungal contamination of food; there are others which could take its place but these might not be any safer.

An interesting observation by Dr Egger and colleagues was that migraine sufferers did not naturally tend to abstain from foods causing their illness, some had a positive craving for them.

These findings constitute substantial evidence in favour of the food intolerance theory and they give migraine sufferers a chance to help themselves by experimenting with their diet. They can try to abstain from three or four suspect items at a time, possibly starting with milk and dairy products. Milk and its products feature predominently in other types of food allergy beside migraine, hence can be regarded as prime suspects. An elimination diet should be kept at least for 3 or 4 weeks and a milkless diet, if possible, should exclude all items containing milk, e.g. chocolates or margarine (the latter usually contains whey).

The finding of Professor Waters[18] that in female migraine sufferers in the 45–64 age group there was lower mortality from all causes than in controls not suffering from migraine, was the subject of much speculation. One suggestion was that the sufferers demanded and received more medical attention than the non-sufferers. Some medications used against migraine (like beta-blockers which have a calming effect) are also used against artery diseases. On the other hand vasoconstrictors (like ergotamine tartrate) have also been tried against migraine. These elevate blood pressure, hence may aggravate artery disease.

There could be a more fundamental explanation, on the assumption that migraine is a food allergy.

Dr J. Ditchfield, in a small-scale survey conducted at Manchester University in 1982, questioned 81 migraine sufferers about their diets. It was found that 27 per cent avoided chocolates and cheese, presumably on account of the propaganda against these items, but more importantly 9 per cent also avoided milk. This was well before the publication of Dr Egger's results. Such instinctive avoidance from an early age may lessen the risk of migraine, but also (more importantly) the risk of eventual death from coronary heart disease (see Chapter 4).

A somewhat related disorder is the so-called irritable bowel syndrome. Likewise a common disorder (the commonest cause for referral to a specialist in gastroenterology), this is characterised by abdominal pains, diarrhoea and/or constipation that sometimes alternate, passage of excessive mucus, and other related symptoms. Many patients also have migraine, or depression, or are excessively anxious. Much work has been done on the pathology of the illness, and it is clear that these patients have a lower threshold for colonic stretching pain than most folk. Many drugs have been tried, with varying success, and most gastroenterologists find irritable bowel syndrome an unrewarding disease to treat and would welcome a simple means to prevent it. By the early 1970s the emerging Fibre Hypothesis had been recruited for use in irritable bowel syndrome, and supplements of wheat bran were recommended on rather limited rationale.

Then in 1982 a group of specialists in Cambridge, UK,[17] reported that an elimination diet avoiding the commonest food provocants – wheat, milk and products, corn, and to some extent tea, coffee, eggs, onions, potatoes, preservatives and citrus fruits – would cure many if not most cases of irritable bowel syndrome, and that the illness could be provoked again by double-blind challenge in most of these. The main body of gastroenterologists in this country have been slow to take up this approach, and in view of the fact that elimination diets cannot be easily prescribed will probably continue to be sceptical, but once again this is largely based on prejudice.

Even more exciting is the suggestion from the Cambridge workers that Crohn's disease will also respond in many instances to the elimination diet approach. Crohn's disease is far from benign; it is a severe form of inflammation that rots away at the intestinal wall and causes much pain and disability. Many patients have sections of intestine removed surgically, as a last resort, and surgery is sometimes complicated by leakage of intestinal contents into the abdominal cavity or even out through the skin. The patient's life is sometimes shortened either by the disease or by its treatment. If the preliminary reports from Cambridge are confirmed, this will be a really exciting breakthrough in medicine.

Returning to migraine and irritable bowel syndrome, many doctors have noted the association of anxiety and depression with these two illnesses. Those who treat them by dietary manoeuvres have frequently noted that as the physical symptoms get better, so do the psychiatric symptoms. This raises the possibility, even to the most unimaginative of medical minds, that classic endogenous depression and or anxiety might also respond to elimination diets, and well-studied cases have indeed been reported in the literature (see Chapter 8).

What Foods Cause Intolerance?

The 'league table' of illness-causing foods in any one country largely reflects the dietary habits of that society. In the UK cow's milk, wheat and other cereal grains, and additives such as chemical preservatives and colourings usually come at the top of the list. Avocado intolerance, on the other hand, is relatively uncommon in the UK (but more common in Israel and California). Goat's milk intolerance is also rather rare in the UK, presumably because goat's milk is a minority enthusiasm, and goat's milk can occasionally be useful for children (though not babies) who are allergic to the cow's variety. Although some foods hardly ever cause intolerance (sago, lamb, pears), there is no such thing as a universally safe food.

Proving Food Intolerance

We have seen that when an illness is reliably provoked, on at least three occasions, by double-blind challenge with a food, that is accepted as proof of food intolerance. But matters are not always so straightforward.

Suppose we were asked to prove, formally, that pregnancy is caused by having sex. The task would not be as easy as we might think. The first problem is that having sex is not *always* followed by pregnancy. A host of other factors are involved. Both partners must be fertile, to begin with, the timing of intercourse must be precise, and many other aspects – nutritional, hormonal, metabolic and perhaps psychological – must also be satisfied. Having sex usually has *no* long-term result, while on the other hand it sometimes gives rise to totally different consequences – one or more venereal diseases, for example. The third problem is the time lapse between the pregnancy and its putative cause – at a distance of possibly several months it is very difficult to trace connections. Let us now suppose, for the sake of the argument, that having sex were only one of the many possible ways of achieving pregnancy; that in a particular woman pregnancy might also be induced, for example, by bicycle riding, eating onions, or reading the works of Proust, and that the chances of becoming pregnant were best if two or more of those activities were indulged in at once. The difficulty of proving *any* connection between sex and pregnancy would be immense. This is the kind of difficulty we face when trying to prove that a particular child's asthma is caused by food intolerance. A definite diagnosis can only be made in cases where the challenges are always positive.

Unfortunately some food sensitivities are variable. One famous case of shellfish allergy was described by Dr R.M. Maulitz and colleagues in 1979,[19] of a marathon runner who had a demonstrable severe allergy to shellfish, but only if he ate them on a day when he had been running. Food challenge was always positive on those days, and negative on other days. Dr D.G. Wraith, of London, describes female patients who are allergic to foods only during the premenstrual period. At other times of the month challenges are negative. Interactions of this type are probably common, but we need to be exceptionally lucky to spot them as in Case 4 above. In such variable sensitivities we can rarely be certain of the diagnosis.

What then of skin tests and blood tests? Alas, all tests can give misleading results. Their only use is to provide clues, when we suspect food intolerance but get no other help from the history and haven't the faintest idea where to start with eliminations. In food intolerance, the proof of the pudding (if proof exists) is in the eating.

Disproving Food Intolerance

All too often the problem is not of isolated episodes of illness, like asthma or urticaria, but of a long-lasting chronic illness that rarely, or never, gets better. Migraine, for example, that afflicts the patient for three days every week, or rheumatism that fills every waking hour with pain and fear. The tantalising hope is that this illness might be entirely curable, cheaply and safely, by a simple change of diet. But then, of course, it might not be. And in any case, *what* change of diet would be needed for this particular patient?

In such circumstances the first requirement is to find out whether *any* dietary manipulation is likely to prove rewarding. If this particular case is never going to respond to dietary manoeuvres, we need to find out sooner and not later.

So the patient is advised to avoid suspect foods. Which foods? Well, does he have a strong *craving* for any particular food or drink? Milk? Coffee? Cheese? What would he feel really deprived of, if he had to avoid it? Many alkaloids and some peptides are addictive, as noted in Chapter 3, so food addiction is a presumptive clue to incomplete digestion of that foodstuff. No clues from the history? Well, avoid *all* foods. Few adults will be damaged by a week on nothing but spring water (tap water is contaminated with traces of various chemicals that can sometimes be responsible for illness in highly sensitive individuals), remembering that teeth must not be brushed, stamps not licked, and gum not chewed. But few adults will seriously contemplate a week of total fasting, the idea being too outrageous. So a restricted diet containing a few foods that very rarely cause problems may be suggested – say, lamb and pears, or sago and turkey. This is sometimes called an 'oligoallergenic diet'. Many suggestions of this kind will be found in the bibliography at the end of this chapter.

If after a week on a severely restricted diet of this kind the patient is no better, we can be reasonably sure that dietary investigations will not profit him. Mind you, we can never be entirely certain of that. It could be argued that the restriction was not carried on for long enough (rheumatic complaints may take several weeks to respond), or else that the illness is also maintained by sensitivity to some airborne material (gases, mites, mould, spores, pollens, etc). Dr Doris Rapp's shoe analogy comes to mind: 'If you have eight nails sticking through the sole of your shoe, your foot will still hurt even if you pull out one or two of them.' Sensitivity to inhalants does exist, of course – hay fever is a classic example. Hence the bizarre air-cleaning manoeuvres that some highly sensitive sufferers are forced to resort to.

It should be noted, in passing, that when patients give up a food or drink that has been damaging their health, they often suffer a period of worsening, lasting several days, before starting to get better. This 'withdrawal syndrome' can also produce new symptoms that the patient does not normally get, especially headaches, nausea and depression, and it can be quite severe. In some ways it is like the withdrawal syndrome that opiate addicts get, and may indeed be caused by a similar mechanism. At any rate patients should be warned to expect it, lest they become discouraged and give up prematurely.

Mechanisms of Food Intolerance

Carl Prausnitz was an immunologist at the University of Breslau, in Germany, in the 1920s and Heinz Küstner was his postgraduate student. Prausnitz was interested in allergy because he suffered from hay fever. Küstner was also allergic, being exquisitely sensitive to fish. Exposure to the slightest dose – even eating parsley that had been chopped on a board previously used for anchovies – caused him to have sneezing, nasal blockage and asthma, grossly inflammed eyes, severe urticaria (hives) all over his body, and after a couple of hours severe vomiting. Attacks would occur within 30 minutes and last for about 12 hours. Curiously, *raw* fish caused him no trouble at all.

Prausnitz injected a small quantity of Küstner's serum into his own skin. He injected some serum from a normal healthy donor into another patch of skin, and some saline into a third. The next day, he injected a small amount of fish extract into the same areas of skin. The patch that had previously received Küstner's serum – but not the other patches – produced a vigorous itchy weal-and-flare reaction, which lasted some hours. The following day Prausnitz ate some cooked fish, and once again the patch of skin that had received Küstner's serum began to itch.

This experiment was tried several times, with different donors and recipients, and usually produced positive results. Prausnitz and Küstner published the results in 1921, stating that 'the state of supersensitivity can be transferred passively to normal persons by the serum of the supersensitive individual'. Strictly speaking they had not transferred the disease, only a positive skin test, but there is little reason overall to doubt their general conclusion. This type of food reaction – an *immediate hypersensitivity* – seems to be brought about by antibodies, passively transferable in the classic fashion from one individual to another, and thus can be classified as a food allergy. Skin tests and blood tests are a good guide to the clinical sensitivities in these illnesses.

Prausnitz, being a Jew, was forced to flee Germany during the 1930s and settled as a penniless refugee in Britain. He became a general practitioner on the Isle of Wight, though he continued to take an active interest on immunological matters until his death. The Prausnitz-Küstner test that he pioneered became the paradigm for allergy of this type, nowadays known as type I hypersensitivity (see below).

Many food intolerance illnesses, however, do not yield readily to explanations of this type. In cases where the symptoms are delayed, following challenge, by many hours (or even days or weeks), the skin tests and blood tests are very poorly correlated with the actual sensitivities of the patient as eventually revealed by elimination dieting and challenges. In these cases we cannot assume that any immunological cause is operating, since none of these illnesses has ever been convincingly transferred to a healthy individual by the patient's blood. We simply do not know the causal mechanisms, although the addictive properties frequently noted (see Case Histories, above) may provide a clue; alkaloids and some food peptides are often addictive (see Chapter 3). Food intolerances in children are commonly of the type I allergy variety, and gradually wane and sometimes disappear as the child grows up. Food intolerances in adults, especially those that first appear in adult life, are rarely type I allergies, and get worse with time rather than better, although after a lengthy avoidance the patient may be able to take occasional small doses of the food without trouble. This latter behaviour is more suggestive of a gradual accumulation of a dietary poison than of an immunological process.

Successful Diagnosis

Suppose that, after a week's fast, or oligoallergenic diet, the patient becomes dramatically better. This is by no means uncommon. Does this prove a diagnosis of food intolerance? Not really. Sudden changes of diet have many consequences. The bacteria in the large bowel (and the average human body contains more bacteria in the bowel than there are cells in the whole of the rest of the body) are drastically changed by *any* alteration of diet. Even fairly minor dietary changes – omission, for example, of milk, yeast, and their products from the average

Western menu – is a powerful jolt to the psyche, not to mention the purse. Family tensions are radically realigned, and the social difficulties can be enormous. A favourable response to diet no more proves food intolerance than a headache, when it responds to aspirin, is proof of aspirin deficiency. An illness that responds to diet only proves that the illness responded to the diet. Mind you, we should not throw the baby out with the bathwater – if a severe chronic illness gets better, few patients are overconcerned to understand precisely why.

Dangers of Elimination Diets

Elimination diets are a nuisance. The hapless sufferer, and his family, are forced to become worriers about food. Every supermarket label must be anxiously scrutinised. Expensive health-food stores must be investigated and patronised, or special sources of supply arranged. Friends must be warned in advance when inviting the patient out to tea, and (since few people care very much about other people's illnesses) the sufferer is frequently faced with the dilemma, when eating out, of either accepting what he's given (and suffering the consequences) or offending his hostess. After a few mutually bruising encounters of this kind the patient stops accepting invitations and becomes lonelier than ever. Introspection and obsessionalism are thus encouraged in people who may have been that way inclined already.

Elimination diets are boring. They may be nutritionally inadequate, so that new symptoms arise due to vitamin deficiency or frank starvation. No-one should begin on an elimination diet unless supervised by a competent dietician. The rest of the family may suffer, not only from the restricted diet but also from the isolation.

So, most doctors require good evidence that the diet is really necessary, before setting the patient on a course from which it may subsequently be difficult to change him. From time to time the patient is encouraged to be challenged with the incriminated foods, to see whether the restriction is still necessary.

Difficulties With, and Prejudices Against Dietary Therapies

Doctors often baulk at food allergies and dietary therapies, even when a dietary origin seems perfectly reasonable and certainly deserving of investigation. One of the many reasons is that dietary advice is complex and time consuming; few can afford the half-hour or so that is needed each time. Sometimes doctors judge the patient incapable of understanding or following the advice. They may think that the illness is not severe enough to warrant such draconian remedies – especially if effective drugs are available. They might be frightened of triggering hypochondria.[20] And in many cases 'common sense' militates against the idea that complex or severe diseases can have such a simple cure, or against the fundamental notion that staples of diet 'full of natural goodness' can possibly be responsible for making some people ill.

So How, Finally, is Food Intolerance Diagnosed and Treated?

With great difficulty. The road towards a firm diagnosis is long and crooked and many patients fall by the wayside. Treatment, once diagnosed, is fraught with problems for the patient and his family. The diagnosis in some cases is impossible, finally, to either prove or disprove. Small wonder that in this vacuum unproven remedies and tests are peddled and promoted as cure-alls. One or more of the claims may yet turn out to be true.

At the end of the day, acknowledging all difficulties and dangers, I am still committed to the 'allergy approach' because I cure many illnesses with it.

Physiology of Digestion

As every school child knows, proteins in the food are masticated and mixed with saliva in the mouth, sterilised and partly digested in the stomach, then fully digested in the small intestine into amino acids by the enzymes of pancreatic and intestinal juices. The amino acids are the basic building blocks of protein. They are absorbed across the wall of the intestine into the portal vein, which carries them to the liver (which detoxicates any poisons left over after the digestion process), then the lungs, and thence into the general circulation for distribution around the body.

Quite how this simple story came to be told is mysterious, as it is quite wrong in one crucial regard. Connheim, in the early years of this century, proved that proteins are not completely digested within the lumen (cavity) of the small intestine. Complete digestion by the enzymes there would take more than a week. The proteins arrive at the absorptive surface (epithelium) of the small intestine mainly in the form of partly digested molecules called oligopeptides, each consisting of several amino acids. Amino acids by themselves are mostly inert and harmless, but oligopeptides often retain toxic or pharmacological activities and are almost always antigenic (see section on Immunology, below). These oligopeptides excite an active immune response in the intestine, and are only finally digested into amino acids during their passage across the epithelium. The immune response in the gut is apparently required before this final stage of digestion can be complete (see reference 12).

A similar process occurs with carbohydrates, with the exception of those complex polysaccharides that evade digestion and are therefore classified as 'fibre'. Fat, on the other hand, is largely taken up in the form of micelles into the lymph, not the blood, and reaches the bloodstream without passing through the liver first (although it is filtered instead by lymph nodes, and also lungs).

Like all bodily processes, digestion can occasionally become defective. Some acute infections, especially gastoenteritis and (in the tropics) measles, leave the digestive mechanisms damaged for some time afterwards. Other environmental insults (drugs, toxins, radiation) can have similar effects. Indeed, the food may itself carry molecules that interfere with digestion (lectins and anti-enzymes: see Chapter 3).

The consequences of defective digestion are several, though they may not all occur at the same time and are not always great enough to cause noticeable problems.

(a) The nutrition of the body may become endangered, including sometimes the proper intake of vitamins or minerals.

(b) Oligopeptides and oligosaccharides formed by partial digestion may exert direct effects – and evoke an immune response that is sometimes self-damaging – on the intestine or liver.

(c) These partially digested molecules may appear in the bloodstream, to exert such effects on other organs of the body.

There is good evidence that food allergic diseases, coeliac disease, atopic (allergic) eczema, inflammatory and infectious bowel diseases are all associated with an unusual degree of permeability ('leakiness') to dietary macromolecules of the intestinal wall and/or liver (see references 1-3, 15). Many small molecules in any case pass freely from the intestine to the bloodstream – this is the rationale for administering drugs in tablet or syrup (or suppository) form.

Allergy

Clemens von Pirquet invented the word *allergy*, in a paper written in 1906, to encompass into a single concept all varieties of phenomena that are brought about by the body's immunological system. The conditions that he sought to bring together were the apparently contradictory events seen in smallpox vaccination (in which a second dose given soon after the first evokes a sharp local reaction although at the same time the person is rendered immune to the disease), syphilis (reinfection likewise provoking a brisk reaction), anaphylaxis, tuberculosis (in which immunity and hypersensitivity go hand in hand) and serum sickness; these phenomena of 'supersensitivity' had to be reconciled with the more usual consequence of vaccination, i.e. immunity. Von Pirquet wrote:

> The vaccinated person behaves towards vaccine lymph, the syphilitic towards the germ of syphilis, the tuberculous patient towards tuberculin, the person injected with serum towards this serum, in a different manner from him who has not previously been in contact with such an agent. Yet he is not insensitive to it. We can only say of him that his power to react has undergone a change. For this general concept of *changed reactivity* I propose the term allergy.

Over the years the meaning ascribed to the word has been narrowed and (in some circles) broadened. Most people now agree that the purely beneficial aspect of immunity – freedom from disease even when exposed to the germs – should not be termed allergy; the process must be self-damaging in some way. On the other hand, many lay people and some doctors have abandoned any link with the immunological conditions listed by von Pirquet and describe *any* adverse effect of an environmental agent as an allergy, irrespective of whether the effect is inborn or acquired and whether immunology is involved or not. Colloquially, to say we are 'allergic' to somebody means that we dislike him. The *Shorter Oxford English Dictionary*, playing safe, gives all three definitions.

Different ways of using words is often at the root of the most acrimonious arguments, and so it is here. Conventional allergists use the narrow definition, meaning a self-damaging immune response; clinical ecologists and most lay folk use the broader definition, and both appeal to von Pirquet for justification. Since his avowed intention when introducing the word was to clarify thinking and thus facilitate research, he would not have been edified to discover, eight decades later, how his invention has served to confuse. A patient declaring himself 'allergic' to (say) industrial pollutants and being referred in due course to an allergist, may be investigated for allergy (of the immunological variety) and found not to have one. The allergist then writes 'This patient does not have an allergy', and everyone remains in the dark. The patient feels foolish, but knows that he is still ill whatever the specialist says. If he had originally used a different word – intolerance, or perhaps sensitivity, and been referred to an environmental toxicologist, he would probably have come away far more satisfied and possibly even made better. So important do words sometimes become.

In this chapter I define allergy as a *self-damaging immune reponse*. Forms of illness that are brought about by exposure to environmental agents (such as foods) but in which the mechanism of action is obscure, I term intolerance or sensitivity. This usage is far from ideal but I am uncomfortable with either of the extreme positions.

Immunological Mechanisms

The body protects itself from infection in many ways. In this context the most relevant are antibodies, T lymphocytes, K cells, complement and phagocytes.

Antibodies are protein molecules that have the ability to bind firmly onto foreign particles or substances called *antigens*. Viruses, bacteria and other parasites all have antigens, as do pollen grains, many drugs, foods and chemicals – in fact pretty well all organic molecules above a certain size that are not the body's own natural components. If the antigen in question is toxic (e.g. viruses, chemicals), the antibody can neutralise it just by binding onto it. Antibodies can also bind simultaneously to two or more different antigens of the same type, thus forming large clumps that are more readily taken up by the body's phagocytes.

Antibodies occur in five main classes, called IgG, IgM, IgA, IgE and IgD. As a broad generalisation antibodies of the IgG and IgM classes (and possibly IgD) have the task of protecting the inner tissues and the bloodstream; antibodies of the IgA and IgE classes protect the surfaces (the skin and mucous membranes).

Antibodies are produced by *plasma cells*, little antibody factories that migrate through the body to whichever sites are in need of their products. Plasma cells are derived from cells called *B lymphocytes*, which are originally formed in the bone marrow.

T lymphocytes (T cells) are also formed in the bone marrow but before use are processed by a gland called the thymus (T for thymus), which lies in the upper part of the thoracic cavity. Mature T cells serve many different functions, of which the most relevant to us is their ability to destroy antigenic cells. These are the body's own cells that have become perverted by infection with viruses, or certain bacteria, or perhaps neoplastic change, and whose cell surfaces have become sufficiently altered as a result to be recognised by the body as foreign. The T cells break open the altered cells, so that the parasites inside can then be attacked by antibodies.

K cells (K for 'killer') also destroy antigenic cells, but only once the cells have first been attached to antibodies. The antibodies focus the attention, as it were, of the K cells onto the target cells.

Complement is the collective name given to a complex system of normal plasma proteins that are called into action ('activated' or 'fixed') whenever antibodies and antigens come together to form immune complexes. Once activated, complement has many functions. By attaching to the immune complex, complement makes the complex more susceptible to the attention of phagocytes (opsonisation). Complement can actually kill, and sometimes destroy, cells to which antibodies have become attached. And most important, complement excites inflammation, that process in which fluid and cells ooze out of the bloodstream into the body tissues. Inflammation is perceived on the surface as swelling, redness, hotness, pain and impaired function of the part. But underneath, the purpose of inflammation is to protect the body tissues from environmental 'insults' such as infection, burns or noxious chemicals, at the same time speeding the repair process. Activated complement also attracts phagocytes to the site where they are most needed.

Phagocytes are the body's scavenger cells, simultaneously acting as soldiers, policemen, executioners and dustbinmen. Most particles that the body wants to get rid of end up as food for a phagocyte. These cells float through the blood and crawl like amoebae between the cells of the static tissues, ingesting and digesting any likely particles – even whole cells – that they come across. *Opsonisation* by complement or by IgG antibodies is the main signal by which they decide whether to engulf a particle or leave it alone. Phagocytes come in many shapes, sizes and colours, each with its own name: macrophages, monocytes, neutrophil polymorphs (shortened to 'neutrophils'), eosinophils and basophils. Some phagocytes remain in the same site most or all of the time – e.g. Kupffer cells in the liver and dust cells in the lungs. Each type of phagocyte has distinct functions in addition to that of phagocytosis itself, but these extra functions need not concern us here.

This lightning review of immunology has of necessity been ruthlessly condensed. The interested reader will find a fuller account in the books cited at the end of this chapter.[8–10]

Mechanisms of Allergy (Hypersensitivity)

Four basic mechanisms are recognised, though others may exist so far undiscovered. All immune responses are basically protective, as we have seen, but most can also cause painful and/or self-damaging effects that we interpret as being 'bad'. When the material that we are protecting ourselves against is something apparently harmless like a foodstuff, the immune reaction is perceived as being inappropriate, or paradoxical, and termed 'hypersensitivity' or 'allergy'.

Type I Allergy

The antibodies in this case are of the IgE class. These are stuck onto the surface of cells called mast cells, which are the body's stores of histamine and other inflammatory chemicals. When the IgE antibodies are presented with the matching antigens they send a signal to the mast cells, which release their contents. The result is inflammation. When the reaction occurs in the mucuous membranes the swelling of the tissues is accompanied by itch and the outpouring of mucus, with violent semi-voluntary expulsive efforts (coughing, sneezing, diarrhoea).

The overall function appears to be the expulsion of antigens from the mucous membranes and skin. The classic example of type I allergy is hay fever, in which the antigen ('allergen') is pollen.

Type II Allergy

The antigen here is frequently a drug. Some of these molecules bind to the surfaces of body cells and alter their chemical structure sufficiently to make them recognisable as foreign by the immune system. Antibodies are formed, of IgG or IgM (sometimes IgD) class, and complement and/or K cells kill the affected cells. If red blood cells are involved, the result is anaemia.

Type III Allergy

This occurs when antigen/antibody complexes are formed that are not efficiently removed by the body's phagocytes. This occurs if the complexes are too small, or if the phagocytes are not working efficiently, or sometimes just because there is too much complex to be disposed of at once. The complexes are trapped in various parts of the body – kidneys, blood vessels, joints, skin, brain – and activate complement, which in turn attracts polymorphs and sets up inflammation. There is evidence that type III allergy occurs in the small intestine in coeliac disease, though not necessarily as a *cause* of the disease.

Type IV Allergy

This is the self-damaging aspect of T cell activity. The cells being attacked are frequently in the skin. The most common examples are contact dermatitis due to industrial chemicals, or sometimes cosmetics. Type IV hypersensitivity is responsible for the tuberculin reaction seen in TB. Experimentally induced type IV reactivity in the intestine of laboratory animals causes a picture remarkably like that of coeliac disease.

The Role of Allergy in Food Intolerance

IgE antibodies (detected in the blood by the radioallergosorbent technique – RAST) against a foodstuff, if found, offer evidence that a type I reaction is occurring or has occurred. They are sometimes found in patients with food intolerance and when they are, the diagnosis of food allergic disease is generally held to be appropriate. Strictly speaking the case is not proven, however, since positive RAST results occasionally occur in people who have no trace of allergic disease. It is after all possible to have an immunological phenomenon that does not manifest itself as a disease. Antibodies of IgG or IgM class against foods are not infrequently found in the general population, and offer evidence that that food has been eaten, but not necessarily that the food has ever been responsible for illness. Likewise, sensitised T cells to certain foodstuffs are also occasionally found, and while these correlate quite well with clinical sensitivity, this is not proof of cause-and-effect. Cases in which demonstrable immunological reactivity against a food has been shown to be the *cause* of a patient's sensitivity to that food are extremely rare, so it could be argued that the term 'food allergic disease' should hardly ever be used (although this is an extreme position[2]).

How Common is Food Intolerance?

No one knows for sure. Estimates in the medical literature range from 0.4 per cent of the Western population to 40 per cent. Many cases do not come to the attention of doctors because the relationship is so obvious and avoidance is so easy. Dr W. Rea of Texas has argued, plausibly, that most people are slightly damaged by food intolerance of one sort or another most of the time, but the damage only amounts to a slight feeling of malaise, tiredness or transient depression, and if these mild symptoms have been suffered for most of the life they are accepted as 'normal'. If Rea is right, the few patients who seek professional help represent the small tip of a very large iceberg.

Is Food Intolerance Becoming Commoner?

It is certainly more in the news, and the diagnosis is therefore made more readily nowadays by both doctors and lay public. Dr K.K. Eaton, a general practitioner in Berkshire, UK, made a careful survey of his practice in 1974 and again in 1979, using the same diagnostic criteria, and noted a pronounced increase in the incidence of various allergies over this five-year period.[7] Food intolerance also showed a moderate increase in incidence, though the difference did not achieve statistical significance. Comparisons of this kind are extremely difficult to do and to interpret, since different doctors use different diagnostic criteria and even a single doctor cannot swear that his ways of thinking have remained totally unaffected by the passage of years. Although many doctors share Dr Eaton's impression that allergies of all kinds are on the increase, it is impossible to be sure if this is true. Many changes have occurred in the lifestyles and environments of Western populations in the last three decades – fashions in infant feeding, industrial pollution, increasing adventurousness in diet and alcohol intake, new drugs – all of which may reasonably be suspected of altering the interaction between the body and its nutrients.

'Total Allergy Syndrome'

This term was reputedly invented by the medical correspondent of the British newspaper, the *Daily Mail*, to describe a well known patient, who is so severely sensitive to foods and air pollutants that she is forced to subsist on very little, and stay indoors breathing filtered air. This lady is certainly not unique. Patients of this kind were presenting at the allergy clinic in Manchester, and being seen by me, many years before the illness became popular in the media.

Like chronic brucellosis (see Chapter 1), the clinical picture is enormously varied from one patient to another, but certain common strands can be perceived in most cases. They have all found by experiment that their illnesses seem to be triggered or aggravated by eating certain foods, drinking certain drinks, breathing certain smells, wearing certain clothes, or having intimate contact with certain people. At first they are delighted to discover that their long-standing ill-health is relieved by giving up a few common foods or activities, but after a few months the symptoms start coming back again and they have to give something else up. The process is repeated until a near-terminal stage is reached. The patient is often female, articulate and attractive, in her thirties. Particularly common symptoms are swellings of the abdomen (or other parts of the body), headaches, sore throats, a sensation of aches and pains and mild fever as if having a nasty dose of flu (but too frequent to be true flu), fluctuating body weight, thirst, and excessive need for rest. The classic 'type I' symptoms of rhinitis, asthma and eczema are no more common in these patients than in the general population. The triggers that they identify are often surprising – tap water, cooking fat, household gas, newsprint, husband or son – quite unlike the housedust and pollens that conventional allergists normally expect to see.

Physical examination and laboratory tests are usually normal except for a tendency to emaciation or obesity, leaving the doctor mystified.

Occasionally false-positive skin tests mislead the unwary. The patient has consulted many doctors in the past, never getting much benefit, and tends to acquire a cynical attitude to the medical profession – one of the diagnostic signs of this syndrome is that the patient makes the doctor feel like an ignorant schoolboy! Not surprisingly, these patients readily acquire an undeserved reputation for being 'difficult'.

Sometimes the picture is complicated by the signs and symptoms of hyperventilation – tingling of lips and hands, with painful spasms of the fingers, anxiety approaching fright, chest pains, and a sensation of breathlessness. Overbreathing for whatever cause, results in a reduced carbon dioxide level in the blood and this is the common factor behind the various symptoms just mentioned. They can be successfully controlled, once the patient is told, by paying careful attention to the breathing or (in severe cases) breathing in and out of a closed paper bag so that the exhaled carbon dioxide is taken in again. Overbreathing is sometimes caused by hysteria, but it is an unwise doctor who concludes that the presence of overbreathing confirms hysteria, or excludes more serious possibilities.

The investigation of 'total allergy syndrome' is difficult, and complicated by mutual distrust between doctor and patient. Both are motivated by the desire to find out if *any* foods can be tolerated, and whether an adequate diet can be established. Since many of the symptoms are subjective, the patient may have difficulty in deciding whether a particular challenge has been positive or negative. Changes in complement levels or immunoglobulin levels sometimes occur after challenge, together with symptoms, but do not prove that the *symptoms* were caused by the challenge. In any case to check these blood levels entails several blood samples a day for several days, which few patients can tolerate. In the majority of cases investigation is unrewarding both for patient and doctor.

Does the 'total allergy syndrome' exist? There is no doubt that the *patients* exist, and are ill, though one may not like the journalistic title. Clinical ecologists prefer to describe these patients are 'universal reactors'. There is no reason to disbelieve the stories that the sufferers tell, any more than one would disbelieve the list of symptoms given by a migraine sufferer (a tale of shimmering castle-wall patterns is very implausible to people who have not experienced them, but are nonetheless not held in serious doubt). Malingerers and hysterics, who invent or imagine their illnesses, characteristically tell very plausible tales and do not go from one doctor to another telling the same outrageous story. In rare cases, a drug or alcohol problem is part of the illness; this should be considered as part of the overall picture and not used by the doctor as a cue to stop thinking.

There is no doubt that some of these patients are made well by admission to a closed-environment 'ecologic unit', in which the air is filtered, building materials and furnishings are carefully chosen to minimise outgassing of vapours, spring water or filtered water is provided and food is prescribed as cautiously as one would prescribe a dangerous drug. Not surprisingly, such units are mainly to be found in North America and are not yet available, even to the very rich, in many other countries. Although improvement of illness in such a controlled environment does not strictly prove chemical or food sensitivity, this is the likeliest explanation. But such detailed investigations can only be done on a very few patients, and investigations outside such a unit are doomed to failure on most occasions. Many doctors in the UK dismiss the syndrome as an invention of the media and disbelieve its existence, but in the absence of satisfactory information this attitude is a prejudice founded on ignorance. This unsatisfactory state of ignorance is likely to last for some time, and in the meantime we are doing nothing, by and large, to help these patients; indeed most of us are helping to make them more miserable.

Can Food Intolerance be Treated?

The most straightforward management is by avoidance, though as we have seen that may have its problems. The drug sodium cromoglycate (Nalcrom) is sometimes very useful. Injection therapy of the kind used for hay fever has mostly been disappointing, though occasional successes have been reported.

Practitioners of the 'Clinical Ecology' school often prescribe 'neutralising doses'. These are arrived at by injecting progressively weaker extracts of the foodstuff into the skin until there is no further growth in size of the weals thus produced. That dose of the extract is then taken, by sublingual drops or sometimes injection, and in many cases, it neutralises the sensitivity. Urine therapy, in which the patient takes a precise dose of his own urine by mouth, also claims successes and – surprisingly – has some theoretical rationale. It is beyond my ability to review the dozens of other 'fringe' methods that are available. Potential clients should be aware that the placebo effect is a very powerful healing force, and accompanies *all* forms of treatment. It is sometimes strong enough to bring about remarkable cures, which are then attributed to whichever therapeutic method was being applied at the time. No rational opinion can be formed as to the efficacy of fringe practices as they have not been scientifically studied.

Can Food Intolerance be Prevented?

There are strong theoretical reasons for believing that *exclusive breast-feeding* for the first 3–4 months of life will protect against food intolerance, but in practice the results of trials have been contradictory.[21] It is surprisingly difficult to obtain an accurate record of babies' feeds, especially for the first few days of life. *Delayed weaning* until after 3–4 months of age should also protect to some extent, especially if weaning takes place gradually over several months. Theoretically the baby should begin weaning by tasting small portions of whatever foods and drinks that the mother is taking, since he should have been gradually prepared to cope with his mother's dietary components during the months of breastfeeding. Pregnant and lactating mothers should not be hectored into taking a pint of milk daily – or to indulge in any dietary excesses – against their own preferences, since some babies can be sensitised by traces of food-derived protein in the mother's milk.[15] It must be confessed that most of this advice is largely based on theory and has not been adequately tested in practice.

References

On Food Intolerance (General)

1. Brostoff, J. and Challacombe, S. (eds.) Food Allergy, *Clinics in Immunology and Allergy* Vol. 2/1 (W.B. Saunders, Eastbourne, 1982).
2. Coombes, R.A.A. (ed.) *The First Food Allergy Workshop* (Medical Education Services, Oxford, 1980).
3. Lessof, M.H. (ed.) *Clinical Reactions to Food* (Wiley, Chichester, 1983).
4. Finn, R. and Cohen, N.H. '"Food Allergy" – Fact or Fiction?' *Lancet* (1978), *1*, 426–8.
5. Buisseret, P.D. 'Common Manifestations of Cow's Milk Allergy in Children', *Lancet* (1978), *1*, 304–5.
6. Pearson, D.J., Rix, K.J.B. and Bentley, S.J. 'Food Allergy: How Much in the Mind?' *Lancet* (1983), *1*, 1259–61.

On Rising Incidence

7. Eaton, K.K. 'The Incidence of Allergy – Has it Changed?' *Clinical Allergy* (1982), *12*, 107–10.

On Immunology

8. Roitt, I.M. *Essential Immunology* (Blackwell, Oxford, 1982).
9. *Clinical Aspects of Immunology* 2nd and 3rd edns (eds. Gell, P.G.H., Coombs, R.R.A. and Lachmann, P.J.) 4th edn (eds. Lachmann, P.J. and Peters, D.K.) (Blackwell, Oxford). *N.B.* The 2nd and 3rd editions contain as an appendix von Pirquet's 1906 paper on allergy.
10. Wright, R. *Immunology of Gastrointestinal and Liver Disease* (Edward Arnold, 1977).
11. Green, F.H.Y. and Freed, D.L.J. 'Antibody-facilitated Digestion and the Consequences of its Failure' in W.A. Hemmings (ed.) *Antigen Absorption by the Gut* (MTP Press, Lancaster, 1978).
12. Freed, D.L.J. and Green, F.H.Y. 'Antibody-facilitated Digestion and its Implications for Infant Nutrition', *Early Human Development* (1977), *1*, 107–12.
13. Prausnitz, C. and Küstner, H. 'Studies on Supersensitivity. Centralblatt fur Bakteriologie, 1. Abt. Origin. (1921) *86*, 160–9. Translated and printed as an appendix to the 2nd edition of *Clinical Aspects of Immunology* (P.G.H. Gell and R.R.A. Coombs (eds.)) (Blackwell, Oxford, 1968), pp. 1298–306.

On Gut Permeability

14. Bjarnason, I., Peters, T.J. and Veall, N. 'A Persistent Defect in Intestinal Permeability in Coeliac Disease Demonstrated by a 51-Cr Labelled EDTA Absorption Test', *Lancet* (1983), *1*, 323–5 Also see references 1–3.

On Breast Milk Contaminated by Traces of the Mother's Diet

15. Miller, V. 'Difficulties and Values of Breastmilk for Atopic Babies' in D.L.J. Freed (ed.) *Health Hazards of Milk* (Baillière-Tindall, Eastbourne, 1984), pp. 113–19.

On Migraine and Irritable Bowel Syndrome

16. Egger, J., Carter, C.M., Wilson, J., Turner, M.W. and Soothill, J.F. *Lancet* (1983), *1*, 865–8.
17. Alun Jones, V., MacLaughlan, P., Shorthouse, M., Workman, E., and Hunter, J.O. 'Food Intolerance: a Major Factor in the Pathogenesis of Irritable Bowel Syndrome', *Lancet* (1982), *2*, 1115–17.
18. Waters, W.E., Campbell, M.J. and Elwood, P.C. 'Migraine, Headache and Survival in Women', *British Medical Journal* (1983), *287*, 1992–3.

Other Topics

19. Maulitz, R.M., Pratt, D.S. and Shocket, A.L. 'Exercise-induced Anaphylactic Reaction to Shellfish', *Journal of Allergy and Clinical Immunology* (1979), *63*, 433–4.
20. Warner, J.O. and Hathaway, M.J. 'Allergic Forms of Meadow's Syndrome (Munchausen by Proxy)', *Archives of Diseases of Childhood* (1984), *59*, 151–6.
21. Walker-Smith, J.A. 'Does Breast Feeding Protect Against Atopic Disease?' in E.L.J. Freed (ed.) *Health Hazards of Milk* (Bailliere Tindall, Eastbourne, 1984), pp. 119–26.

Support Groups and Useful Addresses

(1) UK
Society for Environmental Therapy
National Society for Research into Allergies
PO Box 45, Hinckley, Leics. LE10 1JY
National Eczema Society
5/7 Tavistock Place, London WC1H 9SR
Action Against Allergy (Chairman A. Nathan Hill)
43 The Downs, London SW20 8HG
This organisation maintains a library of 'self-help' allergy books.
Foodwatch (for pure foodstuffs and information)
High Acre, East Stour, Gillingham, Dorset SP8 5JR

For names of doctors specialising in allergy:
British Society for Allergy and Clinical Immunology
(Hon. Sec. Dr C.A.C. Pickering, Wythenshawe Hospital, Manchester M23 9LT)
British Society for Clinical Ecology
(Hon. Sec. Dr R. Finn, Royal Liverpool Hospital Liverpool L7 8XP)

(2) USA and Canada
Society for Clinical Ecology (Sec. Dr Phyllis Saifer)
1561 Hawthorne Terrace, Berkeley, California 91470
American Academy of Allergy
611 East Wells Street, Milwaukee, Wisconsin 53201
New England Society for Allergy
Dr H.B. Freye, 41 East Main Street, Mystic, Connecticut 06335
Canadian Society for Allergy and Clinical Immunology
CAE, 350 Sparks Street, Suite 602, Ottawa, Ontario, Canada K1R 7S8

(3) International
International Association of Allergology (Sec. Dr J.T. McCarthy)
1390 Sherbrook, Montreal, PQ, Canada H3G 1K2
European Academy of Allergology and Clinical Immunology (Sec. Dr J. Jamar)
52 Boulevard de la Cambre, Brussels 1050, Belgium

8 DIET AND MENTAL ILLNESS

V. Rippere

The idea that food may cause susceptible people to become mentally disturbed has an old and respected place in medical history, but it is only recently that scientists have begun to analyse the underlying mechanisms which enable foods to provoke psychological symptoms. Accordingly, work in this important area is as yet far from complete, but there are now a number of reasonably well understood forms of food-induced psychiatric and neurological disorder as well as others which are not yet so well understood. Thus it is known that foods may affect mental functioning because they contain drugs – such as alcohol or caffeine – which affect the central nervous system. They may also affect psychological function because they do not contain adequate amounts of the nutrients needed for proper development and/or operation of the brain. Or foods may affect mental well-being because they contain poisonous substances, either intrinsic to them or occurring as additives or contaminants, which may interfere with the integrity of the brain and nervous system. Moreover, as is recently coming to be more widely recognised, foods and their additives may cause allergies, intolerances, and/or addictions that are capable of affecting mental functioning. Foods may also be partially digested to substances with drug-like actions that can affect brain function. Or they may not be properly metabolised because certain individuals inherit the lack of particular enzymes that are needed to break down and make use of certain food constituents in the body. Either the build-up of improperly metabolised chemicals or other consequences of enzyme deficiencies are capable of affecting brain function. Moreover, foods may affect brain function indirectly because of their immediate effects on the pancreas, the organ which is responsible for controlling the level of glucose – the brain's chief source of energy – in the blood. If certain foods cause the pancreas to overreact and secrete too much insulin, the blood sugar level will fall too low and the brain will be deprived of its energy substrate; this deprivation results in mental symptoms. And finally, foods contribute to determining the level of certain neurotransmitters formed in the brain and these effects may possibly contribute to mental disorder.

From this brief enumeration of the main mechanisms underlying the effects of food on mental function and dysfunction, it is clear that the situation in any given case is potentially quite complex. Although the relationships between all these different sorts of mechanisms have not yet been worked out, it is reasonable to suppose that they are not necessarily mutually exclusive. Indeed, it seems unlikely on *a priori* grounds that, say, consuming excessive amounts of caffeine should protect a person against food-borne mercury poisoning or that having diet-induced hypoglycaemia should prevent the effects of a poorly nourishing diet. On the contrary, experience suggests that food-induced symptomatology in some people results from the simultaneous operation of different mechanisms. There is also evidence that being badly nourished makes people more susceptible to the adverse effects of certain poisonous fungi that contaminate grain crops such as corn or rice.[1] Unfortunately, however, most research is concerned with only one of the many possible underlying mechanisms at a time, which probably leads to gross underestimates of the proportion of people in the population whose mental health is adversely affected by their diet.

Now let us consider each of the mechanisms mentioned earlier. For reasons of limited space, the discussion must be indicative rather than exhaustive.

Psychological Symptoms Caused by Food-borne Drugs: the Case of Caffeinism

As was noted in the discussion of the alkaloids in Chapter 3, coffee, tea, and cola drinks contain the alkaloid caffeine. Though caffeine is classified as a stimulant drug with chief actions on the central nerous system (CNS), it has known effects on other systems of the body, including the cardiovascular system, smooth and striated muscle, gastric secretions, diuresis, and metabolic rate. Within the CNS, caffeine has powerful stimulatory effects on the cortex, medulla, and spinal cord.[2] The drug's effects on performance have been extensively studied,[3–5] but despite the fact that reports of the adverse effects of excessive consumption have been appearing in the medical press for over 150 years,[6] it is only recently that caffeine intoxication, also known as caffeinism, has been formally acknowledged as a form of organic mental disorder in its own right.[7]

There are two syndromes of caffeinism, one resulting from poisoning of various degrees through excessive consumption and the other resulting from addiction through regular consumption. The two syndromes are not mutually exclusive; regular coffee and tea drinkers may also tend to drink these beverages to excess.

Caffeine poisoning has both a mild and a severe form. The mild form, which may occur after consumption of as little as 250 mg (equivalent to perhaps two cups of strong coffee), may be clinically indistinguishable from a functional anxiety state. The symptoms include restlessness, nervousness or anxiety, excitement, flushed face, diuresis, insomnia, and possibly cardiovascular symptoms such as tachycardia (very rapid pulse) or palpitations. The syndrome is diagnosed on the basis of a recent history of caffeine consumption, but some detective work may be necessary if the sufferer has taken caffeine-containing over-the-counter medications (such as painkillers or cold remedies) in addition to or instead of caffeinated drinks. Caffeinism was rediscovered as a cause of mental disturbance in the 1970s when an American psychiatrist realised that some of the chronic, treatment-resistant putatively anxious patients he was seeing were in reality suffering from chronic mild coffee poisoning.[8]

At levels of consumption over about 1 g, a toxic confusional state may occur. This syndrome is characterised by outright delirium, muscle twitching, a rambling flow of thought and speech, periods of inexhaustibility, agitation, and serious disturbances of heart rhythm. Unlike alcohol intoxication, where acute excessive consumption must be paid for with a hangover, caffeine-induced delirium has been found to pass off spontaneously in about 6 hours if no further caffeine is taken.[9]

Caffeine addiction does not require large amounts of the drug to be consumed so long as regular doses are taken. Thus a 3-cups a day person may become just as addicted as a 10-cups a day person, but a modest coffee or tea drinker is probably less likely than a heavy consumer to realise that addiction is present.[10] Caffeine addiction has been studied both experimentally[11,12] and epidemiologically.[13,14] The symptoms of withdrawal include severe headache, possibly accompanied by nausea and vomiting, running nose, lowering of mood, drowsiness, yawning, disinclination to work and inability to work effectively, irritability, nervousness, anxiety, restlessness, lethargy, and muscle tension. It does not seem to be known whether the severity of the full-blown withdrawal syndrome is proportional to the level of previous consumption. The symptoms may continue for several days and are relieved either by prolonging abstention until they wear of spontaneously or by taking caffeine. The effectiveness of many compound analgesics may be as much due to their caffeine content as to the analgesic proper.

In addition to causing its own species of psychopathology, excessive caffeine has also been found to exacerbate preexisting psychopathology in schizophrenics[15] and to be capable of precipitating psychotic episodes in susceptible people.[16] Increased use of caffeine has been found in psychiatric patients to be associated with increased levels of depression as well as of anxiety and also with increased smoking and tranquilliser consumption.[17] These findings suggest that an addictive tendency may transcend the specific addictants employed. In any event, it is clear that our most common social beverages may contribute substantially to psychopathology in some people. The magnitude of the problem may be gauged from the recent finding that 60 per cent of a sample of unselected psychiatric patients were consuming caffeine in excess of 750 mg per day.[18] Psychiatric inpatients reported higher levels of caffeine consumption than outpatients, who in turn reported more than general medical patients and non-patients. It was suggested that above this level of consumption, drinkers may no longer habituate to the drug's pharmacological effects; above this level, there was a virtually linear relationship between amount of caffeine consumed and degree of sympatomatology.

In view of these findings, we may be permitted to wonder why psychiatric inpatients in Britain are allowed regularly to consume toxic amounts of caffeine on the hospital wards. In some cases, their everyday habit of drinking tea, coffee, or coke must be contributing either to the condition for which they are being treated or to its resistance to treatment. Application of existing knowledge about the adverse effects of excessive caffeine consumption on mental functioning could lead to reduction of morbidity and increased efficacy of treatment.

Mental Illness Arising from Nutritional Deficiencies: the Case of Ascorbic Acid Deficiency

Just as the diet may contribute to mental disturbance because of substances it contains, so it may also contribute because of substances it does not contain. There are several syndromes of mental disturbance that are commonly accepted as resulting from deficiencies in specific nutrients. The most familiar are associated with inadequate intake of vitamins in the B-complex, since these were the first to be isolated and systematically investigated. They include beriberi and the Wernicke-Korsakoff syndrome of alcoholism (thiamine), pellagra (niacin), and pernicious anaemia (vitamin B_{12}).[19–22] Much of our knowledge of deficiency diseases has come from research in the first half of the twentieth century, but the real credit for the discovery of nutrient deficiency disease probably goes to James Lind, a Scots physician who in 1753 published *A Treatise of the Scurvy*,[23] in which he described the studies that had led him to the conclusion that the cause of scurvy, the scourge of the world's navies and merchant seamen throughout the past 300 years and known since the Middle Ages at least, was the lack of certain vital elements of diet. Lind also showed that the condition could be both treated and prevented by daily rations of the juice of fresh lemons and oranges.

Although it was not until the 1930s that the constituent of citrus juice responsible for its therapeutic efficacy was identified, Lind's empirical treatment was adopted in 1795, the year after his death, by the British Admiralty, which decreed that henceforth sailors in the British Navy were to be given a daily dose of lime juice. The Admiralty decree effectively marked the end of scurvy amongst British sailors. But the British merchant marine had to endure another 70 years of scurvy, as lime juice rations were not made mandatory until 1865.[24]

Lind's discovery of an effective means of preventing and alleviating scurvy nearly 200 years before vitamin C was isolated in the laboratory illustrates an important point about empirical dietary treatments, namely that they may be perfectly sound even though the chemical means for their effectiveness are not yet clear. The fact that his vital discovery was to languish through 48 years of sterile academic debate on the efficacy of lime juice in scurvy before being put into widespread use foreshadows the reception which his observations on the mental symptoms of scurvy have encountered subsequently.

Classical scurvy, as described by Lind, was characterised by initial pallor, which, as the disease developed, turned 'more darkish or livid'. Subsequently, victims developed a 'universal lassitude, with a stiffness and feebleness of the knees upon using exercise', breathlessness on exertion, itching, swelling, and bleeding of the gums, with offensive breath, dry, rough skin, a tendency to develop bruising, oedema of ankles and legs, skin ulcers at the site of bruising, reduced resistance to infections, fever, diarrhoea, highly coloured, foul-smelling urine, harmorrhages, and finally death. But in addition to these physical and constitutional symptoms, Lind noted, characteristic psychological features: the patients were 'much dejected, and often low spirited'. These symptoms, like the rest, short of death, were found to improve when citrus juice was added to the diet.

This observation is one which, though it has been made repeatedly in many forms by subsequent investigators, the world at large seems reluctant to acknowledge. Several reports of low vitamin C levels in psychiatric patients have appeared,[25-27] and psychiatric symptoms in human subjects experimentally deprived of ascorbic acid have also been reported.[28] Humans with naturally occurring scurvy have been reported to be 'depressed, resentful, and uncooperative'[29] or 'uncertain, disturbed, and aggressive'[30] and to show rapid improvement in their mental state after ascorbic acid treatment. Normal subjects with raised psychopathology scores on a mental illness screening measure have been reported to have lower intakes of ascorbic acid than subjects scoring 0 on the measure.[31] But despite the consistency in these findings, only a few formal trials of vitamin C in treatment of mental disorder have been published – and then with an interval of 20 years between them.

In the first trial, 40 chronic psychiatric inpatient males, mainly schizophrenics, were given either 1 g/day of ascorbic acid or of placebo for 3 weeks, under double-blind conditions. The 20 patients receiving ascorbic acid showed significant decreases in their self-rated depression and in observer-rated symptoms of depression, mania, and paranoia. An average of 6 days was required for patients to become saturated with vitamin C; in normal subjects 1-2 days are required. In addition to their diagnosed mental illnesses, these patients were also suffering from subclinical scurvy. When their deficiency state was remedied, they showed 'an improvement in overall personality functioning'.[32]

In the second double-blind trial of vitamin C in depression, 12 manic and 12 depressed patients were given either placebo or 3 g of ascorbic acid in the morning of two consecutive days. The global severity of their illness was rated both before and hourly for 6 hours afterwards. When patients were given ascorbic acid, they were rated as significantly less ill at 3, 4, and 5 hours than after placebo and reductions in severity were also significantly greater after ascorbic acid.[33]

In this study, no mention was made of possible ascorbic acid deficiency as a reason for the patients' improvement on vitamin C. The study was conducted within the framework of a theory that an excess of dietary vanadium, a trace mineral, may contribute to the causation of manic-depressive illness through its effects on the sodium pump, a mechanism involved in the regulation of impulses through the nerves. Vitamin C was used because of its known ability to reverse the effects of experimentally induced vanadium poisoning in animals. This theory raises new possibilities for the mode of action of vitamin C in alleviating – and perhaps preventing? – depression. It joins the suggestion that high-dose vitamin C may, like the phenothiazine tranquillisers such as chlorpromazine (Largactil), block receptors for the neurotransmitter dopamine in the brain[34] in the array of unanswered questions concerning the role of nutrients and their deficiencies in higher nervous function. These questions include the important issue of how high a daily dose is needed for optimum mental functioning in the psychiatrically healthy as well as the psychiatrically ill and whether a dose of this order is realistically obtinable from food. At the rate of two formal treatment trials in the 231 years since Lind's treatise appeared, these questions may well take milennia to find an answer.

Neurological Symptoms from Food-borne Poisons: Lathyrism, Ginger Paralysis and Minamata Disease

The 1981 epidemic of neuromuscular disease precipitated by contaminated oil in Spain drew the world's attention once again to the often forgotten and dismal fact that foods may affect behaviour because they contain poisons with specific effects on the nervous system. These poisons may be naturally occurring constituents of the food, deliberate additives, or unintended contaminants. The neurological lesions produced by these food-borne toxins may be transient, permanent, or lethal. We may briefly examine one example of each kind.

Lathyrism

Lathyrism illustrates the case of neurological damage arising from natural plant toxins. The chick pea (*Lathyrus sativus*) from which the disease takes its name, contains several toxins, described in Chapter 3, some of which have a pathogenic effect on bones, while others, notably propionic acid, is a neurotoxin.[36] The fact that a monotonous diet of chick peas produces spastic paralysis was known to Hippocrates[37] some two and a half thousand years ago, but this knowledge is insufficient to prevent occasional poisoning epidemics. For instance in 1954 in a remote rural part of India a heavy flood left a thick layer of silt and sand in the fields which up till then had been used for rice paddy. The inhabitants planted the drought-resistant chick-pea instead, which became their dietary staple for 3 or 4 months of the year instead of being eaten only occasionally if at all.

Early in 1960 an epidemic of lathyrism came to the notice of the local health authorities. The early signs of the disease were painful spasms and cramps in the calf muscles and tingling sensations in the legs. After 3-15 days of these prodromal symptoms the patients developed spastic paralysis of the lower limbs, either suddenly, following some exertion, or gradually. Low back pain was common and over half reported precipitancy of micturition. When a prevention campaign was mounted and the villagers were encouraged to replace their lathyrus field with paddy, the epidemic came to an end.[35]

Ginger Paralysis

The case of so-called 'ginger paralysis' illustrates the possibility of serious neurological damage occurring through deliberate, though perhaps unwitting, adulteration of food with a neurotoxic substance.

During the American Prohibition era of the 1930s, fluid extract of Jamaica ginger was widely used as a substitute for alcohol. But as the raw material was expensive, some enterprising bootleggers produced a reasonably convincing imitation and flavoured the beverage with 2 per cent of a chemical called triorthocresyl phosphate (TOCP). Though not itself an insecticide, TOCP is chemically related to the organic phosphorus insecticides, which are highly neurotoxic. It has been used in industry as a plasticiser and in recovering phenol residues from gas plant effluents.[38] It was known in the 1930s to be neurotoxic because when phosphocreosote, a closely related substance, had been used at the turn of the century to treat pulmonary tuberculosis, it had produced a syndrome of paralysis.[38]

Beginning in March and April of 1930, cases of paralysis of the lower limbs began to appear simultaneously in several different American cities. At the Cincinnati General Hospital alone, more than 400 cases were seen in a 6-month period.[39] When the epidemic had passed, it was estimated that approximately 20,000 cases had occurred in the United States.[40]

The clinical picture and course of the illness make sobering reading. Among the first symptoms were abdominal cramps, nausea, and vomiting, followed by prolonged diarrhoea. Within 7-14 days after consuming the poisoned ginger drink, patients developed cramping pain in the calves, followed by numbness and tingling in the legs and finally progressive muscular weakness, first in the legs and then in the arms. Some were so severely disabled that they were unable to feed themselves. Muscle wasting occurred. The weakness and pain usually progressed for about two months, after which slow improvement of the weakness and pain might begin to occur. In severe cases, death from bulbar palsy supervened before the stage of improvement was reached.

At autopsy, demyelination of the nerve sheaths and lesions of the anterior horns of the spinal cord were found. Later evidence also suggested involvement of the pyramidal tracts and the capillaries were also found to be damaged. The illness was characterised as 'a severe polyneuritis with disability especially evident in the motor functions'.[39]

A further episode of TOCP poisoning occurred in Liverpool in November and December 1945, with cotton seed oil used in cooking as the vehicle.[38] The 1981 outbreak of toxic oil poisoning in Spain is only one of a long and depressing series of episodes of neurological disease resulting from adulteration of foods with neurotoxins.

Minamata Disease

Minamata Disease exemplifies the case of neurological damage occurring as a result of unintended contamination of food when toxic metal residues of industrial processes find their way into the food chain.

The cause of the disease, as already described in Chapter 3, was the discharge of large amounts of mercuric chloride and sulphate, which were used as catalysts in a chemical factory, into Minamata Bay.[41] The inorganic mercury compounds in the effluent, as subsequent investigation revealed, where changed into organic mercury by bacteria in the mud at the bottom of the sea. That was absorbed by plankton. Shellfish and tiny fish eat the contaminated plankton who, in their turn, are eaten by larger fish and those by still larger fish. At each stage in the food chain the level of contamination gets higher, a process known as biomagnification. Humans eating the larger fish ingest the toxic accumulation.[43]

The onset of Minamata disease is usually accompanied by fever and general malaise. Later numbness develops in the extremities, sometimes around the mouth, often with slurring of speech. Unsteady gait, deafness, and impairment of vision are common. Difficulty in swallowing and excessive salivation are noted in some victims. Insomnia, emotional instability, taking the form of either depression or euphoria, mental confusion, drowsiness and stupor, are further symptoms. In the original outbreak death occurred in up to a third of the cases and many less severely affected victims remained incapacitated to some degree.[41] Autopsy findings showed cell degeneration in the granular layer of the cerebellum, with other lesions in the basal ganglia, hypothalamus, cortex, midbrain, and spinal cord.[42]

Mental Symptoms Arising from Food Allergy, Addiction and Intolerance

Mental symptoms may occur when people who are specifically sensitive to particular foods and/or their additives are exposed to them. Several different underlying mechanisms, most of them as yet poorly understood, have been distinguished and we may look at some of the major ones.

Cerebral Allergy

Allergic reactions in brain tissue were produced experimentally in monkeys over 40 years ago.[44] Since then there has been increasing attention to the possibility that patients with naturally occurring mental symptoms might be suffering from antibody-mediated hypersensitivity to environmental agents, including foods. A growing body of evidence indicates that patients suffering from schizophrenia, depression, and alcoholism have high rates of antibodies, higher than in control groups of other psychiatric patients or normals.[45–50] Although no control group was used, some 45 per cent of 220 depressed children were found to have a history of allergies,[51,52] though these seemed to be mostly to organic inhalants. These findings are highly suggestive.

But the discovery that more patients than normals have antibodies to foods does not prove that allergy to these foods is responsible for their mental symptoms. The evidence needed to demonstrate a causal role is improvement of the symptoms when the suspected food (or foods) is removed from the diet and recurrence of the symptoms when the food is reintroduced, preferably under double-blind conditions. Evidence of changes in antibody levels supports the interpretation, as is illustrated in the following case.

A 14-year old schoolgirl began to develop mental symptoms: irrational bouts of crying and hysteria, withdrawing to her room and episodes of hearing voices. In addition, she experienced weakness and nausea. She was found to have a history of childhood milk sensitivity, which had then produced gastrointestinal symptoms. She had adhered to a milk-free diet for several years and developed normally. The mental disturbance started after she had lapsed from the milk-free diet. When this history came to light, she was put back on a milk free diet and her clinical state improved. She was then challenged with milk and placebo at 2-weekly intervals. During one of the milk challenges, she was given disodium cromoglycate, a drug which blocks immediate hypersensitivity reactions. During each challenge, she was assessed clinically and her total IgE antibody levels were measured. It was found that she showed no reaction to placebo but had a severe clinical reaction and a sharp rise in her IgE level when milk was taken. With the drug given concurrently with milk, her clinical response was attenuated.[53] An oral preparation of the same drug has been reported to produce improvement of mental symptoms in food allergic patients.[54]

A second type of cerebral allergy to foods appears to have a different basis. This type of reaction, which is less well documented, is thought to be due to irritation in the brain mediated by inflammatory substances known as kinins.[55] Their release is thought to be provoked by the presence of partially digested peptides (large protein molecules) derived from food. The foods are poorly digested because repetitive consumption of a few foods, as occurs in food addiction, leads to diminished efficiency of digestive enzyme production in the pancreas. During provocative food tests in patients with this sort of disorder, it has been shown that exposure to small amounts of reactive foods produces clinical symptoms accompanied by a steep drop or rise in blood sugar level, whether or not the food is a carbohydrate. One 30-year-old man was reported to develop depression and extreme fright alternating with a comatose state 2 hours after a test meal of cream cheese, with a very low blood sugar level of 20 mg per 100 ml of blood. The reaction was relieved with vitamins, adrenocortical extract, and sugar. These abnormal blood sugar responses as well as the clinical reaction to incriminated foods may be prevented or attenuated by prior administration of proteolytic enzymes. A 27-year-old woman developed a blood sugar of 400 mg/100 ml one hour after a test meal of raisins accompanied by tension, trembling, irritability and unprovoked anger. During a second raisin test when enzymes were given, her blood sugar was 120 mg/100 ml one hour afterwards and no symptoms occurred.[56]

Food Addiction

Food addiction, also known as 'masked allergy', was first systematically described in the 1940s[57] and has subsequently been elaborated,[58] but many of the basic phenomena were known to Hippocrates.

In masked allergy, the person experiences an adverse reaction when first exposed to the food. Repeated exposure leads to a phase of adaptation or tolerance, which may last for years. During the adapted phase, the person feels better rather than worse after consuming the food but is otherwise fairly symptom-free. When this adaptation breaks down, the 'high' following exposure lasts for a progressively shorter period, then giving way to a 'low', represented by the emergence of withdrawal symptoms. These may take the form of almost any type or level of pathology, from minor, localised symptoms to widespread constitutional reactions. The highs may also become higher. That is, the person becomes more and more highly stimulated by exposure. At this point of the addiction, exposure to the addictant often increases in frequency. A state of chronic illness supervenes when tolerance breaks down entirely.[58]

Common mental symptoms resulting from masked allergy include a state of 'brain fag', mental 'dopiness', inability to think clearly, low or high mood, mood swings, anxiety, panic attacks, headache and migraine, poor concentration, tension, irritability, fatigue, episodes of sudden tiredness and somnolence after eating, sounds in the ears, giddiness, weepiness, and eating binges. Other symptoms have been found in individual cases and patients with mental symptoms commonly also have multiple somatic symptoms.[59] Several single or double blind studies have corroborated the relationship of these sorts of symptoms to exposure to incriminated foods.[60–63] It has been estimated that 30 per cent of people attending general practitioners in Britain have symptoms due to hidden addictions to food and sensitivity to chemicals and that another 30 per cent have symptoms partly due to these causes.[64]

While, theoretically, any food may be involved, in practice certain foods seem to be more likely than others to cause problems. In British psychiatric patients, the most commonly incriminated foods seem to be wheat and other cereal grains, milk, tea, coffee, and sugar,[65] which are amongst the most common staples of the British diet. We have already examined addiction to coffee and tea in an earlier section and as we will look at the possible effects of habitual consumption of wheat and milk later, we may consider sugar addiction here as an example.

An excellent phenomenological account of sugar addiction appeared in the *Lancet* in 1963.[66] The author, a doctor finding himself some 2 stone overweight, describes his experience as follows:

> Patterns of overeating vary from person to person. My problem was sugar added to cereals and beverages. To my own concern and that of my wife, I discovered I was consuming over 2 lb of sugar a week in this form, and that the amount was rapidly increasing. Part of this was the result of a lifelong 'sweet tooth': I had always been fond of sweet things because of their taste. But a disturbing feature of my recent craving was that it was increasingly powerful and progressive.

> If fought, it resulted in most unpleasant symptoms.
>
> On stopping beverage and cereal sugar, I suffered from sweating, abdominal pains, and a liability to syncope. My mental condition was impaired, and I had headache and subjective head noises. My temper was uncertain. I was continuously apprehensive, and very difficult to live with. These symptoms were immediately relieved by taking sugar. If withdrawal continued, the symptoms settled within two weeks, but it would be disagreeable to repeat the experience.
>
> In summary, I was eating more and more sugar, and its withdrawal caused the intensely unpleasant symptoms of endogenous hyperinsulinism. My problem was not excess weight but a true sugar addiction.

This case example illustrates many of the characteristic features of food addiction – long-standing predilection for the offending food, increasing consumption as tolerance broke down, a prolonged withdrawal syndrome relieved by reexposure to the food and a relationship between food addiction and hypoglycaemia, which we touched upon earlier in this section and will consider again at a later stage.

Adverse Reactions to Food Additives

The idea that chemical additives in food may adversely affect mental and behavioural functioning in susceptible individuals has achieved international prominence in the past 10 years.[67] Although there are now literally thousands of individual additives, however, only two kinds – artificial food dyes and monosodium glutamate – have been studied in any detail from the point of view of behavioural toxicity in humans and many of the available studies are methodologically questionable, since they tend to use as 'placebos' substances with known reactivity in relation to the effects under study.[68] However, it is accepted that tartrazine (yellow food dye No. E102), can cause allergic symptoms of a somatic nature in allergic individuals,[69] and one well-controlled double-blind study showed convincing behavioural deterioration in two hyperactive schoolgirls in their classrooms after a 1 mg dose of tartrazine but not placebo.[70] Adequate doses of mixed food dyes have been shown to produce deterioration in hyperactive children's performance on a laboratory learning task.[71] What is not known is whether these effects are mediated by allergic or by pharmacological mechanisms and some evidence exists to support each possibility.[72,73] It may be that in some children the reaction is allergic and in others the dyes have drug-like effects.

Mental Symptoms Arising from Neuroactive Peptides Formed from Foods

In the mid-1960s it was reported that there was a positive correlation between hospital admissions for schizophrenia and changes in wheat consumption in Scandinavia during the second World War.[74] This finding led to several investigations of the hypothesis that a diet free of cereal grains and milk, of the kind that is known to help sufferers from coeliac disease, might also benefit schizophrenics and this hypothesis has received confirmation in a number of well-conducted studies.[75-77]

These findings raised the question of a possible mechanism mediating the observed effects. The evidence on food antibodies in schizophrenics mentioned earlier makes food allergy a strong possibility in some cases. But the hypothesis that has received the most attention is the possibility that schizophrenics are reacting to neuroactive peptides formed in the body from constituents of wheat gluten and casein, the protein in milk.[78,79] The suggestion that some psychiatric patients may be producing drug-like chemicals in their gut from the everyday foods they eat has considerable, if as yet indirect support. It has been shown that when rats are fed radioactively labelled α-gliadin derived from wheat, significant amounts of protein-bound radioactivity appear in their brain.[80] This finding shows that a considerable amount of the wheat protein metabolites cross the blood-brain barrier and enter the brain. These molecules were also shown to retain some of the antigenic properties of the parent substance, so the finding provides support for the food allergy hypothesis as well as for the peptide hypothesis.

The effects of two different peptides have been examined. The first is a particular acidic fraction derived by enzymatic digestion from wheat gliadin and contains peptides rich in glutamine, glutamic acid, and proline.[81] When given to rats by direct injection into the brain, this polypeptide was found to cause stereotyped movements, catalepsy, 'chewing in air', and seizures, coming on after a long latent interval. Whether this particular polypeptide is the culprit in schizophrenia remains an open question, but the results of the study certainly show that digestion products of gliadin can produce abnormal behaviour. The second type of peptides that have been studied are known as exorphins, which are derived by pepsin digestion of wheat gluten and casein.[82-84] These peptides have been shown in numerous *in vitro* preparations to behave very much like the brain's own endogenous opiates, the endorphins. However, direct studies of the behavioural effects of exorphins in animals do not yet seem to have appeared and their role in abnormal behaviour still requires further investigation.

Mental Problems from Inborn Errors of Metabolism Affecting Tolerance for Dietary Constituents: the Case of Galactosaemia

Over 100 diseases caused by genetically transmitted metabolic errors have been identified. These errors usually take the form of enzyme abnormalities or deficiencies, which lead to biochemical anomalies with adverse effects on body tissues, including the central nervous system.[85]

Galactosaemia is such as inborn error of metabolism. First described in 1908, it is estimated to affect between 1:40,000 to 1:60,000 births.[86] The condition is inherited as an autosomal recessive. It involves deficiency or absence of the enzyme galactose-1-phosphate uridyl transferase, which prevents the normal conversion of dietary galactose, contained in milk, into glucose. As a result of this metabolic block, galactose-1-phosphate accumulates in the tissues, where it is thought to be responsible for producing the damage that leads to symptoms.[87] Hypoglycaemia resulting from reduced availability of glucose is also thought to contribute to certain acute symptoms such as convulsions.[85]

The severity of galactosaemic symptoms varies from one case to another.[88] In neonates and young infants, they include vomiting, diarrhoea, failure to gain weight, liver enlargement, jaundice, and cataracts. Many infants die if left untreated and the survivors are commonly mentally handicapped. Cataracts, cirrhosis of the liver, learning difficulties, and emotional problems are also found.[86,89]

Treatment of galactosaemia involves elimination of dietary galactose, which requires evidence of products containing milk and lactose, starting as early in life as possible and continuing for several years at least. Early introduction of a galactose-free diet leads to prompt clearing of the physical symptoms, but if it is not started until after mental retardation has become manifest, normal intellectual development is not restored. However, IQ has been found to fall off progressively with increasing age at the start of treatment,[90] so it may be beneficial even if not completely protective. Early introduction of the diet with strict compliance has been found to be associated with normal, and in a few cases, above average intellectual development, but strict compliance is also associated with higher parental IQ, so that interpretation of the findings is not entirely straightforward.[86,90,91] Slight to moderate mental handicap seems to be the most usual outcome.[86]

Personality as well as intellectual functioning is reportedly impaired in galactosaemic children, who, when young, are described as shy and sensitive with minor neurotic traits such as thumb sucking, nail biting, and bed wetting.[86] At school they are described as restless, listless, withdrawn, as having difficulties in concentration and in making friends.[89] And as adolescents they are characterised as unusually stormy.[86] The mechanisms mediating their reported difficulties in social adjustment are thought to be multiple and are not well understood.

Overt behaviour disorder may be associated with galactose intolerance in the absence of mental handicap. A 16-year-old girl with a childhood history of minor neurotic traits became socially maladjusted when she began commercial training. Multiple erroneous diagnoses, ranging from psychopathy to epileptic automatism, were made before she was finally diagnosed as having a deficiency of galactose-1-phosphate uridyl transferase activity. But in her case – which, unlike cases of classical galactosaemia, was not associated with physical abnormalities or a history of milk intolerance in childhood – the mechanism to which her episodes of wandering off and bouts of somnolence and negativism were attributed was profound hypoglycaemia after consumption of lactose in milk. On a galactose-free diet, she made an excellent recovery.[92]

This case may represent a different syndrome from classical galactosaemia, but the girl nonetheless illustrates the possibility of considerable behaviour disruption resulting from the interaction of a metabolic error with particular dietary constituents.

Reactive Hypoglycaemia as a Cause of Mental Symptoms

A state of low blood sugar developing after meals in non-diabetics illustrates yet another way in which dietary intolerance may influence brain function and lead to mental symptoms.[93]

Two syndromes of hypoglycaemic symptoms have been differentiated.[94] The first is a neuroglycopenic syndrome usually found with fasting hypoglycaemia of gradual onset but also reported to occur in the course of extended glucose intolerance tests,[95] the symptoms of which may include headache, mental dullness, fatigue, mental confusion, memory disturbance, and even, in extreme cases, seizures and coma.[94] These manifestations result when the brain is deprived of adequate amounts of its energy substrate. The second is the adrenergic syndrome, the symptoms of which include a sense of vague ill-health, anxiety, panic, depersonalisation, accompanied by hunger, palpitations, restlessness, tremor, and nervousness.[96] Sweating and weakness may also occur. These symptoms result chiefly from the secretion of adrenaline and other counter-regulatory hormones into the blood by the adrenal medulla in response to the falling blood sugar concentration in an effort to mobilise stored glycogen from the liver.[97]

Both syndromes are relevant to psychiatric patients, since many of them do not eat adequate breakfasts and consume a large quantity of refined carbohydrates the rest of the time, either in consequence of their addictions to these foods or because of insufficient knowledge, motivation, or funds to consume better diets. This pattern of eating may be associated with neuroglycopenic symptoms throughout the morning followed by anxiety and panic attacks or depersonalisation a few hours after lunch. It does not seem to be necessary for blood glucose levels to be objectively extremely low for these sorts of symptoms to occur in relationship to this sort of eating pattern as long as the blood sugar levels are below the individual's own personal fasting level. It has been shown experimentally in normals that they may be manipulated by changing the nutritional composition of isocaloric breakfast meals or by giving only unsweetened black coffee for breakfast.[98,99]

High proportions of hypoglycaemics have been reported in samples of newly referred psychiatric patients.[100–103] Similarly, high rates of mental symptoms have been noted in patients with hypoglycaemia.[100,105] But despite the consistency of these findings, the condition appears to be very much underdiagnosed in Britain, most probably because clinicians do not look for it. This oversight is unfortunate because there is general agreement that treatment with a high-protein, low carbohydrate diet (and avoidance of obvious precipitants such as caffeine and alcohol) is rapidly effective.[105] In some cases, patients who suffer from psychological symptoms that are not commonly associated with hypoglycaemia, such as obsessional ruminations, may benefit, as the following case[106] illustrates.

After several years of conventional psychological and pharmacological treatment, a 26-year-old man with a 15 year history of obsessional ruminations was offered dietary treatment as a last resort before leucotomy was considered. On an elimination diet alone he made little progress, but after a high-protein breakfast was added to his regimen he began to improve dramatically and after 7 months was obsession-free.

This improvement was maintained during a 23-month follow-up and he reported that he was able to reintroduce all foods except alcohol with impunity. However, earlier in his course, while he was testing foods after a shorter period of avoidance, he noted that some produced exacerbations of his symptoms. As these foods – egg, pork, and tiger nuts – are not noted as sources of concentrated processed carbohydrate, the patient's observations lend support to the food allergy hypothesis of the origin of hypoglycaemia that we noted earlier. Further support also came from the fact that the first of two glucose tolerance tests he underwent showed grossly abnormal results but after a longer period on his diet the results of a second test were less abnormal, which suggests that prolonged adherence to the diet improved the underlying hypoglycaemia as well as his food tolerance and clinical symptoms.

Although further work is needed to elucidate the role of food intolerance in hypoglycaemia, enough is already known to benefit many patients – if only this knowledge is applied in practice.

Mental Functioning Affected by the Formation of Neurotransmitters from Dietary Precursors

In the past 15 years it has come to be recognised that diet may affect mental functioning through its contribution to altering the levels of neutrotransmitters formed in the brain. Previously it was believed that, apart from the effects of food-borne toxins and those of nutrient deficiencies, the blood-brain barrier effectively insulated the brain from the vagaries of short-term, diet-induced chemical fluctuations. But it is now known that brain levels of serotonin and acetylcholine and also possibly dopamine and adrenaline vary considerably with changes in dietary levels of their precursors and other dietary factors, such as the amount of carbohydrate consumed.[107,108]

To date, the possible aetiological implications of these findings have not been worked out in any detail. Their main application has been in the use of high doses of purified nutrients such as tryptophan or choline in the treatment of brain diseases and symptoms that are thought to be of non-nutritional origin, such as Parkinson's disease, insomnia, schizophrenia, depression, Huntingdon's disease, Alzheimer's disease, and Friedreich's ataxia, among others.[107] Much of this work is as yet still quite preliminary and results of different studies tend to be conflicting, possibly because some of the conditions in question, such as depression, are not biochemically homogeneous and research subjects are selected for participation on the basis of clinical and historical rather than biological features. Future research will no doubt determine the significance of these discoveries.

Discussion

The material reviewed in this chapter indicates that foods and their constituents and contaminants are capable of causing mental and neurological disorders of a variety of types, in a variety of ways, and under a variety of conditions. Given such extreme diversity, generalisations about diet-induced mental illness are hazardous, but a few may nonetheless be made. One is that while some diet-induced disturbances of mental function may be completely reversible upon removal of the cause, others may cause permanent structural damage to the nervous system and others still may lead to death. In view of the gravity of some mental and neurological conditions of dietary origin, the field ought not be dismissed as either trivial or quirky. There is not any room for doubt that for some people food may be extremely hazardous to mental health and the general opprobrium which falls on the field and those working in it may be the cause of considerable iatrogenic disease, arising from the failure to apply existing knowledge to the benefit of patients. This point leads us to the second generalisation, namely that most, if certainly not all, of the afflictions we have examined here are in principle preventable by the application of existing knowledge. Many were just as preventable long before the mechanisms which produce them were known, preventable, that is, on a purely empirical basis. And yet, though in some cases the mechanisms are now reasonably well understood, the conditions continue to occur, while basic research delves deeper and deeper into their mechanisms. The fact that people continue to suffer from avoidable diet-induced mental dysfunction, deformity, and even death indicates that the main task for future investigators is in the realm of applied rather than basic medical and behavioural science, at the level of both individuals and populations. If existing knowledge were applied wherever it is relevant, there might be very few victims of diet-induced mental diseases left to study.

References

Introduction

1. Schoental, R. 'Mouldy Grains and the Aetiology of Pellagra: the Role of Toxic Metabolites of *Fusarium*', *Biochemical Society Transactions* (1980), *8*, 147–50.

Caffeine

2. Ritchie, J.M. 'Central Nervous System Stimulants. The Xanthines' in L.S. Goodman and A. Gilman (eds.) *The Pharmacological Basis of Therapeutics* 5th Edn. (New York, Macmillan, 1975), pp. 367–78.
3. Weiss, B. and Laties, V.G. 'Enhancement of Human Performance by Caffeine and the Amphetamines', *Pharmacological Reviews* (1962), *14*, 1–36.
4. Calhoun, W.H. 'Central Nervous System Stimulants' in E. Furchgott (ed.) *Pharmacological and Biophysical Agents and Behaviour* (Academic Press, New York and London, 1977), pp. 181–268 (especially pp. 221–40).
5. Sawyer, D.A., Julia, H.L. and Turin, A.C. 'Caffeine and Human Behaviour: Arousal, Anxiety, and Performance Effects', *Journal of Behavioural Medicine* (1982), *5*, 415–39.
6. Cole, J. 'On the Deleterious Effects Produced by Drinking Tea and Coffee in Excessive Quantities', *Lancet* (1832–3), *2*, 274–8.
7. American Psychiatric Association, *Diagnostic and Statistical Manual of Mental Disorders* (3rd edn), DSM-III. (1980), American Psychiatric Association, Washington, DC.
8. Greden, J.F. 'Anxiety of Caffeinism: A Diagnostic Dilemma', *American Journal of Psychiatry* (1974), *131*, 1089–92.
9. Stillner, V., Popkin, M.K. and Pierce, C.M. 'Caffeine-induced Delirium During Prolonged Competitive Stress', *American Journal of Psychiatry* (1978), *135*, 855–6.
10. Rippere, V. 'Ecological Agoraphobia. II. Caffeinism – Prevalence and Correlates', *Newsletter of the Society for Environmental Therapy* (1983), *3* (3), 10–16.
11. Dreisbach, R.H. and Pfeiffer, C. 'Caffeine-withdrawal Headache', *Journal of Laboratory and Clinical Medicine* (1943), *28*, 1212–19.
12. White, B.C., Lincoln, C.A., Pearce, N.W., Reeb, R. and Vaida, C. 'Anxiety and Muscle Tension as Consequences of Caffeine Withdrawal', *Science* (1980), *209*, 1547–8.
13. Goldstein, A. and Kaizer, S. 'Psychotropic Effects of Caffeine on Man. III. A Questionnaire Survey of Coffee Drinking and its Effects on a Group of Housewives', *Clinical Pharmacology & Therapeutics* (1969), *10*, 477–88.
14. Goldstein, A., Kaizer, S. and Whitby, O. 'Psychotropic Effects of Caffeine in Man. IV. Quantitative and Qualitative Differences Associated with Habituation to Coffee', *Clinical Pharmacology & Therapeutics* (1969), *10*, 489–97.
15. Mikkelsen, E.J. 'Caffeine and Schizophrenia', *Journal of Clinical Psychiatry* (1978), *39*, 732–6.
16. McManamy, M.F. and Schube, P.G. 'Caffeine Intoxication. Report of a Case the Symptoms of Which Amounted to a Psychosis', *New England Journal of Medicine* (1936), *215*, 616–20.
17. Greden, J.F., Fontaine, P., Lubetsky, M. and Chamberlin, K. 'Anxiety and Depression Associated with Caffeinism Among Psychiatric Inpatients', *American Journal of Psychiatry* (1978), *135*, 963–6.
18. Galliano, S. 'Caffeine Consumption in a British Population', *Newsletter of the Society for Environmental Therapy* (1983), *3* (1), 5–8.

Vitamin Deficiencies

19. Davidson, S., Passmore, R., Brock, J.F. and Truswell, A.S. *Human Nutrition and Dietetics*, 7th edn (Churchill Livingstone, London, Edinburgh, 1979).
20. Lishman, W.A. *Organic Psychiatry. The Psychological Consequences of Cerebral Disorder* (Blackwell Scientific Publications, Oxford, London, 1978).
21. Srikantia, S.G. 'Endemic Pellagra' in A. Neuberger and T.H. Jukes (eds.) *Human Nutrition. Current Issues and Controversies* (MTP Press, Lancaster, 1982).
22. Wiener, J.S. and Hope, J.M. 'Cerebral Manifestations of Vitamin B12 Deficiency', *Journal of the American Medical Association* (1959), *170*, 1038–41.
23. Lind, J. *A Treatise of the Scurvy*. Edinburgh, printed by Sands, Murray and Cochran for A. Miller (1753).
24. Pauling, L. *Vitamin C, the Common Cold and the Flu* (W.H. Freeman, San Francisco, 1976).
25. Thorpe, F.T. 'Some Observations on Vitamin C Deficiency in Acute Mental Disorder', *Journal of Mental Science* (1938), *84*, 788–800.
26. Gregory, I. and Paul, R.H. 'Nutritional Deficiencies in Patients Admitted to Mental Hospital', *Canadian Medical Association Journal* (1959), *80*, 186–9.
27. Reading, C.M. 'Letter to the Editor', *Journal of Orthomolecular Psychiatry* (1981), *10*, 29–34.
28. Kinsman, R.A. and Hood, J. 'Some Behavioural Effects of Ascorbic Acid Deficiency', *American Journal of Clinical Nutrition* (1971), *24*, 455–64.
29. Cutforth, R.E. 'Adult Scurvy', *Lancet* (1958), *1*, 454–6.
30. Milner, G. 'Malnutrition and Mental Disease', *Lancet* (1962), *1*, 191.
31. Cheraskin, E., Ringsdorf, W.M. Jr. and Sisley, E.L. *The Vitamin C Connection. Getting Well and Staying Well with Vitamin C* (Thorsons, Wellingborough, 1983).
32. Milner, G. 'Ascorbic Acid in Chronic Psychiatric Patients', *British Journal of Psychiatry* (1963), *109*, 294–9.
33. Naylor, G.J. and Smith, A.H.W. 'Vanadium: a Possible Aetiological Factor in Manic-depressive Illness', *Psychological Medicine* (1981), *11*, 249–56.
34. Thomas, T.N. and Zemp, J.W. 'Inhibition of Dopamine Sensitive Adenylate Cyclase from Rat Brain Striatal Homogenates by Ascorbic Acid', *Journal of Neurochemistry* (1977), *28*, 663–5.

Lathyrism

35. Chaudhuri, R.N., Chhetri, M.K., Saha, T.K. and Mitra, P.P. 'Lathyrism: A Clinical and Epidemiological Study', *Journal of the Indian Medical Association* (1963), *41*, 169–73.
36. Conning, D.M. 'Systemic Toxicity Due to Foodstuffs' in D.M. Conning and A.B.G. Lansdown (eds.) *Toxic Hazards in Food* (Croom Helm, London, 1983).
37. Anonymous 'The Cause of Lathyrism', *Lancet* (1953), *2*, 447–8.

Ginger Paralysis

38. Hotson, R.D. 'Outbreak of Polyneuritis Due to Orthocresyl Phosphate Poisoning', *Lancet* (1946), *1*, 207.
39. Airing, C.D. 'The Systemic Nervous Affinity of Triorthocresyl Phosphate (Jamaica Ginger Palsy)', *Brain* (1942), *65*, 34–47.
40. Anonymous 'Thousands of Cases of "Jamaica Ginger Paralysis"', *Journal of the American Medical Association* (1930), *95*, 1029.

Minamata Disease

41. McAlpine, D. and Araki, S. 'Minamata Disease. An Unusual Neurological Disorder Caused by Contaminated Fish', *Lancet* (1958), *2*, 629–31.

42. Takeuchi, T., Morikawa, N., Matsumoto, H. and Shiraishi, Y. 'A Pathological Study of Minamata Disease in Japan', *Acta Neuropathologica* (1962), *2*, 40–57.
43. Adams, R. and Murray, F. *Minerals: Kill or Cure?* (Larchmont Books, New York, 1977).

Food Allergy, Intolerance, and Addiction

44. Kopeloff, L.M., Barbera, S.E. and Kopeloff, N. 'Recurrent Convulsive Seizures in Animals Produced by Immunologic and Chemical Means', *American Journal of Psychiatry* (1942), *98*, 881–902.
45. Dohan, F.C., Martin, L., Grasberger, J.C., Boehme, D. and Cottrell, J.C. 'Antibodies to Wheat Gliadin in Blood of Psychiatric Patients: Possible Role of Emotional Factors', *Biological Psychiatry* (1972), *5*, 127–37.
46. Mascord, I., Freed, D. and Durrant, R. 'Antibodies to Foodstuffs in Schizophrenia', *British Medical Journal* (1978), *1*, 1351.
47. Hekkens, W.Th.J.M. 'Antibodies to Gliadin in Serum of Normals, Coeliac Patients and Schizophrenics' in G. Hemmings and W.A. Hemmings (eds.) *The Biological Basis of Schizophrenia* (MTP Press, Lancaster, 1978).
48. Hekkens, W.Th.J.M., Schipperin, A.J.M. and Freed, D.L.J. 'Antibodies to Wheat Proteins in Schizophrenia: Relationship or Coincidence?' in G. Hemmings (ed.) *Biochemistry of Schizophrenia and Addiction. In Search of a Common Factor* (MTP Press, Lancaster, 1980).
49. Gowdy, J. 'Immunoglobulin Levels in Psychotic Patients', *Psychosomatics* (1980), *21*, 751–6.
50. Sugerman, A.A., Southern, D.L. and Curran, J.F. 'A Study of Antibody Levels in Alcoholic, Depressive and Schizophrenic Patients', *Annals of Allergy* (1982), *48*, 166–71.
51. Ossofsky, H.J. 'Endogenous Depression in Infancy and Childhood', *Comprehensive Psychiatry* (1974), *15*, 19–25.
52. Ossofsky, H.J. 'Affective and Atopic Disorders and Cyclic AMP', *Comprehensive Psychiatry* (1976), *17*, 335–46.
53. Denman, A.M. 'The Relevance of Immunopathology to Research into Schizophrenia' in G. Hemmings (ed.) *Biochemistry of Schizophrenia and Addiction. In Search of a Common Factor* (MTP Press, Lancaster, 1980).
54. Vaz, G.A., Tan, L.K.-T. and Gerrard, J.W. 'Oral Cromoglycate in Treatment of Adverse Reactions to Foods', *Lancet* (1978), *1*, 1066–8.
55. Bell, I.R. 'A Kinin Model of Meditation for Food and Chemical Sensitivities: Biobehavioural Implications', *Annals of Allergy* (1978), *35*, 206–15.
56. Philpott, W.H. and Kalita, D.K. *Brain Allergies. The Psychonutrient Connection* (Keats Publishing, New Canaan, Connecticut, 1980).
57. Rinkel, H. 'Food Allergy. The Role of Food Allergy in Internal Medicine', *Annals of Allergy* (1944), *2*, 115–24.
58. Randolph, T.G. 'The Descriptive Features of Food Addiction. Addictive Eating and Drinking', *Q.J. Stud. Alc.* (1956), *17*, 198–224.
59. Rippere, V. 'Prevalence of Ecological Disorders in Psychiatric Patients. II. Symptoms, Prevalence and Pointers', *Newsletter of the Society for Environmental Therapy* (1982), *2*, 7–13.
60. Finn, R. and Cohen, H.N. '"Food Allergy": Fact or Fiction?' *Lancet* (1978), *1*, 426–8.
61. King, D.S. 'Can Allergic Exposure Provoke Psychological Symptoms? A Double-blind Test', *Biological Psychiatry* (1981), *16*, 3–19.
62. Brown, M., Gibney, M., Husband, P.R. and Radcliffe, M. 'Food Allergy in Polysymptomatic Patients', *The Practitioner* (1981), *225*, 1651–4.
63. Egger, J., Carter, C.M., Wilson, J., Turner, M.W. and Soothill, J.F. 'Is Migraine Food Allergy? A Double-blind Controlled Trial of Oligoallergenic Diet Treatment', *Lancet* (1983), *2*, 865–9.

64. Mackarness, R. *Not All in the Mind* (Pan, London, 1976).
65. Rippere, V. 'The Diet of Psychiatric Patients', *Newsletter of the Society for Environmental Therapy* (1982), *2*, 12–17.
66. Anonymous 'Obesity and Sugar Addiction', *Lancet* (1963), *1*, 768.

Food Additives

67. Feingold, B. *Why Your Child is Hyperactive* (Random House, New York, 1975).
68. Rippere, V. 'Placebo-controlled Tests of Chemical Food Additives: Are They Valid?' *Medical Hypotheses* (1981), *7*, 819–23.
69. Neuman, I., Elian, R., Nahum, H., Shaked, P. and Creter, D. 'The Danger of 'Yellow Dyes' (Tartrazine) to Allergic Subjects', *Clinical Allergy* (1978), *8*, 65–8.
70. Rose, T.L. 'The Functional Relationship between Artificial Food Colours and Hyperactivity', *Journal of Applied Behavioural Analysis* (1978), *11*, 439–46.
71. Swanson, J.M. and Kinsbourne, M. 'Food Dyes Impaire Performance of Hyperactive Children on a Laboratory Learning Task', *Science* (1980), *207*, 1485–7.
72. Tryphonas, H. and Trites, R. 'Food Allergy in Children with Hyperactivity, Learning Disabilities and/or Minimal Brain Dysfunction', *Annals of Allergy* (1979), *42*, 22–7.
73. Conners, C.K., Goyette, C.H. and Newman, E.B. 'Dose-time Effect of Artificial Colours in Hyperactive Children', *Journal of Learning Disabilities* (1980), *13*, 48–52.

Peptides

74. Dohan, F.C. 'Cereals and Schizophrenia. Data and Hypothesis', *Acta Psychiatrica Scandinavia* (1966), *42*, 125–52.
75. Dohan, F.C., Grasberger, J.C., Lowell, F.M., Johnston, H.T., Jr. and Arbegast, A.W. 'Relapsed Schizophrenics: More Rapid Improvement on a Milk and Cereal-free Diet', *British Journal of Psychiatry* (1969), *115*, 595–6.
76. Dohan, F.C. and Grasberger, J.C. 'Relapsed Schizophrenics: Earlier Discharge from the Hospital after Cereal-free, Milk-free Diet', *American Journal of Psychiatry* (1973), *130*, 685–8.
77. Singh, M.M. and Kay, S.R. 'Wheat Gluten as a Pathogenic Factor in Schizophrenia', *Science* (1976), *191*, 401–2.
78. Dohan, F.C. 'Schizophrenia: are Some Food-derived Peptides Pathogenic?' in G. Hemmings and W.A. Hemmings (eds.) *The Biological Basis of Schizophrenics* (MTP Press, Lancaster, 1978).
79. Dohan, F.C. 'Hypothesis: Genes and Neuroactive Peptides from Food as Cause of Schizophrenics' in E. Costa and M. Tabucchi (eds.) *Neural Peptides and Neuronal Communication* (Raven Press, New York, 1980).
80. Hemmings, W.A. 'The Entry into the Brain of Large Molecules Derived from Dietary Protein', *Proceedings of the Royal Society of London, Series B* (1979), *200*, 175–92.
81. Dohan, F.C., Levitt, D.R. and Kushnir, L.D. 'Abnormal Behaviour after Intracerebral Injection of Polypeptides from Wheat Gliadin', *Pavlov Journal of Biological Science* (1978), *13*, 73–82.
82. Zioudrou, C., Streaty, R.A. and Klee, W.A. 'Opioid Peptides Derived from Food Proteins. The Exorphins', *Journal of Biological Chemistry* (1979), *254*, 2446–9.
83. Zioudrou, C. and Klee, W.A. 'Possible Role of Peptides Derived from Food Proteins in Brain Function' in R.J. Wurtman and J.J. Wurtman (eds.)

Nutrition and the Brain. Vol. 4. *Toxic Effects of Food Constituents on the Brain* (Raven Press, New York, 1979).

84. Klee, W.A. and Zioudrou, C. 'The Possible Actions of Peptides with Opioid Activity Derived from Pepsin Hydrolysates of Wheat Gluten and of Other Constituents of Gluten in the Function of the Central Nervous System' in G. Hemmings (ed.) *Biochemistry of Schizophrenia and Addiction. In Search of a Common Factor* (MTP Press, Lancaster, 1980).

Galactosaemia

85. Adams, R.D. and Lyon, G. *Neurology of Hereditary Metabolic Diseases of Children* (McGraw Hill, London, 1982).
86. Fischler, K., Koch, R., Donnell, G. and Graliker, B.V. 'Psychological Correlates in Galactosaemia', *American Journal of Mental Deficiency* (1966), *71*, 116–25.
87. Gairdner, D.M.T. 'Disorders of Galactose Metabolism. Galactosaemia' in Sir Ronald Bodley Scott (ed.) *Price's Textbook of the Practice of Medicine* (Oxford University Press, Oxford, 1978).
88. Holzel, A. 'Galactosaemia', *British Medical Bulletin* (1961), *17*, 213–16.
89. Komrower, G.M. and Lee, D.H. 'Long-term Follow-up of Galactosaemia', *Archives of Dieases of Childhood* (1970), *45*, 367–73.
90. Donnell, G.N., Collado, M. and Koch, R. 'Growth and Development of Children with Galactosaemia', *Journal of Pediatrics* (1961), *58*, 836–44.
91. Komrower, G.M., Schwarz, V., Holzel, A. and Goldberg, L. 'A Clinical and Biochemical Study of Galactosaemia. A Possible Explanation of the Nature of the Biochemical Lesion', *Archives of Diseases of Childhood* (1956), *31*, 254–64.
92. Hansen, O. 'A Case of Behaviour Disorder with Impaired Carbohydrate Metabolism', *Scandinavian Journal of Clinical and Laboratory Investigation* (1966), *18*, 103–11.

Hypoglycaemia

93. Harris, S. 'Hyperinsulism and Dysinsulinism', *Journal of the American Medical Association* (1924), *83*, 729–33.
94. Permutt, M.A. 'Postprandial Hypoglycaemia', *Diabetes* (1976), *25*, 719–33.
95. Hale, F., Margen, S. and Rabak, D. 'Postprandial Hypoglycaemia and 'Psychological' Symptoms', *Biological Psychiatry* (1982), *17*, 125–30.
96. Marks, V. and Rose, F.C. *Hypoglycaemia* (Blackwell Scientific Publications, Oxford, 1965).
97. Ensink, J.W. and Williams, R.H. 'Disorders Causing Hypoglycaemia' in R.H. Williams (ed.) *Textbook of Endocrinology* (Saunders, Philadelphia, 1974).
98. Orent-Keiles, E. and Hallman, L.F. *The Breakfast Meal in Relation to Blood Sugar Values* (US Department of Agriculture, Circular No. 827, 1949), Washington, DC.
99. Thorn, G.W., Quinby, J.T. and Clinton, M.J. 'A Comparison of the Metabolic Effects of Isocaloric Meals of Varying Composition with Special Reference to the Prevention and Postprandial Hypoglycaemic Symptoms', *Annals of Internal Medicine* (1943), *18*, 913–19.
100. Hoffman, R.H. and Abrahamson, E.H. 'Hyperinsulinism – a Factor in the Neuroses', *American Journal of Digestive Diseases* (1949), *16*, 242–7.
101. Landmann, H.R. and Sutherland, R.L. 'Incidence and Significance of Hypoglycaemia in Unselected Admissions to a Psychosomatic Service', *American Journal of Digestive Diseases* (1950), *17*, 105–8.
102. Salzer, H.H. 'Relative Hypoglycaemia as a Cause of Neuropsychiatric Illness', *Journal of the National Medical Association* (1966), *58*, 12–17.

103. Beebe, W.E. and Wendel, O. 'Preliminary Observations of Altered Carbohydrate Metabolism in Psychiatric Patients' in D. Hawkins and L. Pauling (eds.) *Orthomolecular Psychiatry Treatment of Schizophrenia* (W.H. Freeman, San Francisco, 1973).
104. Harris, S. 'The Diagnosis and Treatment of Hyperinsulinism', *Annals of Internal Medicine* (1936), *10*, 514–33.
105. Freinkel, N. 'Hypoglycaemic Disorders' in P.B. Beeson and W. McDermott (eds.) *Cecil's Textbook of Medicine*, 14th edn. (W.B. Saunders, London, 1975).
106. Rippere, V. 'Dietary Treatment of Chronic Obsessional Ruminations', *British Journal of Clinical Psychology* (1983), *22*, 314–16.

Neurotransmitter Precursors
107. Growdon, J. 'Neurotransmitter Precursors in the Diet: Their Use in the Treatment of Brain Diseases' in R.J. Wurtman and J.J. Wurtman (eds.) *Nutrition and the Brain*. Vol. 3, (Raven Press, New York, 1979).
108. Wurtman, R.J. 'The Effect of Diet on Brain Neurotransmitters' in G. Hemmings and W.A. Hemmings (eds.) *The Biological Basis of Schizophrenia* (MTP Press, Lancaster, 1978).

9 IS OLD AGE A DIET-RELATED DISEASE?

S. Seely

Obviously not. Whatever we eat, our ultimate fate is old age and death. A living animal is a complex, improbable organisation which has to defend its high degree of order against forces of nature tending to equalise it with its environment by converting it into a simple, random conglomeration of matter. In addition, predators and parasites are in constant readiness to destroy a weakening organism. Lastly it may not be to the advantage of the species to let individuals outlive their usefulness. When old animals become unproductive competitors for limited natural resources, nature, in its unsentimental way, may take measures to eliminate them.

To some extent, however, old age is a diet-related disease. If it were possible to live under ideal conditions, which would include an ideal diet, we would still become old and would finally die, but probably a goodly number of years later than now. We might also be able to use our allotted span to better advantage. Mental deterioration in the elderly, for example, is largely due to the narrowing of cerebral arteries by the accumulation of atherosclerotic plaques. Atherosclerosis is probably diet-related, hence an ideal diet, if we knew what it was, would help to preserve mental faculties.

Aging is a complex and still only incompletely understood process. One of its symptoms is the slow accumulation of an inert substance, lipofuscin, in tissue spaces, notably in the heart. This substance is insoluble in any solvent the body can produce, it is so stable that it cannot be broken down and there is no carrier capable of removing it. In other words, no living organism can eliminate all its waste products and make good all its wear and tear. Inert waste products do little harm to a sessile organism, like a plant, but to a motile organism they present a ballast and may become obstacles in internal transport. If the chemical process of which lipofuscin is the endproduct, were fully understood, it might be clear whether the avoidance of certain foods could minimise its accumulation, but much further development is needed before this can be achieved.

Another symptom of the aging process is the oxidative cross-linking of protein fibres, resulting in loss of elasticity and increasing rigidity of tissues. An interesting theory by Kon[1] suggests that the agent mainly responsible for the oxidative process is iron. Ionic iron hydrolyses into insoluble aggregates and catalyses the oxidative process which cross-links biomolecules and produces activated oxygen. Iron in the body is needed only for the haemoglobin of red blood corpuscles. Surplus iron is scavenged by a large carrier molecule, ferritin. Owing partly to its size and partly to its cuboid shape, there are tissue spaces which are inaccessible to it. It is in such spaces where hydrolysed iron can aggregate. The process is of great complexity, because the body defends itself partly by the metabolic turnover of the affected tissues which are continually catabolysed and replaced before irreversible crosslinkages occur, and partly by the enzymatic deactivation of oxygen. On the other hand, the process may be promoted by metabolic disturbances, toxicants, oxidants etc. If the theory is correct, it contains a hint of the involvement of the diet, but we are still a long way from knowing whether the diet could be modified to minimise the risk. On an equal diet women in their reproductive period accumulate less surplus iron than men. This could be partly responsible for their longer life expectation in all advanced countries.

To some extent the animal body can be regarded as a mechanism for energy conversion and as such, the harder it is used, the sooner it wears out. Small homeothermal animals need an enormous amount of energy to keep their core temperature at a constant level, big animals live relatively cheaply in terms of energy expenditure. Thus the basal metabolic rate of the mouse is 160 cal per gram of body weight per day, that of the rat 130, of the dog 35, of man 24 and of the elephant 13. Man's metabolic rate increases 8 times between rest and intense physical effort, so that the basal rate of the mouse is as high as that of a man engaged in fairly hard physical exercise and possibly higher than that of an elephant working to the limit of its capacity. The lifespans of animals are proportional to their total lifetime energy outputs. Thus the lifespan potential of the mouse of 2.5 years, of the rat is 5, of the domestic cat and dog 16, of the lion and tiger 28, of the hippopotamus and orang-utan 50, of the elephant 70 and of the finback whale 80 years. Man's long life is due to his low energy expenditure. In the animal word man is among the moderate-sized animals, but his energy needs are much lower than of his equal-sized contemporaries, partly on account of the use of machines reducing the need for physical exertion, and partly on account of the use of clothes and the heating of dwelling houses, which reduce the energy needs for the maintenance of constant body temperatures. Thus a 65 kg man with a daily net intake of 3,000

Cal expends 46 calories per gram of bodyweight per day, not quite twice as much as his basic metabolic rate of 24 cal/g/day. It is known from the measurement of energy needs in various activities, that energy expenditure increases to about 70 cal/g/day in light exercise, such as walking on level ground at 4–5 km per hour, and to over 100 cal, more than 4 times the basal rate, in moderate exercise, such as walking on level ground at 6–7 km per hour. The daily intake of 3,000 Cal, therefore, covers the needs of a 65 kg man who spends about half his day in a state of basal metabolism and the other half in leisurely walking. It seems clear that few wild animals can earn their daily bread with so little effort.

These considerations support the view that the quantity of dietary intake is just as important as its composition. Note for example, that lipofuscin tends to accumulate in muscles, particularly in the hardest working of them, the heart. In terms of an analogy organs of metabolism correspond to the refinery where crude oil is processed to yield petrol, muscles are the motors which convert the petrol into mechanical work. By the time the petrol reaches the motor, it is immaterial what raw materials it originated from, only its quantity matters. This should not be taken to mean that overeating is not a risk factor, but that aging is an inevitable consequence of using the body as a mechanism of energy conversion and would take place even on an ideal diet. On this basis a sedentary life is more conducive to long life than an active one, supported by the fact that slow-moving, lethargic animals, like turtles, live longer than more active ones.[2]

Lastly it is possible to regard old age like any other disease in that respect that an epidemiological survey can correlate its geographical peculiarities with factors like total calorie intake, or the consumption of various types of food. Table 91. shows life expectation at birth in various countries, using the latest available data,[3] together with total calorie intake in those countries. There is a modicum of negative correlation with calorie intake in advanced countries. If developing countries had also been included in the table, it would be seen that the correlation between dietary intake and longevity is parabolic. Inadequate nutrition is associated with short life, adequate nutrition with long life, but after an optimum level a further increase in total calorie intake probably tends to shorten life.

The expectation of life at birth shown in Table 9.1 is the average for men and women. If male and female life expectation tables had been shown separately, it would be seen that the life expectation of women exceeds that of men in advanced countries by 5–8 years. The relevant

Table 9.1: Life Expectation at Birth

Country	Expectation of life at birth, years	Total calorie intake per day
Japan	76.9	2,520
Holland	76.2	3,200
Norway	76.1	3,100
Sweden	76	2,820
Switzerland	76	3,400
France	75	3,200
Spain	74.9	2,700
Canada	74.7	3,140
Australia	74.6	3,100
Denmark	74.5	3,160
England & Wales	74.2	3,160
US	74.1	3,340
Italy	74.1	3,200
Germany	73.6	3,780
Finland	73.4	3,030
Austria	72.8	3,240
New Zealand	72.8	3,210
Belgium	72.6	3,260
Ireland	72	3,550
Portugal	70.8	3,240
Yugoslavia	70.6	3,210

figures for a few countries are US 70.1-78.1, UK 71.2-77.2, Germany 70.2-76.9, France 70.8-79.1, Japan 74.1-79.6. Beside the countries shown in Table 9.1 two more countries with a remarkable record of longevity are Iceland, male-female average 76.7 years, and Hong-Kong, 76.4 years. The good record of Far-Eastern countries, like Japan and Hong-Kong, is presumably an advocacy for a comparatively simple diet and a comparatively low calorie intake. The other group of countries remarkable for their longevity are those of Northern Europe, Iceland, Norway, Sweden. Whether the table can be correlated with the consumption (or avoidance) of certain foods, still remains to be seen.

References

1. Kon, S.H. 'Biological Autoxidation 1. Decontrolled Iron: an Ultimate Carcinogen and Toxicant', *Medical Hypotheses* (1978), *4*, 445-53.
2. Seely, S. 'The Evolution of Human Longevity', *Medical Hypotheses* (1980), *6*, 873-82.
3. *World Health Statistics Annuals*. World Health Organisation, Geneva (1983).

INDEX